Patient-Centered Medicine

From the reviews of prior editions:

"This book is a tour de force synthesizing 12 years of open, faithful, and persistent inquiry, teaching, and practice by the family medicine faculty at the University of Western Ontario. The result is a complete package for transforming clinical practice and the education of clinicians."

W.L. Miller in *Families, Systems, & Health*

"It provides its targeted audience/reader with a detailed explanation of the background to the patient-centred method . . . Whilst the book focuses on the work of medical practitioners, it will be of value to any health care practitioner who is interested in developing their consultations. It will also be of value to anyone interested in the concepts of power and agenda setting in the patient/ professional relationship."

Sue Cradock in *Practical Diabetes International*

The Patient-Centered Clinical Method (PCCM) has been a core tenet of the practice and teaching of medicine since the first edition of *Patient-Centered Medicine – Transforming the Clinical Method* was published in 1995. This timely fourth edition continues to define the principles underpinning the patient-centered method using four major components, clarifying its evolution and consequent development, and it brings the reader fully up to date. It reinforces the relevance of the method in the current much-changed realities of health care in a world where virtual care will remain common, dependence on technology is rising, and societal changes away from compassion, equity, and relationships toward confrontation, inequity, and self-absorption.

Fully revised by its highly experienced author team ensuring wide interest and written for those practising now and for the practitioners of the future, this new edition will be welcomed by a wide international audience comprising all health professionals from medicine, nursing, social work, occupational therapy, physical therapy, pharmacy, veterinary medicine, and other fields.

Patient-Centered Medicine
Transforming the Clinical Method

Fourth Edition

Moira Stewart, Judith Belle Brown,
W Wayne Weston, Thomas R Freeman, Bridget L Ryan,
Carol L McWilliam, and Ian R McWhinney

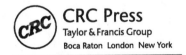

CRC Press
Taylor & Francis Group
Boca Raton London New York

CRC Press is an imprint of the
Taylor & Francis Group, an **informa** business

Fourth edition published 2024
by CRC Press
2385 NW Executive Center Drive, Suite 320, Boca Raton, FL 33431

and by CRC Press
4 Park Square, Milton Park, Abingdon, Oxon, OX14 4RN

CRC Press is an imprint of Taylor & Francis Group, LLC

ISBN: 978-1-032-49623-8 (hbk)
ISBN: 978-1-032-48059-6 (pbk)
ISBN: 978-1-003-39467-9 (ebk)

DOI: 10.1201/9781003394679

Typeset in Minion Pro
by Apex CoVantage, LLC

Dedication

This book is dedicated to Joseph H Levenstein, MD, for his inspiration to us and his outstanding contribution to the practice of medicine. We are grateful to Dr Levenstein for introducing us to the patient-centered clinical method during his time as a Visiting Professor in our department in 1981–1982.

We also dedicate this book to the late Ian R McWhinney, MD, who invited Joseph to come to Western University as a Visiting Professor and provided him and all of us with an intellectually stimulating and nurturing environment in which to co-create the ideas in this book.

Contents

Preface

Patient-Centered Medicine – Transforming the Clinical Method is in its fourth edition. The book's longevity attests to the enduring nature of its messages: the importance of caring for the person in context, partnering equally with patients, and creating compassionate relationships with patients. This book stresses key aspects of patient-centered care: it integrates biomedicine with humanistic medicine; it embraces the emotional level of the patient's experience; and it shares power with the patient.

The patient-centered clinical method has been a core tenet of many health professions since the first edition of *Patient-Centered Medicine – Transforming the Clinical Method* in 1995. The aim of this fourth edition is to reinforce not merely the relevance of the method but its essential nature: in the current much-changed realities of health care where virtual care will remain common, dependence on technology is rising, and society is leaning away from compassion, equity, and relationships toward confrontation, inequity, and self-absorption. This book makes the case that patient-centered care is an important force counteracting these negative influences and has abiding value as an anchor during troubled times. In this edition, the four components of the patient-centered clinical method remain intact. The four components are: exploring health, disease, and the illness experience; understanding the whole person in context; finding common ground; and enhancing the patient–clinician relationship.

In Part One, the fourth edition amplifies the two basic principles of the patient-centered clinical method: sharing power (equity in relationships) and emotional engagement with patients (empathy and compassion). It compares the patient-centered clinical method with other models such as goal-oriented care, person-centered approaches, relationship-centered care, narrative medicine, evidence-based medicine, and shared decision-making. Misconceptions about the patient-centered clinical method are addressed. The current method is placed in historical context in two ways: its evolution over the past 40 years in Chapter 1 and, in Chapter 2, its place in the context of medical history over the centuries.

In Part Two, this book features some important additions to the presentation of the four components: it includes the patient's voices with first-person narratives; it presents cases from around the world (Nigeria, the Netherlands, Brazil, Singapore, Canada) introducing clinicians and patients with a wide variety of social and cultural characteristics; it emphasizes the integration of the biomedical aspects with the patient's experiences as an essential facet of the patient-centered clinical method in comparison with other models; it discusses the value of non-verbal communication and the physical examination; it describes the patient-centered clinical method as a potential solution to complexity in medicine; and it highlights empathy, compassion, and continuity of relationships.

Part Three deals with enacting patient-centered principles in current contexts, some of which enhance patient-centeredness but some inhibit its practice. We have chosen to feature two current contexts. Chapter 8 considers team-based care. Chapter 9 tackles patient-centered care in relation to new technologies such as electronic health records, patient portals, and virtual care.

In Part Four, learner-centered teaching stresses professional identity formation, perceptions of burnout, and issues surrounding international medical graduates and other learners with diverse cultural backgrounds. The case presentation teaching tool is reinforced.

In Part Five, chapters on research findings stress how patient and clinician outcomes are positively influenced by patient-centeredness. Patient-centered care may be helpful in counteracting clinician burnout as well as enhancing patient reported outcomes. Two chapters on measurement present the newest versions of widely used measures created by this authorship team.

In the final chapter, we summarize key messages of relevance to the current context of patient care, teaching, and research. We make recommendations for enhanced humanistic care, for greater emphasis on learner-centered teaching and professional identity formation, and for a multifaceted research agenda to further our understanding of patient-centered care.

Acknowledgements

We thank the Department of Family Medicine and its chair, Dr Scott McKay, our colleagues at the Centre for Studies in Family Medicine and its director, Dr Amanda Terry, of Schulich School of Medicine and Dentistry, Western University, for providing a supportive environment in which to write this book. In particular, we want to express our gratitude to Dr Brian KE Hennen, Chair of the Department of Family Medicine (1987 to 1999), and Chair Dr Thomas R Freeman (1999 to 2011) for their encouragement of scholarly activities. We are indebted to our patients and research participants who generously shared their stories of suffering and coping with suffering; our colleagues who shared their stories of caring for patients, exposing both their failures and their triumphs; and our students, in the Master of Clinical Science and Doctoral programs of the Department of Family Medicine, who stimulated our thinking on patient-centered care and encouraged us to clarify the concepts.

Evelyn Levy has been stellar, contributing her exceptional coordination skills and attention to detail in completing the multiple drafts of the manuscript. Leslie Meredith created the excellent diagrams.

We would like to extend our sincere thanks to Jo Koster and her incredible team at CRC Press/Taylor & Francis. They have all been fabulous to work with.

Finally, we would like to express our heartfelt appreciation for all the support and encouragement provided by our families, in particular Nate and Amy Freeman, Craig Brown, Sharon Weston, David Markle, and Emma Markle.

Authors

Moira Stewart, PhD, is a Distinguished University Professor Emeritus at the Centre for Studies in Family Medicine at Western University Canada and the Dr Brian W Gilbert Tier 1 Canada Research Chair in Primary Health Care Research (2003–2017). Dr Stewart has published widely on the topic of patient-centered care. She has edited, with colleagues, an international series of eight books applying the patient-centered clinical method to such topics as serious mental illness, pregnancy and childbirth, prescribing, palliative care, substance abuse, chronic fatigue, eating disorders, and chronic myofascial pain. She was Co-Principal Investigator of a National Team Grant on patient-centered innovations for persons with multimorbidity. She was the inaugural Principal Investigator on a CIHR Strategic Training Grant on interdisciplinary primary health care research called TUTOR-PHC. Dr Stewart created a researchable database of the electronic medical record data, called DELPHI, with approximately 50 family physicians in Southwestern Ontario. She works closely with policy-makers on her research. Dr Stewart received the James Mackenzie Medal of the Royal College of General Practitioners (2004), the College of Family Physicians of Canada Family Medicine Researcher of the Year Award (2007), and the Martin J Bass Recognition Award, Department of Family Medicine (2008). She is co-recipient of the Dean's Award of Excellence – Team Award at the Schulich School of Medicine & Dentistry (2010), the College of Family Physicians of Canada Lifetime Achievement Award in Family Medicine Research (2012), and the Maurice Wood Award for Lifetime Contribution from the North American Primary Care Research Group (2017).

Judith Belle Brown, PhD, is a Professor in the Centre for Studies in Family Medicine, the Department of Family Medicine, Schulich School of Medicine & Dentistry at Western University, London, Ontario, Canada. She is the Chair of the Master in Clinical Science (MClSc) and PhD programs in Family Medicine at Western, both of which are offered via distance education. She is the Co-Chair of TUTOR-PHC, an interdisciplinary research training program. Dr Brown has been conducting research on the patient-centered clinical method for over four decades and has presented papers and conducted workshops both nationally and internationally on this topic. She has edited, with colleagues, an international series of eight books applying the patient-centered clinical method. The series elaborates the patient-centered principles on such topics as serious mental illness, pregnancy and childbirth, prescribing, palliative care, substance abuse, chronic fatigue, eating disorders, and chronic myofascial pain. Dr Brown was made an honorary member of the College of Family Physicians of Canada in 1996. She is the is co-recipient of the College of Family Physicians of Canada Best Original Research Article Award (2009), the Dean's Award of Excellence – Team Award for the Centre for Studies in Family Medicine (2010), one of the Top 20 Pioneers of Family Medicine Research in Canada (2015), the Dean's Award of Excellence – Schulich Leadership Award for Graduate/Postgraduate (2015), the College of Family Physicians of Canada Family Medicine Researcher of the Year (2016), and the College of Family Physicians of Canada Outstanding Family Medicine Research Article Award (2016).

W Wayne Weston, MD, CCFP, FCFP, is Professor Emeritus of Family Medicine at the Schulich School of Medicine & Dentistry, Western University, Canada. After graduating from the University of Toronto in 1964, he practiced in the small village of Tavistock, Ontario, for 10 years before joining the faculty at Western University where he contributed to research and teaching of the patient-centered clinical method. He taught a graduate course on teaching and learning for 30 years as part of the Master of Clinical Science in Family Medicine at Western. He has published over 200 book chapters and articles in such journals as *Canadian Family Physician, Canadian Medical Association Journal, Academic Medicine, Medical Teacher, Medical Education, Families, Systems and Health,* and the *Canadian Medical Education Journal.* As an award-winning leader in faculty development, he provided over 400 presentations and workshops for faculty on many topics – including patient-centered interviewing, problem-based learning, and clinical teaching – in Canada, New Zealand, Scotland, the United States, the United Arab Emirates, and Kazakhstan. He received the Dean's Award of Excellence for Teaching (2001), the Douglas Bocking Award for Excellence in Medical Teaching (2005) from the Schulich School of Medicine & Dentistry, and the prestigious 3M Award for Excellence in University Teaching in Canada (1992). He was the first recipient of the Ian R McWhinney Family Medicine Education Award (1998) and the Canadian Association for Medical Education Award for Distinguished Contribution to Medical Education (2001). He had a key role in creating the Center for Education Research and Innovation at Western.

Thomas R Freeman has been a full-time faculty member in the Department of Family Medicine, Schulich School of Medicine & Dentistry, at Western University since 1989 and was appointed Professor Emeritus in May 2019. He remains active as a research adjunct professor at the Centre for Studies in Family Medicine. He is the Past Chair of the Department of Family Medicine at Western and Past City-Wide Chief, Department of Family Practice, London Health Sciences Centre and St. Joseph's Health Care, London. He practiced comprehensive family medicine for 40 years. He was a Visiting Scholar at the Robert Graham Center for Policy Studies in Family Medicine and Primary Care in Washington DC in 2013. His current research interests are the nature and outcome of common symptoms in family practice, vaccine data quality, and virtual care. He has published in the *Canadian Medical Association Journal, Canadian Family Physician, Family Practice,* and *BMC Health Services Research* and has received funding from the Canadian Institutes of Health Research, Physicians' Services Incorporated Foundation, the Ministry of Health and Long-Term Care, and Health Canada. He is a co-author on *Patient-Centered Medicine – Transforming the Clinical Method* and *McWhinney's Textbook of Family Medicine.* He has delivered invited plenary addresses in Canada, New Zealand, Japan, and Türkiye. He co-teaches the Foundations in Family Medicine course in the graduate programme of the Department of Family Medicine. He received an Award of Excellence from the College of Family Physicians of Canada in 2008, and a Dean's Award of Excellence for Lifetime Achievement in 2020.

Bridget L Ryan, PhD, is an Epidemiologist and Associate Professor at the Centre for Studies in Family Medicine, and the Departments of Family Medicine and Epidemiology and Biostatistics at Western University, London, Ontario, Canada. Dr Ryan was a contributor to the third edition of this book. Her research focuses on patient-centered primary care, persons with multimorbidity, and patient engagement with healthcare technology. She is an Adjunct Scientist at ICES, Ontario, Canada, where she conducts research using health administrative data focused on those with multimorbidity. Dr Ryan has published on the epidemiology of multimorbidity in Ontario including the prevalence of multimorbidity and its relationship with mortality, and she led a systematic review on the incidence of multimorbidity. She has published on patients' and clinicians' attitudes toward the adoption of patient portals and on the uptake of virtual visits by family physicians in London and Middlesex County, Ontario, during the COVID-19 pandemic. She held an AMS Fellowship in Compassion and Artificial Intelligence from the AMS Healthcare Group, where she explored how best to deliver virtual care that is compassionate. She is Principal Investigator on a CIHR grant where patients and family physicians are co-creating a model of virtual and in-person primary care. She is Co-Principal Investigator on a CIHR grant developing primary care-based digital tools to support family physicians and patients to talk about social isolation and health. Along with Dr Amanda Terry, she leads DELPHI, a researchable database containing de-identified primary electronic medical records from practices in Southwestern Ontario.

Carol L McWilliam*, MScN, EdD, is a retired Professor in the Arthur Labatt Family School of Nursing, Faculty of Health Sciences, at Western University, London, Canada. She conducts research in the areas of health promotion, health services delivery, and relationship building, with a focus on patient-professional and inter-professional communication. She makes a unique contribution to the field as a qualitative research methodologist, with work published in *Social Science and Medicine, Family Medicine, Patient Education and Counseling, Journal of Advanced Nursing, International Journal of Quality in Health Care,* and *International Journal of Health Promotion.*

Ian R McWhinney*, OC, MD, FCFP, FRCP, (1926–2012) was Professor Emeritus in the Department of Family Medicine at Western University, Canada. He was born in Burnley, Lancashire and educated at Cambridge University and St. Bartholomew's Hospital Medical School. For 14 years, he was a General Practitioner in Stratford-on-Avon. In 1968, he was appointed Foundation Professor of Family Medicine at Western University. He retired in 1992 and had a post-retirement appointment in the Centre for Studies in Family Medicine. His most recent books are a third edition of *A Textbook of Family Medicine,* published in 2009, and *A Call to Heal,* published in 2012.

---

* These authors' words in the Fourth Edition are identical to the third Edition. The authors' description therefore remains unchanged from the Third Edition.

Contributors

IkeOluwapo O Ajayi
Consultant Family Physician
Family Medicine Department
University College Hospital
and
Professor
Department of Epidemiology
    and Medical Statistics
College of Medicine
University of Ibadan
Ibadan, Nigeria

Lorraine Bayliss
Patient Partner
Ontario SPOR SUPPORT Unit
and
TUTOR-PHC Training Program
Ontario, Canada

Lynn Brown*
Social Worker
WestBridge Associates Counselling
    and Consulting Services
London, Ontario, Canada

Vera Henderson*
Family Practice Nurse
Middlesex Centre Regional Medical Clinic
Ilderton, Ontario, Canada

Juul Houwen
Family Physician
WGC Lindenholt
Department of Primary and Community
    Care
Radboud University Medical Center
Nijmegen, The Netherlands

Jennifer K Johnson
Family and Hospitalist Physician
Georgian Bay General Hospital
Midland, Ontario, Canada
and
Adjunct Professor
Department of Family Medicine
Schulich School of Medicine & Dentistry
Western University
London, Ontario, Canada

Britta Laslo
Family Physician
Hamilton, Ontario, Canada

Barry Lavallee*
Acting Director
University of Manitoba's Centre for
    Aboriginal Education
Centre for Human Rights Research
University of Manitoba
Winnipeg, Manitoba, Canada

Eng Sing Lee
Family Physician, Senior Consultant
National Healthcare Group Polyclinics
and
Assistant Professor (Clinical Practice)
Department of Global and Population
    Health
and
Director of Family Medicine and Primary
    Care Programme
Lee Kong Chian School of Medicine
Nanyang Technological University
Singapore

Omolara Lewechi-Uke
Consultant Family Physician
Federal Medical Center
Abeokuta, Nigeria

Peter Lucassen
Retired Family Physician
Senior Researcher Department of Primary
    and Community Care
Radboud University Medical Center
    (Radboudumc)
Nijmegen, The Netherlands

Melad Marbeen
Family Physician
Oxford Medical Centre
and
Adjunct Professor
Department of Family Medicine
Schulich School of Medicine & Dentistry
Western University
London, Ontario, Canada

Leslie Meredith
Research Associate
Centre for Studies in Family Medicine
Schulich School of Medicine & Dentistry
Western University
London, Ontario, Canada

Joan Mitchell*
Nurse Practitioner
Byron Family Medical Centre
London, Ontario, Canada

William R Phillips
Professor Emeritus of Family Medicine
University of Washington
Seattle, Washington, USA

Sudit Ranade
Chief Medical Officer of Health
Yukon Territory
and
Assistant Professor, Department of
    Family Medicine
Adjunct Professor, Master of Public
    Health Program
Schulich School of Medicine & Dentistry
Western University
London, Ontario, Canada

Nisanthini Ravichandiran
Family Physician, Lecturer
Department of Family and Community
    Medicine
University of Toronto
Toronto, Ontario

Caroline Villa Martignoni Rebicki
Family Physician
Sociedade Brasileira de Medicina
    de Família
Brazil
and
Resident Physician
Department of Family and Community
    Medicine
UT Health San Antonio, Texas

Olivia Reis
Family Physician
Regina Family Medicine Unit
Regina, Saskatchewan
and
Assistant Professor
Department of Family Medicine
University of Saskatchewan College of
    Medicine
Saskatoon, Saskatchewan

Christine Rivet*
Associate Professor
Department of Family Medicine
Ottawa, Ontario, Canada

Lynn Shaw*
Occupational Therapist, Associate
    Professor, Field Chair
Occupational Science
School of Occupational Therapy
Faculty of Health Sciences
Western University
London, Ontario, Canada

---

* These contributors' words in the Fourth Edition are identical to the Third Edition. The contributors' description therefore remains unchanged from the Third Edition.

PART ONE

Overview

Introduction

MOIRA STEWART, JUDITH BELLE BROWN, W WAYNE WESTON,
THOMAS R FREEMAN, BRIDGET L RYAN, AND CAROL L MCWILLIAM

In the face of world turmoil, cultural seismic shifts, ubiquitous and often inadequate technology, and a life-altering pandemic, health care is in something close to free fall. To be part of the renewal of a safe and nurturing society, health care will need to cleave to the importance of caring, connection and coordination.

It has been 10 years since the third edition of this book. Is the patient-centered clinical method still relevant given the massive problems facing society? In our view, patient-centered health care is even more relevant today in helping to swing the pendulum back from divisiveness toward healing and hope.

In the 1980s, when the patient-centered clinical method was first conceptualized and used in research and education, it was at the periphery of medicine.[1-6] Indeed, many educators and researchers viewed patient-centered medicine as a "soft science" – caring and compassion were acknowledged to be important aspects of humanitarian care, but few people were aware of the pivotal role of patient-centered communication in modern scientific medicine. In the first edition of this book, we described the full patient-centered clinical method, with the goal of placing it at the epicenter of clinical practice and medical education.[7]

In the 1990s, the patient-centered clinical method was embraced by many groups of medical students, residents, graduate fellows, community physicians, and health profession faculties across North America, Europe, Türkiye, the United Arab Emirates, Argentina, Brazil, Australia, New Zealand, Japan, and Southeast Asia. The patient-centered clinical method formed the basis of many medical education curriculae internationally, at both the undergraduate and the graduate level.[8] Furthermore, the patient-centered clinical method served as the guide for the summative evaluation of postgraduate training in several countries.[9, 10] Research, focusing on the patient-centered clinical method, exploded; international studies reinforced not only the patients' desire for, and satisfaction with, patient-centered care[11, 12] but also the positive impact of such care on patient outcomes, health care utilization, and costs of care.[13-15] These studies supported an emerging international definition of patient-centered care.[16]

Nonetheless, commitment to patient-centeredness waned in the 2010s as it competed with many other forces in health care including a utilitarian model of efficient transactions and an infatuation with technology as a panacea.[17]

More recently though, there has been a resurgence of interest in patient-centered, compassionate, and whole person care: a reawakening of how it works in our current society.[17-19]

DOI: 10.1201/9781003394679-2

Our goal, in launching this fourth edition, is to place the patient-centered clinical method in the current world context and provide constructive information and encouragement.

THE PATIENT-CENTERED CLINICAL METHOD

In this book the patient-centered model and method is described and explained. A program of conceptual development, education, and research, which has been underway for the last four decades, provides the material. Although the program took place in the context of family medicine, its messages are relevant to all disciplines of medicine and to other healthcare professions, such as nursing, social work, physiotherapy, and occupational therapy. The overarching framework is the model. The way of implementing the framework reflects the clinical method. This book presents both a framework and its implementation, the patient-centered clinical method.

Patient-centered care presupposes two stances in the mindset of the clinician. First, the hierarchical notion of the professional being in charge and the patient being passive does not hold here. To be patient-centered, the clinician must be able to empower the patient and share the power in the relationship, and this means renouncing control that traditionally has been in the hands of the professional. This is the moral imperative of patient-centered practice. In adopting these values, the practitioner will experience the direction the relationship can take when power is shared. Second, maintaining an exclusively objective stance in relation to patients produces an unacceptable insensitivity to human suffering. The clinician must also engage the patient at the emotional level. To be patient-centered requires a balance between the subjective and the objective, a bringing together of the mind and the body.

The evolution of the patient-centered clinical method from the six components presented in 1995 to the four components introduced in 2013 is described in the third edition on pages 5 and 6.

In this book, therefore, we describe the four interactive components of the patient-centered clinical method, summarized in Box 1.1 and illustrated in Figure 1.1.

The first three interactive components encompass the encounters between patient and clinician. The fourth component focuses on the ongoing relationship that forms the foundation on which the interactions occur. Although distinct components are used to facilitate teaching and research, patient-centered clinical practice is a holistic concept in which components interact and unite in a unique way in each patient–clinician encounter and relationship.

The goal of the first component of the patient-centered clinical method is to explore disease and patients' perceptions of health and illness. In addition to assessing the disease process by history and physical examination, the clinician actively seeks to enter into the patients' worlds to understand both the perceptions of health (its meaning to patients and their aspirations or life goals) and the unique experience of illness (the patients' feelings about being ill, their ideas about the illness, how the illness is affecting their functioning, and, lastly, what they expect from the clinician).

The second component is the integration of these concepts (health, disease, and illness) with an understanding of the whole person. This includes an awareness of the multiple aspects of the patients' lives, such as personality, developmental history, life cycle issues, and the multiple contexts in which they live.

The mutual task of finding common ground between patient and clinician is the third component of the method and focuses on three key areas: defining the problem, establishing the goals of treatment, and identifying the roles to be assumed by patient and clinician.

The fourth component emphasizes that each contact with the patient should be used to build on the patient–clinician relationship by including compassion, empathy, a sharing of power, healing, and hope. To do so requires a focus on the self of the patient and the clinician, self-awareness, mindfulness and practical wisdom, as well as an appreciation of unconscious aspects of the relationship such as transference and countertransference.

BOX 1.1: The Four Interactive Components of the Patient-Centered Clinical Method

1. Exploring Health, Disease, and the Illness Experience:
   - unique perceptions and experience of health (meaning and aspirations)
   - history, physical, lab
   - dimensions of the illness experience (feelings, ideas, effects on function, and expectations).

2. Understanding the Whole Person:
   - the person (e.g., life history, personal and developmental issues)
   - the context (e.g., family, employment, social support, culture, community, and ecosystem).

3. Finding Common Ground:
   - problems and priorities
   - goals of treatment and/or management
   - roles of patient and clinician.

4. Enhancing the Patient–Clinician Relationship:
   - compassion and empathy
   - power
   - healing and hope
   - self-awareness and practical wisdom
   - transference and countertransference.

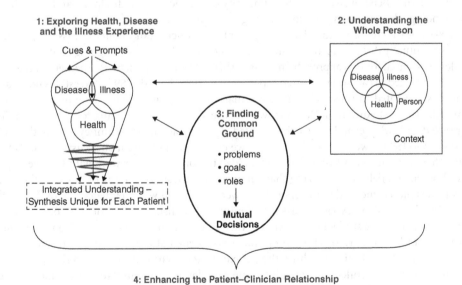

Figure 1.1 The Patient-Centered Clinical Method – Four Interactive Components

A BRIEF HISTORY OF THE PATIENT-CENTERED CLINICAL METHOD AT WESTERN UNIVERSITY

Early Ideas: The Department of Family Medicine at Western University, London, Ontario, Canada, began work on the patient–doctor relationship at its inception with the arrival in 1968 of the inaugural chairperson, Dr Ian R McWhinney. His work elucidating the "real reason" the patient presented to the doctor[20] was inspired by Balint[21] and set the stage for explorations of the breadth of all patient problems – whether physical, social, or psychological – and of the depth, the meaning of the patient's presentation. The research of his PhD student Moira Stewart was guided by these interests and focused on eliciting patients' discomforts, worries, and disturbances in daily living and social problems.[22-24]

Ideas from Practice: Dr Joseph Levenstein from South Africa was invited by McWhinney to be a visiting professor for 1 year (1981–1982) and was a powerful catalyst, bringing with him an idea from his practice.[25] He had been challenged by a clinical clerk in his office to explain "what are you doing when you meet each patient?" He had no answer. So, he audiotaped 1000 visits and focused on the ones that he thought had been successful in which, he concluded, he had identified and addressed each patient's unique expectations, needs, and fears. Levenstein's idea galvanized the department in the academic year of 1981–1982, and all the clinical faculty members met Joseph regularly to debate these ideas and view videotaped examples. Following Joseph's departure, Dr W Wayne Weston was chosen by McWhinney to lead a faculty development process for a year (mid 1982–1983). Weston said, "We changed Joe's model of 'expectations, needs, and fears' to Feelings (including fears), Ideas, Function and Expectations (Component 1)."

Reflection and Definition: The patient-centered clinical method evolved further through the work of the department's Patient–Doctor Communication Group at Western University who hammered out language to best describe the ideas, coming from the clinicians who Weston was facilitating, which later became Components 2, 3, 4, 5, and 6. For example, the group considered not only the patients' presenting problems but also their context of life cycle, family, work, and community. Dr Judith Belle Brown noted the similarity of her social work discipline and medicine in understanding "the person in situation," taking into consideration human development and context. Next came the consideration of how the patient and clinician talk about these issues; prioritize them; and mutually discuss treatment approaches, goals, and roles. The ongoing relationship was considered essential for this approach and was enshrined as a component. Refinement of the ideas over 3–5 years[26] led to two series of three papers each in 1986[1, 3, 4] and 1989.[2, 5, 6] Weston said, "Based on insights generated in these sessions, I summarised our progress with diagrams to illustrate the model." The first edition of the book was published in 1995.[7] Preparing for the first edition, we grappled with what exactly was being created, and here again, McWhinney led the thinking. Was this a model? Or was it a method? Were we creating a multi-item checklist for students to follow? There was much confusion. We were guided by comparing our work with George Engel's biopsychosocial model[27] and realizing that a model does not suggest a way of practice; therefore, our work was more a method than a model. We were impressed with Pendleton's book[28] from the United Kingdom, which described "tasks," not minute checklists, so we wrote the components as injunctions to guide the student or clinician in their quest for an approach to caring for patients.

Teaching and Advocacy: Teaching programs were created at the residency and undergraduate medicine levels, including teaching the patient-centered clinical method to the residents in family medicine with a collection of readings and role playing, and numerous presentations were made to students, residents, and faculty around the world. Students in the department's graduate program (MClSc in family medicine) wrote theses on the topic from South Africa, Nigeria, Japan, and Singapore. Brown led the advocacy at the College of Family Physicians of Canada for the method to be used to guide the scoring rubric of the certification examination including training examiners and writing the case scenarios based on the patient-centered clinical method.[9]

Research: Research measures were developed in the 1980s and, over the next three decades, Stewart led a multi-method research program including a cohort study, randomized trials, and qualitative studies.[29-44] Dr Bridget L Ryan joined the research program in 2013.

Unique in Medicine: A program of conceptual development arising from practice and then enveloping teaching and research covering four decades is unique in medicine. One facet supported the other with teaching insights assisting in conceptual development and with research findings informing teaching and concepts.

THE PATIENT-CENTERED CLINICAL METHOD IN RELATION TO OTHER MODELS OF PRACTICE

Models of practice are valuable in several ways: first, they guide our perceptions by drawing our attention to specific features of practice; second, they provide a framework for understanding what is going on; and third, they guide our actions by defining what is important. A productive model will not only simplify the complexity of reality but also focus our attention on those aspects of a situation that are most important for understanding and effective action. The dominant model in medical practice, since the early 20th century, has been labeled "the conventional medical model." No one would question the widespread influence of the conventional medical model, but it has often been challenged for oversimplifying the problems of sickness.[45, 46] Engel describes the problems with the conventional medical model this way:

> It assumes disease to be fully accounted for by deviations from the norm of measurable biological (somatic) variables. It leaves no room within its framework for the social, psychological, and behavioral dimensions of illness. The biomedical model not only requires that disease be dealt with as an entity independent of social behavior, it also demands that behavioral aberrations be explained on the basis of disordered somatic (biochemical or neurophysiological) processes.[47]

Balint and colleagues[48, 49] introduced the term "patient-centered medicine" and contrasted it with "illness-centered medicine." An understanding of the patient's complaints based on patient-centered thinking was called "overall diagnosis," and an understanding based on disease-centered thinking was called "traditional diagnosis." Others elaborated the approach.[50-53] Patient-centered medicine[21] aligns with the work of Rogers[54] on client-centered counseling, Newmann and Young[55] on total person approach in nursing, and the "Two-Body Practice" in occupational therapy.[56]

Epstein et al.[57] have described, compared, and contrasted five approaches to patient–doctor communication. Stewart[19] has updated a review of patient-centered concepts based on reviews of the many frameworks arising in the past decades.* In Table 1.1, six reviews since 2000 are compared. While there is considerable detail in the table, there are two key findings. First the headings (in bold) use different language across the six reviews. However, second, one can see quite similar concepts in the subheadings (in italics). For example, across the first row, one repeatedly sees the words "patient experience" and "patient preferences" and "patient perspective."

* This paragraph and Table 1.1 and Table 1.2 are reproduced with permission from:

Stewart M. Evidence on Patient-Centeredness, patient-centered systems, and implementation and scaling of whole person health. Commissioned paper for the National Academies of Sciences, Engineering and Medicine, Health and Medicine Division, Consensus Study Report – Achieving Whole Health – A New Approach for Veterans and the Nation, Editors: Krist AH, South-Paul J, and Meisnere M, 2023. https://doi.org/10.17226/26854. Reproduced with permission from the National Academy of Sciences, Courtesy of the National Academies Press, Washington, DC.

Table 1.1 Six Approaches to Patient-Centered Concepts*

Patient-Centered Clinical Method Patient at the Centre	Mead & Bower, 2000[76]	Institute of Medicine, 2001[77]	Morgan & Yoder, 2012[78]	Langberg et al., 2019[79]	Sturgiss et al., 2022[58]
Exploring Health, Disease and the Illness Experience – Symptoms, Signs, Laboratory results – Patient's meaning of what health is and aspirations for life – Patient's illness experience including feelings, ideas, function and expectations	**Biopsychosocial** – Social and psychological factors – full range of difficulties – health promotion **Patient as Person** – Patient's experience – eliciting patient expectations, feelings, ideas	**Respectfulness to Patients' Values, Preferences and Expressed Needs #1**	**Individualized Care** – unique needs, preferences, and health concerns **Holistic Care** – physical, cognitive and psychosocial functioning **Respectful Care** – strengths and abilities	**Biopsychosocial** – involving physical, cognitive, emotional, behavioural, social and spiritual domains **Patient-as-Person** – uniqueness of each patient – patient perspective – patients experience illness differently – explore both the disease and the illness experience	**Biopsychosocial** – social determinants of health **Patient as a Person** – strengths based
Understanding the Whole Person in Context – Patient as a person – An individual developmental trajectory and personality – A family, social support and work – Community and culture	**Patient as Person** – within his or her unique context	**Involving Family and Friends for Decision making and Support #6**	**Individualized Care** – Personality **Holistic Care** – responding to the needs of the whole person in context – the family, cultural and religious context	**Biopsychosocial** – "holistic", "whole person" **Patient-as-Person** – patient experience differs depending on current life situation	**Biopsychosocial** – social determinants of health **Patient as a Person** – person as part of a collective – spirituality, cultural needs

Finding Common Ground
– *Mutual discussion between the patient and clinician of*
  – *the nature of the problems*
  – *the goals*
  – *the roles of each*
– *Reaching mutual agreement*
 	
Sharing Power and Responsibility
– *encourage patient involvement in care*
– *recognise patient's preferences*
Therapeutic Relationship
– *common understanding of goals and requirements of treatment*
	Providing Information, Communication and Education #3
	– *so patients can be properly equipped to take part in medical decisions*
	Ensuring Physical Comfort, #4
		Individualized Care
		– *an individual Care Plan*
		Respectful Care
		– *patients' preference*
		– *supporting goals*
		Empowering Care
		– *self-confidence*
		– *participation in decision-making*
			Sharing Power and Responsibility
			– *encouraging patient participation*
			– *shared decision-making*
			– *empowerment*
			– *common ground*
				Sharing Power
				– *seen as equals*
				– *empowerment*
				Sharing Responsibility

Enhancing the Patient–Clinician Relationship – *Surfacing emotion* – *Compassion, caring, empathy and trust* – *Power in the relationship* **Sharing Power and Responsibility** – *egalitarian relationships*	**Providing Emotional Support #5** – *relieving fear and anxiety*	**Respectful Care** – *listening* – *autonomy* – *effective communication*	**Sharing Power and Responsibility** – *egalitarian partnership* – *respect for patient autonomy*	**Therapeutic Relationship/ Bond/Alliance** – *compassion* – *emotional engagement*

(Continued)

Table 1.1 Six Approaches to Patient-Centered Concepts (Continued)

Patient-Centered Clinical Method Patient at the Centre	Mead & Bower, 2000[76]	Institute of Medicine, 2001[77]	Morgan & Yoder, 2012[78]	Langberg et al., 2019[79]	Sturgiss et al., 2022[58]
- Continuity of the relationship and constancy - Engendering healing and hope - Clinician self-awareness - Transference and counter-transference	**Therapeutic Relationship** - empathy, congruence and unconditional positive regard - develop the emotional context in consultations			**Therapeutic Alliance** - valuing the relationship - constructive relationship - respectful communication - mutual respect	
	The Doctor as Person - doctor and patient influence each other - attention to cues to the affective relationship	**Co-ordinated and Integrated Care #2**		**The Doctor as Person**	**Provider as Person** - professional clinical responsibilities - advocate for the patient
				Co-ordinated Care - Accessibility, - Co-ordination and continuity - A care pathway	**Co-ordinated Care, Access, Continuity of Care**

* Table 1.1 is reproduced with permission from:

Stewart M. Evidence on Patient-Centeredness, patient-centered systems, and implementation and scaling of whole person health. Commissioned paper for the National Academies of Sciences, Engineering and Medicine, Health and Medicine Division, Consensus Study Report – Achieving Whole Health – A New Approach for Veterans and the Nation, Editors: Krist AH, South-Paul J, and Meisnere M, 2023. https://doi.org/10.17226/26854. Reproduced with permission from the National Academy of Sciences, Courtesy of the National Academies Press, Washington, D.C.

Table 1.2 Four Common Elements and Two Less Common Elements of Patient-Centered Conceptual Frameworks

1) Patient Experience (thoughts and feelings)
2) Person in Context (especially family)
3) Discussion of Goals, Preferences and Shared Decisions
4) Relationship including Empathy, Emotion and Sharing Power
5) Clinician as Person
6) Co-ordination

Reproduced with permission from Stewart 2023, NASEM Report.

Using the words of the subheadings, Table 1.2 shows the four most common concepts plus the two less commonly included concepts arising from the literature on patient-centered frameworks from 2000 to 2022, indicating more similarities than differences in the definition of patient-centeredness. A worldwide definition, foreshadowed by earlier authors,[16] seems to be quite clear now; both Sturgiss et al.[58] and Table 1.2 support this clarity in the definition.

Four other frameworks for improving care and education have become prominent in the past decades and can be compared and contrasted with the patient-centered clinical method: shared decision-making, narrative medicine, goal-oriented care, and evidence-based medicine.

Stewart and Phillips compare and contrast the patient-centered clinical method with shared decision-making in Box 1.2.

BOX 1.2: Patient-Centered Clinical Method (PCCM) and Shared Decision-Making (SDM)

Moira Stewart and William R Phillips

To help bring SDM[74, 75] and PCCM into a complementary alliance, we compare and contrast the two concepts in Table 1.3. The following text elaborates on the rows in Table 1.3.

The two clinical approaches often occur in different clinical contexts. SDM usually focuses on selected clinical encounters and specific decisions, often about testing or treatment. PCCM embraces continuous, comprehensive care across multiple encounters, problems, and decisions. SDM can separate treatment decisions from the rest of the work done by patient and clinician.

SDM is most easily applied when the question is straightforward, high-quality evidence is available, and clinical guidelines are broadly accepted. PCCM, on the other hand, is most valuable in the assessment of the patient and their problems, understanding their views, and building a healing relationship.

If the clinical question is clear and high-quality evidence is available to inform decisions, SDM can be reasonably straightforward. It is an essential clinical skill. In many situations, however, the evidence does not exist or is unclear, or the patient does not accept evidence-based recommendations. This is particularly common in primary care practice serving unselected patients with undefined problems, often complicated by

Table 1.3 Comparing Patient-Centered Clinical Method with Shared Decision-Making

Comparing Patient-Centered Clinical Method with Shared Decision-Making		
Dimension	**PCCM** **Patient-Centered** **Clinical Method**	**SDM** **Shared Decision-Making**
Context Scope	Comprehensive care	Clinical encounter
Time Course	Throughout care	At selected decision points
Clinical Situation	When assessment, understanding, and partnership are needed	When a decision needs to be made, usually about testing or treatment.
Strongest Setting	When context is important, question is unclear, patients' experiences deserve exploration	When evidence is available, guidelines are clear, options are defined
Goals Commitment	To the patient	To evidence-based practice
Objectives	Explore patient emotions, ideas and context Find common ground Build relationship	Reach a decision. Empower patient choice Educate patient
Skills Information gathering	Elicit the patient's world view	Assess the patient's values on risks and benefits of each decision
Communication	Listening	Explaining

multimorbidity, polypharmacy, and myriad social factors. Guidelines often address such challenges by suggesting the clinician shift to a patient-centered approach. The strategy is to ask the patient's ideas or expectations to move the decision forward or motivate the patient to adhere to recommendations. However, this comes late in the interaction and possibly without the benefit of an ongoing relationship built through a shared history of patient-centered care. The PCCM would explore patient emotions, ideas, and context earlier in the course of care and at a deeper level, not just to make a specific decision but also to guide care from a partnership built on common ground.

The goals of the two approaches can also be different. In PCCM, the commitment of the clinician is primarily to the patient. In SDM, the commitment can be focused on evidence-based practice. With an elderly patient, for example, the PCCM might mean that there will be no shared decision-making if the patient clearly wishes to rely on the clinician's recommendation with no discussion. SDM implies the goals are sharing and deciding, quite different from the PCCM goals of understanding. This is a major philosophical difference: advocacy for the patient versus advocacy for sharing the decision.

The objectives of SDM usually focus on reaching a clinical decision, which often includes educating the patient and – when done expertly – it can empower patient

choice. The objectives of PCCM more broadly engage the tasks of understanding the patient, finding common ground, and building a relationship to guide care,
including clinical decisions. SDM is often transactional, while PCCM aims to be more
relational.

The PCCM empowers clinical care beyond situations when the evidence is murky or
the patient is hesitant. There are many reasons a patient might be reticent about a particular evidence-based intervention. Understanding the patient's view of the options may
require a broad undertaking, a shared discussion of the patient's and clinician's perception of the problems, roles, and goals of care. It requires respect for patients' autonomy.
Such a discussion may redefine the tasks for both the patient and physician. For example, a patient balks at the doctor's prescription offered for her headache because she
saw an uncle die from a stroke after taking that medication. A patient with cancer, when
encouraged to describe his motivation, says that his main goal in life at this stage is to
dance at his daughter's wedding. Such revelations can change the work of the clinician
and patient in meaningful ways.

In addition, the PCCM explicitly invites the clinician to build a relationship and knowledge over time. When that clinician sees the patient in hospital with serious pneumonia,
she will be better prepared to offer the care needed to reach the patient's goals, aspirations, and preferences for care.

The two approaches also require different yet complementary clinical skills.
SDM requires expertise in evidence-based medicine, applying the best evidence
to patient care and patient education. Communication skills are essential to both
approaches. SDM focuses more on explaining, while PCCM more heavily emphasizes
listening.

The PCCM includes four interactive components, of which finding common ground
is most similar to SDM. Importantly, in PCCM, finding common ground is linked to the
other three components, and the visit/conversation with the patient may weave back and
forth from one component to another. In the PCCM, the shared decision-making process
fits within – not isolated from – the broader context of care.

Turning to narrative medicine, two current definitions help us compare and contrast it to the
patient-centered clinical method. Narrative medicine is "the capacity to skillfully receive the
accounts persons give of themselves – to recognize, absorb, interpret and be moved to action by
the stories of others."[59] "The mission of narrative medicine has been to restore humanity, imagination and moral engagement to the medical world."[60]

Narrative medicine, in common with the patient-centered clinical method, stresses the
patient's particular story (Components 1 and 2 of the patient-centered clinical method) revealed
in the context of an ongoing patient–clinician relationship (Component 4). The two approaches
also seek to enhance the clinician's comfort in engaging patients at an emotional level. Narrative
medicine relates to Component 3, "Finding Common Ground," as a process of the patient and
clinician co-constructing the patient's story to promote both understanding and change. One
difference is that narrative medicine separates itself from the tasks of conventional medicine,
in contrast to the patient-centered clinical method, which includes medical tasks as part of its
work.

Another approach is goal-oriented care, which is similar to the patient-centered clinical method, in that it seeks to integrate its work with medical tasks, especially of prevention and chronic illness care:

> Goal-oriented care is not about asking patients what they want and helping them get it. Goals, objectives and strategies are, wherever possible, developed and agreed upon by patient and physician. Patients contribute information about needs, desires, resources, values, and preferences. Physicians contribute information about medical options, obstacles and probabilities. Care plans are developed by considering all of this information.[61]

Both Mold and De Maeseneer[62] stress that the process of clarifying goals is "an end in itself"[63] and is "of utmost importance."[64] Goal-oriented care is more strengths-based than problem-based, stating that the "problem-oriented approach tends to dehumanize care and underestimate the importance of therapeutic relationships."[65] This is the most striking contrast to the patient-centered clinical method; goal-oriented care is strongly strengths-based while the patient-centered clinical method incorporates both a problem-focus and attention to patients' goals to obtain an integrated understanding.

There are several areas of similarity of the goal-oriented care and the patient-centered clinical method. One is the way health is defined by both as "the meaning of health to the patient and the patients' ability to realize aspirations and purpose in their lives" (Chapter 3 of this book on Component 1); and "health is the ability to successfully face . . . challenges and capitalize on . . . opportunities."[66] A second similarity is the emphasis, in Component 1 of the patient-centered clinical method, on the effects of function on patients' lives. A third similarity is that both approaches stress the "mutual discussion of problems, roles and goals" (Chapter 6 of this book) and the determination of "capabilities, roles and responsibilities."[67]

Another way of viewing practice is evidence-based medicine, sometimes characterized as the "hard science" of medicine while the patient-centered clinical method is the "soft" side of it. This is to misrepresent both evidence-based medicine and the patient-centered clinical method, which, in truth, have significant areas of confluence.

The early writings describing evidence-based medicine make clear that it is not intended to replace clinical judgment. Clinical decision-making is described as taking into account three elements: the evidence, patient particulars, and patient preference.[68, 69] Evidence-based medicine has made tremendous strides in describing and putting into practice a method for acquiring the best available evidence about an issue in health care. It is not itself a clinical method, although it does inform the clinician. Research on the patient-centered clinical method has made clear that finding common ground between both the physician's and the patient's perspectives is key to a successful clinical outcome.

Evidence-based medicine assists the physician in assessing the quality of the information. It is not a substitute for clinical judgment or clinical intuition, which arise out of a specific interaction between a particular patient and a particular clinician. The patient-centered clinical method describes a method for ensuring that the patient's particulars and preferences are taken into account and an agreed plan arrived at. From this vantage point, the patient-centered clinical method incorporates or subsumes evidence-based medicine.

The many models we have described in this chapter, including the patient-centered clinical method, all set out to make the implicit in patient care, explicit. While models help clarify the basics, they never completely capture what happens in reality. The tacit knowledge of the clinician and patient are not captured in the models, which are, by definition, oversimplifications.

Stewart[70] stated that while "models do help in teaching and research they fail to capture the indivisible whole of a healing relationship."

VALUE OF THE PATIENT-CENTERED CLINICAL METHOD

In order to convince colleagues, education committees, and policy-makers of the value of transitioning to a patient-centered approach, one needs to be able to answer the essential questions: Does it work? Do patients want it, and why? Can it work in the face of new technologies?

Chapter 9 provides the reader with a view of how patient-centered care transpires in a highly technological world.

Chapter 14, on the contributions of qualitative and mixed methods studies, describes examples elucidating patient-centered care.

Chapter 15 covers the most up-to-date quantitative literature on the effect of patient-centered care on patient reported outcome measures as well as on clinician well-being.

COMMON MISCONCEPTIONS ABOUT THE PATIENT-CENTERED CLINICAL METHOD

It is incumbent on us as authors to be clear about what the patient-centered clinical method is and what it is not.

Some readers have the impression that the patient-centered clinical method focuses primarily on the patients' psychosocial issues versus their diseases, on patient–clinician communication and being nice to patients. On the contrary, it is fully integrated into the clinical tasks of health professionals; biomedicine is part of the patient-centered clinical method. The reader will have noted the Disease circle in the diagram in Figure 1.1, indicating the inclusion of the knowledge, methods, and tasks of biomedicine. This notion sets the patient-centered clinical method apart from other models of patient-centeredness represented in the literature.

Others have called being patient-centered an abdication of the health professional's role, acquiescing to patients' demands and rigidly adhering to the notion that the patient makes all decisions. The patient's "right to choose" becomes the "central feature" of healthcare.[71] On the contrary, being patient-centered aligns with flexibility, encouraging patients' voices on whether and when they will share in decisions. This alignment of the patient-centered clinical method and shared decision-making in the minds of readers is persistent; we attempt to be clearer in their similarities and differences, as can be seen in Table 1.3.

Another false impression that we authors have left in the reader's mind is that there are two agendas competing in an interaction between a patient and a clinician; rather, in the patient-centered clinical method, there is a developing partnership to tackle the tasks of solving problems at hand and the co-creation of a plan.

In addition, the acronym FIFE (feelings, ideas, function, and expectations) can be very useful for students as they are learning to inquire about the patient's illness experience. However, it can also be dangerous if it becomes an appendage to the conventional review of systems: "Any visual problems – blurred vision ... ?" "What do you feel about this?" "How are your bowels – any constipation; diarrhea ... ?" "Any ideas about what is causing this?" Thus "FIFEing" the patient, as we have heard students remark, becomes just another interviewing technique or an additional step in their review of systems and does not reflect a genuine interest in and concern about the patient's unique illness experience and does not encourage attentive listening.

Having said that, sometimes patients' expectations are very clear and straightforward. They want treatment for their athlete's foot or completion of a medical form for insurance purposes.

Thus it is not always essential to explore, in-depth, patients' perceptions of health or their illness experience. What is essential is that doctors listen to patients' cues and prompts in order to make appropriate and sensitive inquiries.

The notion that patient-centeredness recommends a single style of practice is worrisome.[72] We find it difficult to present a diagram and an approach and, at the same time, avoid giving the impression that a standard approach is recommended. Nonetheless, a standard approach is not recommended; rather, the diagrams are a guide, and the goal is different conversations with different patients.

The argument that a physician does not need to be patient-centered in all visits – for example, when a patient presents a straightforward problem – is supported by the description of visits as falling into types: routines, rituals, or dramas.[73] Arguing in favor of the view that physicians are not patient-centered all the time is our own result that physicians with low average scores on patient-centeredness show small standard deviations for these scores, perhaps revealing a more rigid and inflexible approach. However, high-scoring physicians show wide standard deviations, suggesting a flexibility in their clinical approach.[5] Nonetheless, our contention is that physicians do not know whether the visit ought to be routine, a ritual, or a drama unless they are patient-centered and ask brief and appropriate questions at the beginning of the visit.

Alongside the notion of a single style of practices is the mistaken idea that the patient-centered clinical method is a set of tasks that do not need to be applied during each visit but, rather, that can be cherry-picked – that is, some used or some discarded.

A brief patient–doctor dialog about a minor sore throat serves as an example.

Doctor: (While reaching for a tongue depressor) Is there anything unusually worrying about this sore throat?
Patient: No. (Pause)
Doctor: Do you think this is anything out of the ordinary?
Patient: No . . . I don't think so.
Doctor: Anything else going on in your life that you want to tell me about today?
Patient: No. Things are great!

Only after such a 5-second interchange can a doctor be sure that this visit is going to be routine as opposed to a drama.

CONCLUSION

In this introductory chapter we have presented the four components of the patient-centered clinical method. We also provided a historical perspective of the evolution of the patient-centered model and of the clinical method that serves to implement the theoretical model. The place of the patient-centered model and clinical method was examined in relation to other conceptual models and current trends in health care. This chapter has pointed to later chapters which provide empirical evidence supporting the adoption of the patient-centered clinical method. In the final sections, challenges in practicing the patient-centered clinical method in the current context were explored, with attention given to some common misconceptions about the patient-centered clinical method.

The following case, covering all four components of the patient-centered clinical method, also places the method in relation to narrative medicine and guidelines from evidence-based medicine. The family physician and patient have known each other for many years.

THE MAN, THE POEM, THE SECRET*

Peter Lucassen

"You are here for the results of your tests, I think?" "Yes, that's correct," he replied. I knew the 62-year-old man sitting in front of me very well and for a long time. We had a warm relationship. Last week, he had consulted me with a lot of complaints, both physical and mental. He had mentioned the word "depressed." A few years ago, he underwent coronary artery bypass surgery and now he was worried that his complaints had a relation with the surgery or with heart problems coming up again. He complained about chronic cough, runny nose, shortness of breath especially during coughing, extra heart beats and frequently a heart rate exceeding 100 beats/minute; during periods in which his heart beat increased, he was tired; further complaints: ice cold fingers, especially during the night, hot feelings in his middle fingers during the day, not-specific chest pain, no pleasure in doing things, passivity, and no interest whatsoever in sex. I knew from previous consultations that his daughter had ended her marriage with a man he considered more a friend than a son-in-law. During the conversation last week he had tears in his eyes. After physical examination I referred him for blood tests, chest X-ray, sinus X-ray and electrocardiography.

'Yeah, I have been looking through results of the tests just before you entered and I can tell you that nothing is wrong. The X-rays of your sinuses and lungs are without any abnormality; your blood tests do not show any abnormality either, and the same goes for the electrocardiography." "That's fine," he replied. "I think that your coughing is caused by your antihypertensive medication. And your other complaints, I don't think that they are caused by some disease. It seems to me that you experience a kind of restlessness or feeling down or something like that." At this point in the consultation, I had to make a choice: do I continue with checking the patient's depression criteria, all the symptoms mentioned in the guideline? Or do I invite him to tell his story? Because he once had told me that he used to write songs and sketches which gave him a lot of fun.

So, I continued: "Some people really get a better understanding of what is going on with them when they write-up the story of their life. Would that be something you could do?" His eyes immediately filled with tears and suddenly he stood up, searched in his pocket and took out a piece of paper. He said: "I wrote a poem, that has to be on my tombstone when I'm dead." I asked him if he would recite the poem for me and he nodded.

> Why?
> Why always in such a hurry
> Why flows my blood so fast
> Why all that turbulence
> Why was I sometimes so fierce
> I long so badly for rest and peace
> At times I found this at the shores of the sea
> But always the turbulence returned
> And everything had to be done in haste
> Now, I've found my peace
> Although leaving hurts me much

> Now, I've found my peace
> Because my turbulence is no more.

He folded the paper and returned it to his pocket. A poem for a tombstone. How do I continue? Is the man depressed and should I try to confirm this diagnosis? And is he suicidal? And should I inquire this? He did not give me an opportunity to continue as he said: "Doctor, if I write-up the story of my life, doctor, I think that you will never want to see me again." I said: "I'm not a judge. I'm here to help people." And again, his eyes filled with tears and he said to me: "Doctor, then I'll have to tell you a secret. I have made one big mistake in my entire life, a big mistake. It should be possible to correct a mistake." And then he started to talk. "It's about 40 years ago, I was 22 years old. I was going steady with the young woman who would become my wife. My wife is part of a big family, she had many brothers and sisters. They lived in the middle of a small village and earned their money with a grocery shop, that part of the house. There were always a lot of people in the house because it was cozy, pleasant and warm. My girlfriend, who was 21 had a younger sister who was 19. The sister often talked with me and asked me to help with her homework. As it was noisy and busy downstairs, we went upstairs. After a while the sister started talking about sexual matters, about how these things were for boys and so on. I became excited and in the end we made love to each other. It happened several times, but after some months I finished with it. Oh, I regret very much what had happened and I swear to you, doctor, that I never touched another woman in my life except my own wife, although I had the chance to do so several times. I'm so sorry, doctor, I'm feeling so guilty." We were silent for a while. I realized that we had run out of time and that several patients would be waiting for me. However, I wanted to know how the story went further, so I asked him: "How did things continue? Your sister-in-law lives in the same small village as you and your wife. What kind of relationship do you have?" "Doctor, we have a good relationship," he told me, "we are on good terms and we never have talked about it." "Thank you, for telling me this," I said, "shall we make a further appointment for next week? "OK," he said.

One week later, I saw him sitting in the waiting room. His appearance was totally different. He looked very happy, he smiled. He told me that he felt very relieved. Very few of his symptoms were still there. He told me that he could go without any help.

I have been his general practitioner for many more years after this confession, but he never showed any signs of severe depression. He has been doing very well since then.

---

* This case was published by Lucassen PL. The man, the poem, the secret. *Patient Educ Couns.* 2009 May 1; 75: 147–8. Reprinted with permission of *Patient Education and Counseling*.

In the following case, we see the patient-centered clinical method being enacted by a public health physician in a brief yet powerful dialogue demonstrating the interaction of all four components.

LOVE IN THE TIME OF HIV

Sudit Ranade

"You know me, Dr R! There isn't much that phases me, but I just feel really uncomfortable seeing this guy by myself."

Those words stayed with me as I walked into the bright, sterile clinic room with the nurse who had asked for my assistance. In front of me, seated in a chair that seemed much too small for him, was a burly, bearded man dressed in a biker style. He had too few teeth for his age, and the ones that remained were broken and stained yellow. He had tattoos covering both of his arms that looked like biker gang insignia. He also had tattoos on his face that looked like teardrops falling from his eyes. I was about to tell this man he had HIV.

I had reviewed the current best practices about how to give this delicate diagnosis, but one look at the situation told me I would need a more human approach than to simply follow the guidelines. The nurse took a seat in the corner. I established his connection to the nurse and my connection to her, to validate a connection between all of us in the room. Then, I asked him what he knew about the reason for his visit: "Well, yuz called me because I had some tests done and I'm here for the results." – Yes.

I thanked him for coming and asked him to tell me more about the tests that had been done. He had a 3-month history of progressive pneumonia that finally involved him being admitted to hospital for several days. The microbiological profile of the pneumonia was unusual (*Pneumocystis jirovecii*, which used to be called *Pneumocystis carnii*). The presence of this infection indicates immune compromise (and was once almost synonymous with AIDS), so an HIV test was done at the hospital. The positive HIV test result was sent to our public health clinic for us to perform contact management, which requires making contact with the original or index case. While we would prefer a diagnosis to be communicated by someone's own physician, in this case his doctor's office was closed for three weeks and we needed to get him started on treatment and begin to follow up on his contacts. I wondered how he would take the news, but I wanted to assess his level of understanding about his illness first.

"One of the tests that they did on your blood in the hospital was an HIV test, and it was done because of the kind of lung infection you had. Were you aware that this test was done?"

"Yup," he replied.

"Can you tell me what you know about HIV?" He replied that he knew it was an infection, but that was about it. I reviewed some basic information about HIV with him, and then said: "Your test result shows me that you have the HIV virus. Normally, our procedure is to retest to make sure it is a true result, and we will retest you but based on what you have told me I think the retest will show us the same thing."

I reviewed with him that we needed to get him on treatment as soon as possible, and that with good adherence to medication and other healthy behaviors he could expect to live for many years. He agreed but seemed lost in thought. "Is there anything that you want to ask or talk to me about?"

"So, how did I get this?" he asked quietly.

OK. I took a deep breath, looked at the nurse, and started: "Good question. Keep in mind that it can be very difficult to pinpoint an exact source, but we know that HIV is transmitted in the blood, so the highest risks are from sharing needles and from unprotected sex with a person who has HIV. So I need to ask you some sensitive questions to help us understand this together – is that ok?" Nod.

"Have you ever injected drugs before?" Head shake *no*. "Just to be clear – you have never?" – "No."

"I understand from what you told our nurse that you have spent some time in jail – sometimes things happen in jail that people don't like to talk about but is there any way you could have been exposed to someone else's blood or body fluids there?" – "No."

"Have you ever had a blood transfusion?" – "No."

"Well, then that leaves sexual activity. Are you sexually active?" Head nod.

"Do you have sex with men, women, or both?" "Women."

"How many sexual partners have you had in the last 2 years?" "Just one – my wife."

I asked some questions about his wife, and whether she had ever used injection drugs, which he denied. Then suddenly he broke down. I had been expecting this (the moment when betrayal is suspected or realized), but I was completely unprepared for what followed. I discussed the need to get his wife tested for HIV:

"You can't!"
"Why not?"
"Because I lost her a few months ago." Crying.
"Lost her? She's . . . dead?" His head nods between sobs.
"I'm so sorry. Can you tell me a bit about her? What was your relationship like?"
"We were great! She stood by me while I was in jail, helped to raise our girls, and we picked right up again when I came out and I have tried to be a better person ever since. She's the only woman I ever loved."
"I'm sorry to ask this, but how did she die?"
"She went to the hospital a few months before me, died there from a lung infection."
Uh-oh.
"Had she lost a lot of weight?" – "Yes."
"Did it all happen fairly suddenly?" – "Yes," he replied.
"Do you know if she was tested for HIV?" "Don't know," he replied. I told him that since she wasn't tested we couldn't know for sure, but it certainly sounded like she could have died from HIV.
Was he sure she didn't inject drugs? – "Yes."
"I don't want to be insensitive, but do you know if she had any other partners?"
"No, she couldn't have, she couldn't have."
My nurse looked very concerned. I wasn't sure what he would do with this, but I knew I needed to check for his suicidality and his support system.
"Sometimes when people are told they have HIV, they go to a very dark place. Are there other people in your family to help you through this?"
"My daughters are great – we're just all trying to deal with it together."
"Have you ever thought about ending your life?"

"No – I would never – my daughters need me too much".
"Ok, we've talked about a lot today. I have to step out to bring you some
  forms to sign that let us get you into treatment. Will you be ok if I do that?"
  Nod.

I left the room to get some consent forms for referral to treatment and came back to reinforce that we were there for him and available to answer his questions at any time. When I re-entered the room, he was wailing like a lost, scared child. It was heartbreaking to witness the effects of his realization of his wife's infidelity while mourning her passing, coupled with the effects of a life-changing diagnosis. In that instant, the man had transformed from a person we had been afraid of to a person we were afraid for. I was terrified for his prospects, his ability to cope with a life-changing diagnosis, and the implications of being betrayed by his only love. Would he be able to find meaning in his circumstances and hope for the future? Would he self-destruct? I was encouraged that he denied suicidality, expressing the importance of being there for his daughters as well as his willingness to share his diagnosis with them. But what would become of him? I was sure there was more to his story, but beyond ensuring he obtained speedy access to HIV treatment, I never found out. When I left the room again, the nurse said: "Thank you! I've never seen that done before but I think you did it well!" As I gave her a half-hearted smile we heard renewed sobbing coming from the clinic room. "Don't worry Dr R, I'll sit with him for a little while more and make sure he's ok before he goes. He knows that he can always call us."
My smile widened a bit as I left, knowing I was leaving him in caring hands.

REFERENCES

1. Brown JB, Stewart MA, McCracken EC, et al. Patient-centered clinical method II. Definition and application. *Fam Pract*. 1986; 3(2): 75–79.
2. Brown JB, Weston WW, Stewart MA. Patient-centered interviewing part II: Finding common ground. *Can Fam Phys*. 1989; 35: 153–157.
3. Levenstein JH, McCracken EC, McWhinney IR, et al. The patient-centered clinical method. 1. A model for the doctor-patient interaction in family medicine. *Fam Pract*. 1986; 3(1): 24–30.
4. Stewart MA, Brown JB, Levenstein JH, et al. The patient-centered clinical method III. Changes in resident's performance over two months of training. *Fam Pract – Int, J*. 1986; 3: 164–167.
5. Stewart M, Brown JB, Weston W. Patient-centered interviewing III: Five provocative questions. *Can Fam Phys*. 1989; 35: 159–161.
6. Weston WW, Brown JB, Stewart MA. Patient-centered interviewing. Part I: Understanding patients' experiences. *Can Fam Phys*. 1989; 35: 147–151.
7. Stewart M, Brown JB, Weston WW, et al. *Patient-Centered Medicine: Transforming the Clinical Method*. Thousand Oaks, CA: Sage Publications; 1995.
8. Stewart M, Ryan BL. *Catalogue of Curricula for Medical Education in Patient-Centered Care*. Report Commissioned and Prepared for the Canadian Medical Association, Ottawa; 2012.

9. Brown JB, Handfield-Jones R, Rainsberry P, et al. The certification examination of the college of family physicians of Canada: IV simulated office orals. *Can Fam Phys.* 1996; 42: 1539–1548.

10. Tate P, Foulkes J, Neighbour R, et al. Assessing physicians' interpersonal skills via videotaped encounters: A new approach for the Royal College of General Practitioners Membership examination. *J Health Commun.* 1999; 4(2): 143–152.

11. Little P, Everitt H, Williamson I, et al. Observational study of effect of patient centredness and positive approach on outcomes of general practice consultations. *BMJ.* 2001; 323(7318): 908–911.

12. Little P, Everitt H, Williamson I, et al. Preferences of patients for patient-centered approach to consultation in primary care: Observational study. *BMJ.* 2002; 322: 468–472.

13. Dwamena F, Holmes-Rovner M, Gaulden CM, et al. Interventions for providers to promote a patient-centered approach in clinical consultations (review). *Cochrane Library,* Issue 12; 2012.

14. Epstein RM, Franks P, Shields CG, et al. Patient-centered communication and diagnostic testing. *Ann Fam Med.* 2005; 3(5): 415–421.

15. Stewart M, Ryan BL, Bodea C. Is patient-centered care associated with lower diagnostic costs? *Health Policy.* 2011; 6(4): 27–31.

16. Stewart M. Towards a global definition of patient centred care. *BMJ.* 2001; 322(7284): 444–445.

17. Hodges BD, Paech G, Bennett J, editors. *Without Compassion, There Is No Healthcare: Leading with Care in a Technological Age.* Montreal: McGill-Queen's Press-MQUP; 2020.

18. Crist A et al. *National Academies of Sciences, Engineering, and Medicine. 2023. Achieving Whole Health: A New Approach for Veterans and the Nation.* Washington, DC: National Academies Press. Doi: 10.17226/26854.

19. Stewart M. *Evidence on Patient-Centeredness, Patient-Centered Systems, and Implementation and Scaling of Whole Person Health.* Commissioned Paper for National Academy of Sciences, Engineering, and Medicine Board on Health Care Services, Health and Medicine Division, Consensus Study: Transforming Health Care to Create Whole Health – Strategies to Assess, Scale and Spread the Whole Person Approach to Health; March 2023.

20. McWhinney IR. Beyond diagnosis. An approach to the integration of behavioural science and clinical medicine. *N. Engl. J. Med.* 1972; 287: 384–387.

21. Balint M. *The Doctor, His Patient, and the Illness.* New York, NY: International Universities Press; 1957.

22. Stewart MA, McWhinney IR, Buck CW. How illness presents: A study of patient behavior. *J Fam Pract.* 1975; 2(6): 411–414.

23. Stewart MA, McWhinney IR, Buck CW. The doctor/patient relationship and its effect upon outcome. *J Roy Coll Gen Pract.* 1979; 29: 77–81.

24. Stewart MA, Buck CW. Physicians' knowledge of and response to patients' problems. *Med Care.* 1977; 15(7): 578–585.

25. Levenstein JH. Whither family medicine? *Can Fam Phys.* 1981 Dec; 27: 1868–1872.

26. McCracken EC, Stewart MA, Brown JB, McWhinney IR. Patient-centered care: The family practice model. *Can Fam Phys.* 1983 Dec; 29: 2313–2316.

27. Engel GL. The clinical application of the biopsychosocial model. *Am J Psychiat.* 1980; 137(5): 535–544.

28. Pendleton D. *The Consultation: An Approach to Learning and Teaching.* Oxford: Oxford University Press; 1984.

29. Brown JB, Stewart M, McWilliam C. Using the patient-centered method to achieve excellence in care for women with breast cancer. *Patient Educ Couns.* 1999; 38: 121–129.
30. Stewart M, Meredith L, Brown JB, Galajda J. The influence of older patient-physician communication on health and health-related outcomes. *Clin Geriatr Med.* 2000; 16(1): 25–36. Communication between older patients and their physicians.
31. McWilliam CL, Brown JB, Stewart M. Breast cancer patients' experiences of patient-doctor communication: A working relationship. *Patient Educ Couns.* 2000; 39: 191–204.
32. Stewart M, Brown JB, Donner A, McWhinney IR, Oates J, Weston WW, Jordan J. The impact of patient-centered care on outcomes. *J Fam Pract.* 2000; 49(9): 796–804.
33. Stewart M, Brown JB, Hammerton J, Donner A, Gavin A, Holliday RL, Whelan T, Leslie K, Cohen I, Weston W, Freeman T. Improving communication between doctors and breast cancer patients. *Ann Fam Med.* 2007 Sep–Oct; 5(5): 387–394.
34. Stewart M. The patient-centered clinical method: A family medicine perspective. *Turk Aile Hek Derg* (Turkish Journal of Family Practice) Dec 2013; 17(2): 73–85.
35. Stewart M, Fortin M, with the PACE in MM Team, Belanger M, Bestard-Denomme L, Bhattacharyya O, Borges DS, Bouhali T, Brown JB, Charles J, Chouinard MC, Emond V, Gallagher F, Glazier RH, Hogg WE, Katz A, Loignon C, Pariser P, Pham T-N, Piccinini-Vallis H, Reichert S, Ryan BL, Sampalli T, Sussman J, Thind A, Wodchis W, Wong ST, Zwarenstein MF, Couture M, Huras PW. Patient-centered innovations for persons with multimorbidity: Funded evaluation protocol. *CMAJ Open.* 2017 May 9; 5(2): E365–72. Doi: 10.9778/cmajo.20160097.
36. Sasseville M, Stewart M, Bouhali T, Fortin M. Relevant outcomes for patient-centered interventions for persons with multimorbidity: Experts' discussion. *Ann Fam Med.* 2017 Jul 1; 15(4): 388–389. Doi: 10.1370/afm.2116.
37. Poitras ME, Maltais ME, Bouhali T, Bestard-Denommé L, Stewart M, Fortin M. What are the effective elements in patient-centered and multimorbidity care? A scoping review. *BMC Health Serv Res.* 2018 Jun 14; 18(1): 446. Doi: 10.1186/s12913-018-3213-8.
38. Ramond-Roquin A, Stewart M, Ryan BL, Richards M, Sussman J, Brown JB, Bouhali T, Bestard-Denommé L, Fortin M. The "patient-centered coordination by a care team" questionnaire achieves satisfactory validity and reliability. *J Interprof Care.* 2019 Sep 1; 33(5): 558–569. Doi: 10.1080/13561820.2018.1554633.
39. Nguyen TN, Ngangue PA, Ryan BL, Stewart M, Brown JB, Bouhali T, Fortin M. The revised patient perception of patient-centeredness questionnaire: Exploring the factor structure in French-speaking patients with multimorbidity. *Health Expect.* 2020 Aug 1; 23(4): 904–909. Doi: 10.1111/hex.13068.
40. Fortin M, Stewart M, Ngangue P, Almirall J, Bélanger M, Brown JB, Couture M, Gallagher F, Katz A, Loignon C, Ryan BL, Sampalli T, Wong ST, Zwarenstein M. Scaling up patient-centered interdisciplinary care for multimorbidity: A pragmatic mixed-methods randomized controlled trial. *Ann Fam Med.* 2021 Mar 1; 19(2): 126–134. Doi: 10.1370/afm.2650.
41. Fortin M, Stewart M. Implementing patient-centered integrated care for multiple chronic conditions: Evidence-informed framework. *Can Fam Phys.* 2021 Apr 1; 67 (4): 235–238. Doi: 10.46747/cfp.6704235.
42. Stewart M, Fortin M, Brown JB, Ryan BL, Pariser P, Charles J, Pham TN, Boeckxstaens P, Reichert SM, Zou GY, Bhattacharya O, Katz A, Piccinini-Vallis H, Sampalli T, Wong ST, Zwarenstein M. Patient-centered innovation for multimorbidity care: A mixed-methods, randomised trial and qualitative study of the patients' experience. *Br J Gen Pract.* 2021 Apr 1; 71(705): e320–e330. Doi: 10.3399/bjgp21X714293.
43. Ngangue P, Brown JB, Forgues C, Ag Ahmed MA, Nguyen TN, Sasseville M, Loignon C, Gallagher F, Stewart M, Fortin M. Evaluating the implementation of interdisciplinary

patient-centered care intervention for people with multimorbidity in primary care: A qualitative study. *BMJ Open.* 2021 Sep 24; 11(9): e046914. Coauthor, doi: 10.1136/bmjopen-2020–046914.

44. Fortin M, Stewart M, Almirall J, Berbiche D, Bélanger M, Katz A, Ryan BL, Wong ST, Zwarenstein M. One year follow-up and exploratory analysis of a patient-centered interdisciplinary care intervention for multimorbidity. *J Comorb.* 2021 Nov 17; 11: 26335565211039780. Coauthor, doi: 10.1177/26335565211039780.

45. Reiser SJ. *Technological Medicine – The Changing World of Doctors and Patients.* Cambridge: Cambridge University Press; 2009.

46. Schleifer F, Vannatta JB. *The Chief Concern of Medicine – The Integration of the Medical Humanities and Narrative Knowledge into Medical Practices.* Ann Arbor: University of Michigan Press; 2013.

47. Engel GL. The need for a new medical model: A challenge for biomedicine. *Science.* 1977 Apr 8; 196(4286): 129–136, 130. Doi: 10.1126/science.847460.

48. Balint M, Hunt J, Joyce D, et al. *Treatment or Diagnosis: A Study of Repeat Prescriptions in General Practice.* Philadelphia, PA: JB Lippincott; 1970.

49. Hopkins P, & Balint Society. *Patient-Centered Medicine: Based on the First International Conference of the Balint Society in Great Britain on "The Doctor, His Patient, and the Illness,"* held on 23rd–25th March, 1972 at the Royal College of Physicians, London. Regional Doctor Publications Ltd. [for] the Balint Society; 1972.

50. Stevens J. Brief encounter. *J Roy Coll Gen Pract.* 1974; 24: 5–22.

51. Tait I. *The History and Function of Clinical Records.* Unpublished MD Dissertation Thesis, University of Cambridge; 1979.

52. Byrne PS, Long BEL. *Doctors Talking to Patients.* London, UK: Her Majesty's Stationery Office; 1984.

53. Wright HJ, MacAdam DB. *Clinical Thinking and Practice: Diagnosis and Decision in Patient Care.* Edinburgh, UK: Churchill Livingstone; 1979.

54. Rogers C. *Client-Centered Therapy – Its Current Practice Implications and Theory.* Riverside Cambridge, MA: Riverside Press; 1951.

55. Newman B, Young RJ. A model for teaching total person approach to patient problems. *Nurs Res.* 1972; 21: 264–269.

56. Mattingly C, Fleming MH. *Clinical Reasoning – Forms of Inquiry in a Therapeutic Practice.* Philadelphia, PA: FA Davis; 1994.

57. Epstein RM, Campbell TL, Cohen-Cole SA, et al. Perspectives on patient-doctor communication. *J Fam Pract.* 1993; 37(4): 377–388.

58. Sturgiss EA, Peart A, Richard L, Ball L, Hunik L, Chai TL, Lau S, Vadasz D, Russell G, Stewart M. Who is at the centre of what? A scoping review of the conceptualisation of 'centredness' in healthcare. *BMJ Open,* 2022 May 2; 12(5): e059400. Doi: 10.1136/bmjopen-2021–059400.

59. Charon R, DasGupta S, Hermann N. *The Principles and Practice of Narrative Medicine.* New York, NY: Oxford University Press; 2017: 1.

60. Launer J. *Narrative-Based Practice in Health and Social Care: Conversations Inviting Change.* New York, NY: Routledge; 2018: 6.

61. Mold JW. *Goal-Oriented Medical Care: Helping Patients Achieve Their Personal Health Goals.* Chapel Hill, NC: Full Court Press; 2020: vi.

62. De Maeseneer J. *Family Medicine and Primary Care: At the Crossroads of Societal Change.* Tielt: LannooCampus Publishers; 2017.

63. Mold JW. *Goal-Oriented Medical Care: Helping Patients Achieve Their Personal Health Goals*. Chapel Hill, NC: Full Court Press; 2020: xxi.
64. De Maeseneer J. *Family Medicine and Primary Care: At the Crossroads of Societal Change*. Tielt: LannooCampus Publishers; 2017: 63.
65. Mold JW. *Goal-Oriented Medical Care: Helping Patients Achieve Their Personal Health Goals*. Chapel Hill, NC: Full Court Press; 2020: v.
66. Mold JW. *Goal-Oriented Medical Care: Helping Patients Achieve Their Personal Health Goals*. Chapel Hill, NC: Full Court Press; 2020: 1.
67. De Maeseneer J. *Family Medicine and Primary Care: At the Crossroads of Societal Change*. Tielt: LannooCampus Publishers; 2017: 63.
68. Haynes RB, Devereaux PJ, Guyatt GH. Physicians' and patients' choices in evidence based practice. *BMJ*. 2002; 324(7350): 1350.
69. Sackett DL, Straus SE, Richardson WS, et al. *Evidence-Based Medicine. How to Practice and Teach EBM (2e)*. New York, NY: Churchill Livingstone; 2000.
70. Stewart M. Towards a global definition of patient centred care. *BMJ*. 2001; 445.
71. Launer J. *Reflective Practice in Medicine and Multi-Professional Healthcare*. Boca Raton, FL: CRC Press; 2022: 172.
72. Lussier MT, Richard C. Because one shoe doesn't fit all. *Can Fam Phys*. 2008; 54: 1089–1092 (Eng), 1096–1099 (Fr).
73. Miller WL. Routine, ceremony, or drama: An exploratory field study of the primary care clinical encounter. *J Fam Pract*. 1992; 34(3): 289–296.
74. Elwyn G, Durand MA, Song J, Aarts J, Barr PJ, Berger Z, Cochran N, Frosch D, Galasiński D, Gulbrandsen P, Han PKJ, Härter M, Kinnersley P, Lloyd A, Mishra M, Perestelo-Perez L, Scholl I, Tomori K, Trevena L, Witteman HO, Van der Weijden T. A three-talk model for shared decision making: Multistage consultation process. *BMJ*. 2017 Nov 6; 359: j4891. Doi: 10.1136/bmj.j4891.
75. Légaré F, Stacey D, Forest PG, Archambault P, Boland L, Coutu MF, Giguère AMC, LeBlanc A, Lewis KB, Witteman HO. Shared decision-making in Canada: Update on integration of evidence in health decisions and patient-centered care government mandates. *Z Evid Fortbild Qual Gesundhwes*. 2022 Jun; 171: 22–29. Doi: 10.1016/j.zefq.2022.04.006.
76. Mead N, Bower P. Patient-centeredness: A conceptual framework and review of the empirical literature. *Soc Sci Med*. 2000 Oct; 51(7): 1087–1110. Doi: 10.1016/s0277-9536(00)00098-8.
77. Institute of Medicine (US) Committee on Quality of Health Care in America. *Crossing the Quality Chasm: A New Health System for the 21st Century*. Washington, DC: National Academies Press (US); 2001.
78. Morgan S, Yoder LH. A concept analysis of person-centered care. *J Holist Nurs*. 2012 Mar; 30(1): 6–15. Doi: 10.1177/0898010111412189.
79. Langberg EM, Dyhr L, Davidsen AS. Development of the concept of patient-centeredness – A systematic review. *Patient Educ Couns*. 2019 Jul; 102(7): 1228–1236. Doi: 10.1016/j.pec.2019.02.023.

2

The Evolution of Clinical Method

IAN R McWHINNEY

The clinical method practiced by physicians is always the practical expression of a theory of medicine, even though it is not made explicit. The theory embraces such concepts as the nature of health and disease, the relation of mind and body, the meaning of diagnosis, the role of the physician, and the conduct of the patient–doctor relationship. The theory and practice of medicine is strongly influenced in any era by the dominant theory of knowledge and by societal values. Medicine is always a child of its time.

In recent times, medicine has not paid much attention to philosophy. When our efforts have been crowned with such great successes as they have in the past century, why be concerned if someone questions our assumptions? Indeed, we often behave as if they are not assumptions but simply the way things are. Crookshank[1] marks the end of the 19th century as the time when medicine and philosophy became completely dissociated. Physicians began to see themselves as practitioners of a science solidly based on observed facts, without a need for inquiry into how the facts are obtained and, indeed, what a fact is.[2] We believe ourselves to be at last freed from metaphysics, while at the same time maintaining a belief in the theory of knowledge known as physical realism.

Although continuous with the Hippocratic tradition of Greek medicine, the clinical method that has dominated Western medicine for nearly 200 years had its main origins in the European Enlightenment of the 17th century. Whitehead[3] called this the century of genius, on whose capital of ideas we have lived ever since. It was the century of Galileo and Newton, of Descartes, Locke, and Bacon. Bacon urged mankind to dominate and control nature, thus lightening the miseries of existence. In *The Advancement of Learning*[4] he provided, as his agenda for medical science, a revival of the Hippocratic method of recording case descriptions, with their course toward recovery or death; and the study of the pathological changes in organs – the "footsteps of disease" – with a comparison between these and the manifestations of illness during life. Clinical medicine at this time was dominated by untested theory ungrounded in bedside observation. The new scientific ideas had recently been applied to medicine by men such as Vesalius and Harvey, but their discoveries had been in anatomy and physiology, not in pathology and clinical science. Medicine was still practiced in ignorance of these discoveries. If Bacon set the agenda for science, it was Descartes who provided the method: the separation of mind and matter, with value residing only in mind; the separation of subject and object; and the reduction of complex phenomena to their simplest components.

DOI: 10.1201/9781003394679-3

Of all 17th-century figures, none has had more influence on science and medicine than René Descartes. In his Traité de l'homme, published in 1634, he wrote: "The body is a machine, so built up and composed of nerves, muscles, veins, blood and skin, that even though there were no mind in it at all, would not cease to have the same functions."[5] Descartes' concept of the body as machine had enormous consequences for medicine. It replaced the vitalist concept of premodern medicine and made possible the basic sciences of medicine and all the benefits they have conferred on us. Descartes' reductionist approach to inquiry, and his separation of *res extensa* from *res cogitans* enabled biology to make great progress. However, the problems left unresolved by Descartes have been gnawing away at the conceptual foundations of medicine and science. The questions include: how can a non-material mind act on a material substance, and what is the relationship between the mind of the observer and the world of phenomena? The philosopher Burtt wrote: "An adequate cosmology will only begin to be written when an adequate philosophy of mind has appeared."[6]

It was in the century of genius that reason was enthroned and modern science was born. However, it was a reason defined as formal logic, divorced from human experience and seeking for universal laws to explain natural phenomena. Mathematics was the model and Newton's Principia was the great exemplar. The idea of nature as a vast machine – including the human body – seemed eminently plausible. The aim was to attain knowledge that was universal and certain. Toulmin describes this as a radical shift in the paradigm of knowledge:

> From 1630 on, the focus of philosophical inquiries has ignored the particular, concrete, timely and local details of everyday human affairs: instead, it has shifted to a higher, stratospheric place on which nature and ethics conform to abstract, timeless, general and universal theories.[7]

In his book *Return to Reason*, Toulmin reminds us that a "universal" was for the Greeks a concept that was true "on the whole" or "generally," but not invariably applicable in every case. "In real-life situations, many universals hold generally rather than invariably."[8] This applies especially in biology and the human sciences.

Since the 17th century, physics has been the model for all sciences. However, physics, writes the biologist Yates[9] is "characterized by uniformity and generality":

> Biology, in contrast, presents diversity and specialness of form and function and sometimes a striking localness of distribution of its objects. Biological systems are *complex*. Physics is a strongly reductionist science and has prospered in that style; [the metaphor of organisms as machines] is false and destructive of conceptual advances in the understanding of complex living systems that self-organize, grow, develop, adapt, reproduce, repair and maintain form and function, age and die.[9] (italics in the original)

Our patients do all these things. They are complex systems – organisms – and our clinical method should enable us to deal with complexity.

THOMAS SYDENHAM

It was in the intellectual climate of the 1600s that there arose the first modern physician to use systematic bedside observation: Thomas Sydenham. Sydenham described the symptoms and course of disease, setting aside all speculative hypotheses based on unsupported theories. He classified diseases into categories – a novel idea at the time – believing that they could be classified by description in the same way as botanical specimens. Finally, he sought a remedy for each "species" of disease, exemplified by the newly introduced Peruvian bark (quinine). His great innovation, however, was to correlate his disease categories with their course and outcome, thus giving them predictive value. His method bore fruit in the distinction, for the first time, of syndromes such as acute gout and chorea. Sydenham was a close friend of John Locke, who took a great interest in his observations, sometimes accompanying him on his visits to patients.

FROM SYDENHAM TO LAENNEC

After Sydenham, the work of classifying diseases was taken up by others, notably Sauvages of Montpellier, a physician and botanist, who sought to group diseases into classes, orders, and genera in the same way that biologists were classifying plants and animals. Biology and medicine were at this time predominantly descriptive sciences. Sauvages was a strong influence on Carl von Linné, the Swedish physician and botanist who was responsible for the Linnaean system of botanical classification – another instance of the connection between medicine and the ideas of the Enlightenment. The groupings of Sydenham's successors, however, were of little practical value because they were not correlated with the course and outcome of disease and represented only random combinations of symptoms with no basis in the natural order.

Sydenham died in 1689 and for the next hundred years no system for classifying diseases proved to be of lasting value. The next great step, and the one that laid the foundations for the modern clinical method, was taken by the French clinician – pathologists in the years after the French Revolution. The political turmoil engendered by Enlightenment ideas was associated with a further application of these ideas to medicine. Laennec, the greatest genius of the French school, described the method:

> The constant goal of my studies and research has been the solution of the following three problems:
>
> 1. To describe disease in the cadaver according to the altered states of the organs.
> 2. To recognize in the living body definite physical signs, as much as possible independent of the symptoms . . .
> 3. To fight the disease by means which experience has shown to be effective: to place, through the process of diagnosis, internal organic lesions on the same basis as surgical disease.[10]

For the first time, clinicians examined their patients, using new instruments such as the Laennec stethoscope. Then they linked together two sets of data: (1) signs and symptoms from the clinical inquiry and (2) the descriptive data of morbid anatomy. At last medicine had a classification system based on the natural order of things: the correlation between symptoms, signs, and the appearance of the organs and tissues after death. The system proved to have great predictive value, and it was further vindicated when Pasteur and Koch showed that some of these entities had specific causal agents. The clinical method based on this system developed gradually during the 19th century, until by the 1870s it had taken the form familiar to us today.

As is always the case, this development in clinical method was associated with a change in the perception of disease. Since classical times, Western medicine has used two different explanatory models of illness.[1, 11] According to the ontological model, a disease is an entity located in the body and conceptually separable from the sick person. According to the physiological or ecological model, disease results from an imbalance within the organism, and between organism and environment; individual diseases have no real existence, the names being simply clusters of observations used by physicians as a guide to prognosis and therapy. According to the latter view, it becomes difficult to separate the disease from the person and the person from the environment.

Each model is identified with a clinical method, the ontological with a conventional or academic, and the physiological with a natural or descriptive method. The natural, concerned with the organism and disease, attempts to describe the illness in all its dimensions, including its individual and personal features. The conventional, concerned with organs and diseases, attempts to classify and name the disease as an entity independent of the patient.

Crookshank,[1] who introduced these terms, also observed that the best physicians in all ages have used a balance of the two methods. The patient-centered clinical method can be seen as the restoration of balance to a clinical method that has gone too far in the ontological direction.

The success of the new clinical method in the late 1800s soon resulted in a dominance of the ontological model, a dominance it has retained ever since. Whereas in former times the word diagnosis often meant the diagnosis of a patient, the aim of diagnosis was now to identify the disease. Disease was located in the body. As in all taxonomies, the disease categories were abstractions that, in the interest of generalization, left out many features of illness, including the subjective experience of the patient.

Figure 2.1 illustrates the process of abstraction. The three irregular shapes represent patients with similar illnesses. They are all different because no two illnesses are exactly the same. The

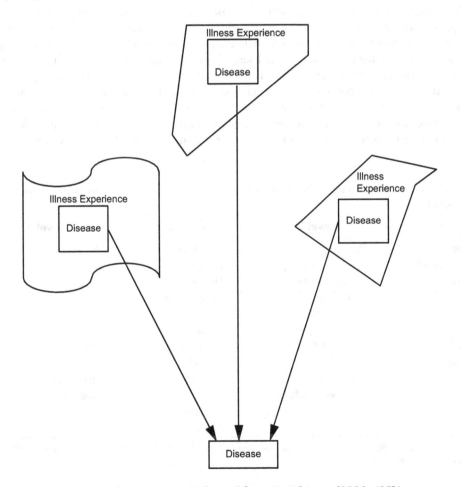

Figure 2.1 The Process of Abstraction (Adapted from McWhinney [2000: 135].)

four squares represent what the patients have in common. In the process of abstraction we take the common factors and form a disease category – multiple sclerosis, carcinoma of the lung, and so on. Abstraction gives us great predictive power and provides us with our taxonomic language. It enables us to apply our therapeutic technologies with precision, but it comes at a price. The power of generalization is gained by distancing ourselves from individual patients and all the particulars of their illness. "A large acquaintance with particulars," said William James, "often makes us wiser than the possession of abstract formulas, however deep".[12] If we look closely, every patient is different in some way. It is in the care of patients that the particulars become crucial. If we are to be healers, we need to know our patients as individuals; they may have their diseases in common, but in their responses to disease they are unique.

With its predictive and inferential power, the new clinical method was highly successful. Indeed, the application of new technologies to medicine depended on it. It had other strengths: it gave the clinician a clear injunction, "identify the patient's disease or rule out organic pathology"; it broke down a complex process into a series of easily remembered steps; and it provided canons of verification – the pathologist was able to tell the clinician whether they were right or wrong.

So successful was the method that its weaknesses only became apparent much later, as its abstractions became further and further removed from the experience of the patient. No abstraction is ever a complete picture of what it represents: it becomes less and less complete as levels of abstraction and power of generalization increase. Table 2.1 illustrates degrees of abstraction in a patient with multiple, fluctuating neurological symptoms. The first and lowest level is the patient's experience before it has been verbalized: his or her raw experience that something is not right. Level 2 is the patient's expressed sensations, feelings, and interpretations, and his or her understanding by the doctor. Level 3 is the doctor's clinical assessment and analysis of the illness: the clinical diagnosis of multiple sclerosis. Level 4 is the definitive diagnosis after an MRI scan. As we increase the levels of abstraction, individual differences are ironed out in the interest of generalization. The lower levels of abstraction are closest to the patient's lifeworld. As we increase the level of abstraction, the danger is that we forget that our abstraction is not

Table 2.1 Levels of Abstraction in a Patient with Multiple, Fluctuating, Neurological Symptoms and Signs

Level 1	Level 2	Level 3	Level 4
Patient's sensations and emotions	Patient's expressed complaints, feelings, interpretations	Doctor's analysis of illness: clinical assessment	MRI scan
Preverbal	Second-order abstraction	Third-order abstraction	Fourth-order abstraction
Illness	'Illness' (doctor's understanding)	'Disease' (clinical diagnosis: multiple sclerosis)	'Disease' (definitive diagnosis: MS)

Source: McWhinney IR: A Textbook of Family Medicine, 2nd ed. p. 77. Reprinted with permission of Oxford University Press, New York.

synonymous with the real world. The diagnosis of multiple sclerosis and the MRI scan are not the patient's experience. To forget this, in Alfred Korzybski's[13] aphorism, is mistaking the map for the territory. Many of the recently published illness narratives have drawn our attention to this weakness.

ILLNESS NARRATIVES

In the past 3 decades, there has been a remarkable increase in the number of books and articles describing personal experiences of illness. These writings, by patients themselves or by their relatives, are often bitterly critical of clinicians and, by implication, of the modern clinical method. Hawkins[14] sees this literature as a possible reaction to a medicine "so dominated by a biophysical understanding of illness that its experiential aspects are virtually ignored." Two themes recur in these stories:

> the tendency in contemporary medical practice to focus primarily not on the needs of the individual who is sick but on the nomothetic condition we call the disease, and the sense that our medical technology has advanced beyond our capacity to use it wisely.[14]

Some illness narratives are written by patients who have a professional perspective as physicians, philosophers, sociologists, or poets. Sacks[15] viewed his experience of a body image disorder from the perspective of an existential neurologist and medical theorist. Stetten[16] found that his fellow physicians were interested in his vision, but not in his blindness. Toombs, a phenomenologist who has multiple sclerosis, noted that the attention of physicians is directed to their patients' bodies rather than their patients' problems of living. The patient feels "reduced to a malfunctioning biological organism."[17] Toombs writes:

> no physician has ever inquired of me what it is like to live with multiple sclerosis or to experience one of the disabilities that have accrued . . . no neurologist has ever asked me if I am afraid, or . . . even whether I am concerned about the future.[17]

Writing of his experience with testicular cancer, Frank,[18] a sociologist, observed that the more critical his illness became, the more his physicians withdrew.

True to its origins in the age of reason, this clinical method was analytical and impersonal. Feelings and the life experience of the patient did not figure in the process. The meaning of the illness was established on one level only – that of physical pathology. The focus was on diagnosis, with much less attention to the detailed care of the patient. In keeping also with its Cartesian origins, it divided mental from physical disorder, bringing the two together in dubious terms such as "functional illness," "psychosomatic disease," and "somatization."[19]

The central idea on which the modern clinical method was based came into being at a time when Enlightenment ideas had become the dominant worldview of the West. Man had become the measure of all things, metaphysics devalued, tradition weakened, progress proclaimed, and knowledge put to practical use for the benefit of mankind. The fruits born by these ideas in our own time include this clinical method and all the benefits and problems of modern medicine.

Modern medicine continues to make great advances, many of them based on the mechanical metaphor. Training these technologies on their target has required diagnostic precision and the modern clinical method has rightly attached great importance to the linear logic of differential diagnosis. However, the promise of new technologies often falls short of expectations when they are applied in the real world of practice. It is here that linear logic meets the logic of complexity. Whether they are preventive, therapeutic, or rehabilitative, the technologies require acceptance by the patient, motivation, cooperation, and often determination. They may require a different way of life and the giving up of lifelong habits or cherished pleasures. The changes must be timely, and consistent with lifetime goals and priorities. The patient must be convinced that their efforts are justified.

Many illnesses are themselves complex and multifactorial, requiring an approach different from the linear logic and targeted technology that can work so well in diseases with a specific etiology. Illnesses such as chronic pain, eating disorders, depression, and addiction have an existential dimension that must be addressed if they are to be understood. Attention must be paid to patients' sufferings, to their emotions, beliefs, and relationships, not only for humanitarian reasons but also because they have an important bearing on the origins of illness.[20]

The patient-centered clinical method is designed to deal with complexity. While using linear logic where appropriate, its essence is the understanding of the patient as a whole, a knowledge of their illness experience, and an attempt to attain common ground. Common ground is the key to therapeutic success, but it is often difficult to obtain. It tests the doctor's ability to motivate the patient by resolving objections, laying doubts to rest, allaying fears, and clearing up misconceptions.[21] The art of persuasion has ancient roots in medicine. The Greeks spoke of a "therapy of the word."[22] Before the Enlightenment, rhetoric – the art of persuasion – was a respected field of study. Its purpose was to take general fundamental principles and apply them in practical situations such as clinical medicine, taking into account all the local circumstances of time and place. The fact that rhetoric is now a derogatory term is a reflection on the limits of our knowledge. The search for common ground should be an exchange and synthesis of meanings. The physician interprets the patient's illness in terms of physical pathology, the name of the disease, causal inferences, and therapeutic choices. The patient interprets it in terms of experience: what it is like for them to suffer from the illness, beliefs about its nature, and expectations of therapy. Ideally, the exchange results in a synthesis of perspectives: they are, after all, different perspectives – concrete or abstract – of the same reality. However, there are some reasons why synthesis may not be achieved – at least initially. For the patient, the encounter with the physician is often emotionally charged. The physician's interpretation or management of the illness may be rejected. The physician may not believe the patient – a disbelief not necessarily conveyed in words. There are a hundred ways of saying, "I don't believe you."

Attaining empathetic understanding requires attention to the patient's emotions. This is something that the modern clinical method does not do in any systematic way. True to Descartes' supposed separation of mind from body,* the method of most clinical disciplines does not include attention to the emotions. Internal medicine attends to the body; psychiatry attends to the emotions. Family practice is one of the few clinical fields that transcend this deep fault line. As long ago as 1926, Crookshank, writing on the theory of diagnosis, noted that the handbooks of clinical diagnosis, which appeared in the early 1900s, "give excellent schemes for the physical examination of the patient while strangely ignoring, almost completely, the psychical [sic]."[23] The price we have paid for the benefits of abstraction is a distancing of doctor from patient. We have justified this to ourselves as objectivity, but to our patients it is often seen as indifference to their suffering.

The teaching with regard to the patient–doctor relationship was "don't get involved." In one respect, fear of the emotions was well founded – to be involved at the level of one's unexamined emotions is potentially harmful. However, what the teaching did not say was that involvement

---

* Contrary to modern assumptions, Descartes did not deny mind-body interactions but maintained that most aspects of affective states are primarily somatic.

is necessary if one is going to be a healer as well as a competent technician. There are right and wrong ways of being involved and the teaching gave no guidance about finding the right way. The teaching was also profoundly mistaken in suggesting that one can encounter suffering and not in some way be affected. Our emotional response may be repressed, but this exacts a heavy price, for repressed emotion may be acted out in ways that are destructive of relationships. There is no such thing as non-involvement and only self-knowledge can protect us from the pitfalls of involvement at the level of our egocentric emotions. Without self-knowledge, moral growth is likely to have shallow roots. This is why the patient-centered clinical method includes attention to the patient–doctor relationship, and, by implication, to the physician's self-awareness. The daily encounter with suffering can evoke strong emotions: helplessness in the face of incurable illness, fear of discussing questions that frighten us, guilt at our failures, anger at our patient's demands, and sadness at the suffering of someone who has become a friend. If we fail to acknowledge and deal with our disturbing emotions, they may be acted out in avoidance of the patient, emotional distancing, exclusive concentration on the technical aspects of care, and even cruelty. Lack of emotional insight can disturb or destroy the relationship between patient and doctor, adding to the patient's sufferings and often leaving the doctor with a sense of failure. It is not easy to look suffering in the face without flinching.

All this implies that we see ourselves no longer as detached observers and dispassionate dispensers of therapy. To be patient-centered means to be open to a patient's feelings. It means becoming involved in a way that was made difficult by the old method. This has the potential for making medicine a much richer experience for us, as well as more effective for our patients. However, there are pitfalls. There are right and wrong ways of becoming involved. There are ways of dealing with some of the disturbing things our new openness will expose us to. Hence, the importance of the knowledge and insight I have referred to. It is through such experiences that students can develop emotionally as well as intellectually.

If we are to recapture our capacity to heal, we will have to transcend the literal-mindedness that seems to follow when we become prisoners of our abstractions. A new clinical method should find room for the exercise of imagination and for restoring the balance between thinking and feeling.

KURT GOLDSTEIN'S HOLISTIC APPROACH TO MEDICINE

Any serious illness or injury sends reverberations throughout the organism. Total attention to the main symptom can miss any attention to a problem brought on by the illness or injury, a problem that turns out to be a change that assists the patient's recovery.

Goldstein describes the holistic approach:

The Organism consists mainly of a detailed description of the new method, the so-called holistic, organismic approach. Certainly, isolated data acquired by the dissecting method of natural science could not be neglected if we were to maintain a scientific basis. But we had to discover how to evaluate our observations in their significance for the total organism's functioning and thereby to understand the structure and existence of the individual person. We were confronted then with a difficult problem of epistemology. The primary aim of my book is to describe this methodological procedure in detail, by means of numerous observations.

The great number of examples from various fields in which the usefulness of the method was to be demonstrated may make the reading of the book at times difficult. But it seemed to me relevant to include such diverse observations since in this way I could exemplify the characteristic feature of the new method, namely, that by using this principle much of what we observe in living beings can be understood in the same manner. This created another advantage. Such diverse material, from the fields of anatomy, physiology, psychology, and philosophy, that is, from those disciplines concerned with the nature of man, were correlated for the reader. In this way he could observe that the method may be useful for the solution of various problems that may, superficially, seem to be divergent and that have, until now, been treated as unrelated.[24]

A DIFFERENT WAY OF THINKING ABOUT HEALTH AND DISEASE

Most difficult of all, perhaps, will be the transition from linear, causal thinking to cybernetic thinking. Linear thinking is deeply ingrained in our culture. The notion of a cause is based on the Newtonian model of a force acting on a passive object, as when a moving billiard ball collides with a stationary one. The action is in one direction only. In medicine, this notion is exemplified by the doctrine of specific etiology – of an environmental agent acting on a person to produce a diseased state.

The notion of cybernetic causation is based on the model of self-organizing systems. The human organism can be viewed as a self-organizing system, maintaining itself by interaction with its environment and by a system of feedback loops from the environment and from its own output. Self-organizing systems have the ability both to renew and to transcend themselves. Healing is an example of self-renewal in which constituent parts are renewed while the integrity of the organization is maintained. Organisms transcend themselves by learning, developing, and growing. Self-organizing systems require energy, but as organizations they are maintained and changed by information. The notion of cause in self-organizing systems is based on the model of information that triggers a process that is already a potential of the system. The response is not the direct result of the original stimulus but the result of rule-governed behavior that is a property of the system. If the process is long term, destabilizing, and self-perpetuating, then the question of cause becomes much more complex than that of identifying the trigger. The trigger that initiated the process may be quite different from the processes perpetuating it. We have to consider the processes in the organism that are perpetuating the disturbance. The key to enhancing healing may be in strengthening the organism's defenses, changing the information flow, or encouraging self-transcendence, rather than neutralizing an agent.

Nonlinear logic is "both-and" rather than "either-or." Perspectives that we regard as opposites can be seen as complementary polarities – different aspects of the same reality. The pitfalls of either-or thinking are exemplified by a leading neurologist's perspective on migraine: "Practitioners should realize that migraine is a neurobiologic, not a psychogenic disorder."[25] Nonlinear logic would say: "Why can it not be both?"

It is self-knowledge that enables us to know where we are on the scale of these complementary polarities: between involvement and detachment, between concrete and abstract, between the particular and the general, or between uncertainty and precision.

THE REFORM OF CLINICAL METHOD

It is not surprising that criticism of the modern clinical method from within the profession has come mainly from fields of medicine that most experience the ambiguities of abstraction and the importance of the patient's life story, notably general practice and psychiatry. In the 1950s Michael Balint, a medical psychoanalyst, began to work with a group of general practitioners, exploring difficult cases and the doctors' affective responses to them. Balint distinguished between "overall" diagnosis and traditional diagnosis; he emphasized the importance of listening and of the personal change required in the doctor; and he introduced new terms such as "patient-centered medicine"; "the patient's offers" and the doctor's "responses"; the doctor's belief in his "apostolic function"; and the "drug doctor" – the powerful influence for good or harm of the patient–doctor relationship. The idea that physicians should attend to their own emotional development as well as the emotions of the patient was revolutionary in its day. In other ways, Balint's method conformed to the dualistic approach of the period. The method was intended to apply only to certain patients with "neurotic illnesses," not to those with straight-forward clinical problems.[26]

In the 1970s Engel,[27, 28] an internist and psychiatrist with a psychoanalytic orientation, used systems theory as a model for integrating biologic, psychologic, and social data in the clinical process. Engel's critique of the modern clinical method focused on the unscientific nature of the physician's judgments on interpersonal and social aspects of patients' lives, based on "tradition, custom, prescribed rules, compassion, intuition, common sense, and sometimes highly personal self-reference."[28]

Any successor to the modern clinical method must propose another method with the same strengths: a theoretical foundation, a clear set of injunctions about what the clinician must do, and canons of verification by which it may be judged. Laín Entralgo attributes the failure of Western medicine to integrate the patient's inner life with the disease to the lack, among other things, of a method – "a technique [for] laying bare, to clinical investigation and to subsequent pathological consideration the inner life of the patient . . . an exploration method – the dialogue with the patient."[29] Balint and Engel both provided a theory, but they were less clear about what the clinician must do and how the process is to be validated. Although Engel emphasized that the verification must be scientific, validation of both models was bound to depend on qualitative methods that were barely accepted as scientific. A model is an abstraction; a method is its practical application; and medicine had to wait longer for the transition to occur. The patient-centered clinical method is an answer to Laín Entralgo's challenge.

Clinical medicine, it seems, took a long time to fall under the domination of the Enlightenment paradigm of knowledge. Although the modern clinical method was concerned with abstractions, until our own time the individual case or series of cases remained the focus of attention for study and for teaching. Our abstractions have been low level, not far removed from experience of patients. In more recent times, however, the development of clinical method can be seen as moving toward increasing levels of abstraction, and an increasing distance from the experience of illness. The fact that a ward round can now be done around the charts rather than around the beds is an indication of how far we have gone.

THE DIFFICULTIES OF CHANGE

It is important not to underestimate the magnitude of the changes implied by the transformation of our clinical method. It is not simply a matter of learning some new techniques, although that is part of it. Nor is it only a question of adding courses in interviewing and behavioral science to the curriculum. The change goes much deeper than that. It requires nothing less than a change in what it means to be a physician, a different way of thinking about health and disease, and a redefinition of medical knowledge.

A glance at any medical school curriculum is usually sufficient to show that it is dominated by the modern paradigm of knowledge. Of course, this kind of knowledge is important, but restoring the balance in medicine requires that it be balanced by other kinds of knowledge: an understanding of human experience and human relationships, moral insight, and that most difficult of accomplishments, self-knowledge. Whitehead criticized professional education for being too full of abstractions, a condition he described as "the celibacy of the intellect,"[30] the modern equivalent of the celibacy of the medieval learned class. Wisdom, he believed, is the fruit of a balanced development. What we need is not more abstractions but, rather, an education in which the necessary abstractions are balanced by concrete experiences, an education that feeds both the intellect and the imagination. Much of this is not the kind of knowledge that can be learned in the classroom or from books, although some of it can. There is now, for example, a rich literature describing personal experiences of illness. If we are to give as much attention to care as we give to diagnosis we will need to feed our imagination with accounts of what it is like to go blind, have multiple sclerosis, suffer bereavement, bring up a handicapped child, and the many other experiences our patients live with. We will need also to know the many practical ways in which life for them can be enriched or made more tolerable.

Human relationships and moral insight, again, are not principally classroom subjects, except insofar as students learn moral lessons from the way they are treated by their teachers. However, once its importance is acknowledged, and time allowed for it, understanding of relationships can be deepened with the help of teachers who are sensitive, reflective, and prepared to expose their own vulnerability. Self-knowledge, by definition, cannot be taught. However, its growth can be fostered by teachers who are themselves embarked on this difficult journey – a journey that is never complete. The patient-centered clinical method is the most recent version of the historic struggle to reconcile two often competing notions of the nature of disease and the role of the physician. The past century has seen the increasing dominance of abstraction and the devaluation of experience. The patient-centered clinical method can be viewed as a move to bring medical practice and teaching back to the center, to reconcile clinical with existential medicine.[31] It may seem paradoxical that the modern clinical method does not have a name. It is simply the way clinical medicine has been taught in the medical schools in modern times. Giving the successor method a name has its dangers – notably, that of conveying different meanings to different people. In this transition period, however, it does seem necessary to have a name for the new method, but when the transition is complete, perhaps it can simply become "clinical method."

The new method should not only restore the Hippocratic ideal of friendship between doctor and patient but also make possible a medicine that can see illness as an expression of a person with a moral nature, an inner life, and a unique life story: a medicine that can heal by a therapy of the word and a therapy of the body.

REFERENCES

1. Crookshank FG. The theory of diagnosis. *Lancet.* 1926; 2: 934–942, 995–999.
2. Fleck L. *The genesis and development of a scientific fact.* Chicago: University Chicago of Press; 1979.
3. Whitehead AN. *Science and the modern world.* San Francisco, CA: Collins, Fontana Books; 1975.
4. Bacon F. The advancement of learning [1605]. In *Primer of intellectual freedom.* Cambridge, MA: Harvard University Press; 1949 Dec 31: 172–192.
5. Foss L. *The end of modern medicine biomedical science under a microscope.* Albany, NY: State University of New York; 2002: 37.
6. Burtt EA. *The metaphysical foundations of modern science,* 2nd ed. Garden City, NY: Doubleday; 1954: 324.
7. Toulmin S. *Cosmopolis: The hidden agenda of modernity.* Chicago, IL: University of Chicago Press; 1992: 34–35.

8. Toulmin S. *Return to reason*. Cambridge, MA: Harvard University Press; 1991: 11.

9. Yates FE. Self-organizing systems. In CAR Boyd (ed). *The logic of life: The challenge of integrative physiology*. New York, NY: Oxford University Press; 1993: 189.

10. Faber K. *Nosography in modern internal medicine* (Jean Martin, Trans.). New York, NY: Paul B. Hoeber, Inc; 1923: 35.

11. Dubos R. *Man adapting*. New Haven, CT: Yale University Press; 1980.

12. James W. *The varieties of religious experience: A study in human nature*. New York, NY: New American Library; 1958: ix.

13. Korzybski A. *Science and sanity: An introduction to non-Aristotelian systems and general semantics*, 4th ed. Lake Bille, CT: International Non-Aristotelian Library Publishing Co; 1958.

14. Hawkins AH. *Reconstructing illness: Studies in pathology*. West Lafayette, IN: Purdue University Press; 1993: 279–284.

15. Sacks O. *One leg to stand on*. London, UK: Gerald Duckworth; 1984.

16. Stetten D, Jr. Coping with blindness. *N Engl J Med*. 1981; 305: 458.

17. Toombs K. *The meaning of illness: A phenomenological account of the different perspectives of physician and patient*. Norwell, MA: Kluwer Academic Publishing; 1992: 106.

18. Frank A. *At the will of the body: Reflections on illness*. Boston, MA: Houghton, Mifflin; 1991.

19. McWhinney IR, Epstein RM, Freeman TR. Rethinking somatization. *Ann Intern Med*. 1997; 126(9): 747–750.

20. Foss L. *The end of modern medicine biomedical science under a microscope*. Albany, NY: State University of New York; 2002.

21. Botelho R. *Beyond advice: Becoming a motivational practitioner*. Rochester, NY: Motivative Healthy Habits Press; 2002.

22. Entralgo PL. *The therapy of the word in classical antiquity*. New Haven, CT: Yale University Press; 1961.

23. Crookshank FG. The theory of diagnosis. *Lancet*. 1926; 2: 934–942, 995–999.

24. Goldstein K. *The organism*. New York: Zone Books; 1995: 18.

25. Olesen J. Understanding the biologic basis of migraine. *N Engl J Med*. 1994; 331(25): 1713–1714.

26. Balint M. *The doctor, his patient, and the illness*. 2nd ed. New York, NY: International Universities Press; 1964.

27. Engel GL. The need for a new medical model: A challenge for biomedicine. *Science*. 1977 Apr 8; 196(4286): 129–136. Doi: 10.1126/science.847460.

28. Engel GL. The clinical application of the biopsychosocial model. *Am J Psychiatry*. 1980; 137(5): 535–544.

29. Entralgo PL. *Mind and body*. New York, NY: PJ Kennedy; 1956.

30. Whitehead AN. *Science and the modern world*. San Francisco, CA: Collins, Fontana Books; 1975: 223.

31. Sacks O. *Awakenings*. London, UK: Pan Books; 1982.

32. McWhinney IR. Being a general practitioner: What it means. *Eur J Gen Pract*. 2000 Jan 1; 6(4): 135–139.

33. McWhinney IR, Epstein RM, Freeman TR. Rethinking somatization. *Ann Intern Med*. 1997; 126(9): 77, 747–750. Reprinted with permission.

PART TWO

The Four Components of the Patient-Centered Clinical Method

INTRODUCTION

JUDITH BELLE BROWN AND MOIRA STEWART

In this Part Two of the book, the four interactive components of the patient-centered clinical method are described in detail. The components are accompanied by case examples from around the world. As well, the components are illustrated by short narratives from patients and caregivers; these are called Patient's Voice or Caregiver's Voice. While each component is, for the most part, described as a discrete entity, the expert clinician weaves among the components throughout the process in response to the patient's expressed needs and concerns and comes to an understanding that is a synthesis unique to each patient.

DOI: 10.1201/9781003394679-4

3

The First Component: Exploring Health, Disease, and the Illness Experience

MOIRA STEWART, JUDITH BELLE BROWN, CAROL L MCWILLIAM, THOMAS R FREEMAN, AND W WAYNE WESTON

OVERVIEW OF THE CHAPTER

There is a long history documenting the failure of conventional medical practice in meeting patients' perceived needs and expectations. Component 1 of the patient-centered clinical method addresses this failure by proposing that clinicians cast a wider gaze, including disease but going beyond disease to include an exploration of health and the illness experience of patients. This chapter marks the clear distinction of the patient-centered clinical method to other models of humanistic health care; it weds the scientific with the humanistic goals.

This chapter is organized as follows. First, the terms used in this chapter are broadly defined: health, disease, and the illness experience; their interconnectedness is described in a diagram. How clinicians follow cues to guide the exploration of disease, health, and illness is covered using a key case of Rex. Next, exploring the disease is presented in detail with a Caregiver's Voice illustrating the physical examination. Then, how clinicians explore health is covered. The illness experience of the patient is examined next, illustrated by a short case and a patient's voice. Related topics such as cues and narratives are probed. The chapter concludes with two cases.

HEALTH, DISEASE, AND ILLNESS

Effective patient care requires attending as much to patients' perceptions of health and personal experiences of illness as to their diseases. *Health*, for the purposes of this chapter, is defined in a way that is akin to the most recent World Health Organization definition of a "resource for living".[1] We define health as encompassing the patients' perception of health and what health means to them and their ability to pursue the aspirations and purposes important to their lives.

Disease is diagnosed by using the conventional medical model by analysis of the patient's medical history and objective examination of their body by physical examination and laboratory

DOI: 10.1201/9781003394679-5

investigation. It is a category, the "thing" that is wrong with the body-as-machine or the mind-as-computer. Disease is a theoretical construct, or abstraction, by which physicians attempt to explain patients' problems in terms of abnormalities of structure and/or function of body organs and systems and which includes both physical and mental disorders.

Illness, for its part, is the patient's personal and subjective experience of sickness: the feelings, thoughts, and altered function of someone who feels sick.

Disease and illness do not always coexist; health and disease are not always mutually exclusive. Patients with undiagnosed asymptomatic disease perceive themselves to be healthy and do not feel ill; people who are grieving or worried may feel ill but have no disease. Patients and practitioners who recognize these distinctions and who realize how common it is to perceive a loss of health or feel ill and yet have no disease are less likely to search needlessly for pathology. However, even when disease is present, it may not adequately explain the patient's suffering since the amount of distress a patient experiences refers not only to the amount of tissue damage but also to the personal meaning of health and illness.

Research has long supported the contention that disease and illness do not always present simultaneously. For some illnesses, patients do not even seek medical advice.[2, 3]

> Many people present with medically unexplained symptoms. For example, more than a quarter of primary care patients in England have unexplained chronic pain, irritable bowel syndrome, or chronic fatigue, and in secondary and tertiary care, around a third of new neurological outpatients have symptoms thought by neurologists to be 'not at all' or only 'somewhat' explained by disease.[4]

In Figure 3.1, the patient with a sensation of being ill but having no disease is in the upper right-hand part of the Venn diagram or in the dark gray portion on the right. There are a variety of reasons for feeling ill but having no disease diagnosis: the problem may be transient; it may be managed so early that it never reaches a diagnosis (e.g., impending pneumonia); it may be a borderline condition that is difficult to classify; the problem may remain undifferentiated; and/or the problem may have its source in factors such as an unhappy marriage, job dissatisfaction, guilt, or lack of purpose in life.[5] Patients falling into the group at the center of Figure 3.1, represented by the medium gray, where disease, illness, and health overlap, would have experiences of ill health (sensory, cognitive, and emotional), a diagnosed disease and perceptions of their health, and what health means to them. For example, it is known that people with chronic disease may rate their health as good or very good despite having the disease. People in the center of the diagram have potential for health-enhancing attitudes and activities. The patient in the portion of Figure 3.1 in light gray in the left-hand overlap would have no feelings of ill health but would have a diagnosed disease as well as perceptions of their health and what health means to them. Patients in the upper left-hand part of Figure 3.1 have a disease that is asymptomatic and also feel their disease interferes with their aspirations and life purposes. Examples of such patients may be those sometimes called partial patients, with high cholesterol, high blood pressure, or high blood sugars (pre-diabetes or early diabetes).

Figure 3.1 is meant to clarify the definitions of disease, health, and illness and to point out where they stand alone and where they overlap. But this is an oversimplification, as Rosenberg has elegantly stated:

> We are never illness or disease, but, rather always their sum in the world of day-to-day experience. Illness and disease are not closed systems, but mutually constitutive and continuously interacting worlds.[6]

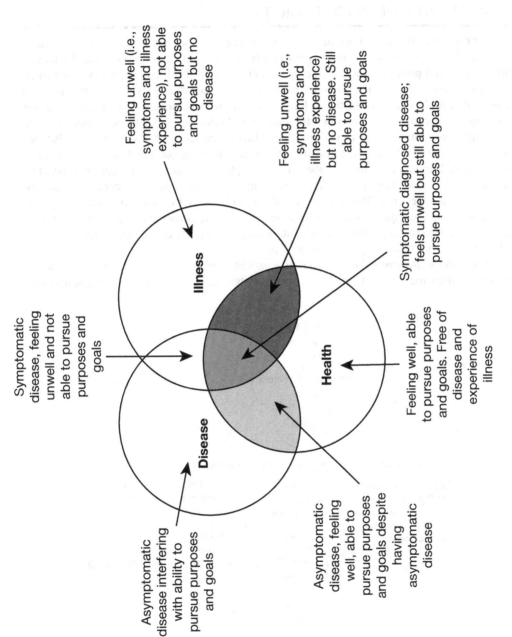

Figure 3.1 Overlap of Health, Disease, and the Illness Experience

We authors are seeking to ensure that Component 1 is not considered only about the illness experience, but rather we seek to reestablish a balance among the three elements of disease, health, and illness.

COMPONENT ONE IN ITS ENTIRETY

To assist the reader in the goal of embracing the whole of Component 1, Figure 3.2 was created. It stresses that the source of the inquiry process is the clinician's ability to elicit and attend to patients' **cues and prompts**. These cues may signal the disease, health, or the illness experience. If the cue refers to disease, it may be a symptom (such as breathlessness) or a sign (such as a unique rash). A physical examination is likely to occur. Investigations and laboratory tests may be ordered. The conversation between the patient and clinician about these disease-oriented topics might veer off in other directions, depending on patients' cues and prompts. Patients might raise an issue related to the meaning of health to them or comment on a life aspiration. Patients often bring up their feelings about their symptoms, an idea about them, their effect on function, or the expectations patients have regarding their care; these four aspects are called the patient's illness experience. The conversation about all these matters need not take a long time because the issues are spontaneously raised by patients. The clinician and patient move to an integrated understanding of the multiple interconnected aspects of the areas to be dealt with and approach a synthesis unique for that patient.

Other authors also stress the need to notice patient cues and to follow them with responses that mirror the patient's words, inviting them to elaborate.[7, 8] There are many examples in the

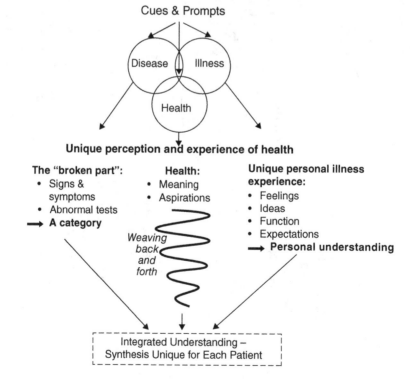

Figure 3.2 Component 1: Exploring Health, Disease, and the Illness Experience

literature of clinicians ignoring cues, by interrupting with their own list of questions, instead of following up on the cue.[7-9] It can be argued that in the case entitled "The Man, the Poem, the Secret" in this book at the end of Chapter 1, the clinician noticed each symptom presentation as a cue to a larger unknown issue and resisted the temptation to medicalize each cue, but rather, they encouraged a broader exploration of the cues. In the case of Rex, coming up later in this chapter, cues are noticed and attended to. Also later in this chapter, details of cues to illness experience are highlighted.

How Can Clinicians Conduct Such an Interview with Patients?

Charon suggests beginning an encounter with a new patient with an invitation:

> I will be your doctor, and so I need to know a great deal about your body, your health, and your life. Please tell me what you think I should know about your situation.[10]

Launer suggests two key questions that help patients take their story into issues of importance to them. One is "What do you mean by '[repeat a phrase used by the patient]'". Another is after a patient raises a particularly difficult problem, again use the patient's words: "So, when things get '[patient's words]' for you, what is it that keeps you going?"[11]

Launer also suggests the use of silence, where "short respectful silences" can be helpful in eliciting "information" and also in exuding a "compassionate attitude".[11]

The following case, about Rex, illustrates the patient-centered clinical method in its entirety; it explicitly describes dimensions of Component 1 (disease, health, and the illness experience – the topic of this chapter), Component 2 (person and context), Component 3 (finding common ground), and Component 4 (the patient–clinician relationship).

CASE EXAMPLE

Mr Rex Kelly was a 58-year-old man who had been a patient in the practice for 10 years. He had been a healthy man with few problems until 8 months ago, when he had a massive myocardial infarction and required triple coronary artery bypass surgery. He was married, with grown children, and he worked as a plumber. He had come to the office for diet counseling about his elevated cholesterol.

The following excerpt from the visit demonstrates the doctor's use of the patient-centered approach. The interaction began with Dr Wason stating, "Hi Rex, I'm glad to see you again. I understand you are back to check on your progress since your heart attack. Is there anything else you would like to discuss today?"

"That's right, doc, I'm sticking to our plan. I'm feeling pretty good about my weight. I'm down 5 more pounds and almost at my goal. I'm wondering how my last cholesterol turned out."

"Congratulations, Rex, you have done really well with the diet and that has helped bring down your cholesterol – it's now almost at the target level, too."

The interview then shifted to Rex's exercise program, and he stated that he had been regularly following his exercise regimen throughout the summer months and was walking up to 4 miles a day. Dr Wason asked, "Will you be able to continue your walking during the winter?"

"I think so," indicated Rex. "I don't mind walking in the winter as long as it's not too cold."

"Yes, you do need to be cautious during the severe weather," replied Dr Wason. Rex looked away and appeared sad. The doctor paused and asked, "Is there something concerning you, Rex?"

"Oh well . . . no," stated Rex quickly. "No, not really." "Not really?" reflected Dr Wason.

"Well," replied Rex, "I was just thinking about the winter and . . . well . . . no, I guess I'll be able to go to the cabin if I just keep warm."

"Why are you concerned that you won't be able to do that, Rex?" asked the doctor.

"Well, I don't know. I'd just miss it if I couldn't participate."

"It sounds as if that activity is important to you," responded Dr Wason. "Well, yes, it has been a very important family activity. We have some land and a little cabin up north of here, and it's really how we spend our winter weekends – the whole family together."

"It sounds as if not being able to participate in something that's been an important family activity would be very difficult for you," reflected the doctor.

"Yes, it would be. I just feel that so many things have been taken away from me that I really would miss not being able to do that."

The doctor responded, "Rex, during the last several months you have experienced a lot of changes and a lot of losses. I sense it has been very difficult for you."

Rex solemnly replied: "Yes, doc, it has. It's been tough. I've gone from being a man who is really healthy and has no problems to having a bad heart attack and a big operation and being a real weight watcher. And I still don't have the energy I used to have and sometimes I worry about having another heart attack. And my wife is worried too – she is always reminding me to be careful and we are both anxious about resuming our lovemaking. It has been a big change, and it has had its tough moments, but I'm alive and I guess that is what matters."

"It seems that you – and your wife too – still have a lot of feelings surrounding your heart attack and the surgery and the changes that have occurred," observed Dr Wason.

"Yes, we have," Rex noted soberly, ". . . we have."

"I'm glad I can tell you that you have passed the most dangerous period after your heart attack and now your risk is quite low. In some ways, because of your better diet and regular exercise, you are healthier than you were before your heart attack. That's good news, but I am concerned about your sadness and wonder if it would be helpful at your next appointment for us to talk about that more, to set aside some time just to look at that?" inquired Dr Wason.

"Yes, it would. It's hard to talk about, but it would be helpful," Rex answered emphatically.

"Are you encountering any problems with sleep or appetite Rex?" asked the doctor.

"No, none at all," stated Rex.

The doctor asked a few more questions exploring possible symptoms of depression. Finding none, he again offered to talk further with Rex at their next visit and suggested it might be helpful to invite his wife to an upcoming appointment. The patient answered affirmatively.

The doctor already knew the patient's medical conditions before the interview began. He picked up on the patient's sadness and his initial hesitancy in exploring how the heart attack had made him fearful. At the same time, the doctor ruled out serious depression by asking a few diagnostic questions and offered the patient an opportunity to explore further his feelings about his health and illness experience. Also, the doctor and patient explored the patient's aspirations for a healthy life, in his case including going to the cabin with his family and resuming lovemaking. The reader will notice that the interview effortlessly weaved among the disease, health, and the illness experience.

By considering the patient's health and illness experience as a legitimate focus of enquiry and management, the physician has avoided two potential errors. First, if only the conventional biomedical model had been used, by seeking a disease to explain the patient's distress, the doctor might have labeled the patient depressed and given him unnecessary and potentially hazardous medication. A second error would have been simply to conclude that the patient was not depressed and move on to the next part of the interview. Had the physician decided that the patient's distress was not worthy of attention, he might have delayed the patient's emotional and physical recovery and the patient's adjustment to living with a chronic disease.

This case also illustrates a synthesis of medical management after a myocardial infarction with attention to the patient's view of health and his illness experience. This patient was following all of the guidelines, but he still did not feel healthy or secure in his body. Also, his fears were shared by his wife, thus compounding his anxiety. Dealing with this patient's experience of health and illness, and including his wife in the discussions, may be helpful in promoting health, alleviating fears, correcting misconceptions, encouraging him to discuss his discouragement, or simply "being there" and caring what happens to him. At the very least, this compassionate concern is a testimony to the fundamental worth and dignity of the patient; it might help prevent him from becoming truly depressed; it might even help him to live more fully.

EXPLORING THE DISEASE

The concept of *disease* is central to the biomedical model, reducing the patient's symptoms and physical findings to externally observable disorders of structure or function. It is materialist and reductionist in nature and has its genesis in the 19th century medical focus on discrete pathological observations, laboratory tests, and technologies such as EKG, EEG, and X-ray. It rose in tandem with, and was a necessary antecedent to, *diagnosis*, the identification of a patient's sickness into a discrete category. The two together, disease and diagnosis, gave rise to what became known as scientific medicine. The continued burgeoning of new medical technologies in the last 100 years helped to solidify this linkage into techno-scientific medicine. The drawbacks to the concept of disease as structured include the observation that, unlike the infectious disease era when it became defined, illnesses are increasingly chronic rather than acute and self-limited. As people age, multiple chronic diseases, multimorbidity, along with the accompanying polypharmacy, become more common. Assigning a disease label identifies what everyone with that diagnosis has in common and leaves out what is unique to each individual patient. The call for the end of the disease era[12] is, however, premature. Disease nosologies remain essential to clinicians, administrators, insurers, specialties, and researchers and to the patients, for whom they provide a linkage between the particular and the general. Rosenberg observes "the clinician can be seen as a kind of interface manager, shaping the intersection, between the individual patient and a collectively and cumulatively agreed-upon picture of a particular disease and its optimal treatment".[13] The meaning of the term disease has evolved from its origins when it relied upon a set of symptoms and signs to, increasingly, the sum of the expanding laboratory, cytological, imaging technologies, and genetics that are relied upon for definition. What remains the case, however, is that it represents the objectively observable components of sickness. Disease pictures are no less real for being the product of technologies "inasmuch as we believe in them and act individually and collectively on those beliefs".[13]

In addition to attention to signs and symptoms and the use of laboratory and imaging, a well-conducted physical examination, pertinent to the patient's symptoms and concerns, is essential for diagnostic or objective purposes as well as for subjective purposes. It conveys to the patient competence, confidence, and thoroughness. Physicians view it as a central element of their professional identity.[14] It continues the process of defining the "broken part" and is necessary to guide further investigations as shown in Figure 3.2. In the biomedical approach the evaluation of subjective symptoms, objective signs, and investigations plus clinical reasoning are aimed at arriving at a tentative or confirmed diagnosis. The patient-centered approach recognizes, in addition, the human value of direct touch as method of communicating empathy and avoiding objectifying the patient. The physical examination serves a healing as well as a diagnostic purpose.[15] The ritual of physical examination helps the clinician focus and provides a direct connection with the patient.[16] The clinician watches the patient's facial expression to detect any discomfort that may be occurring. Listening carefully to the patient continues during the examination, not only for any discomfort being created but also for what is sometimes revealed verbally. Many clinicians have found that important feelings and memories come to patient consciousness when parts of the body are touched.

Though complete physical examinations on asymptomatic individuals are no longer recommended, the examination of a symptomatic patient provides opportunity for the clinician to detect unrelated problems such as suspicious skin lesions or the early signs of a parkinsonian gait. Periodic physical examinations are necessary for well childcare (as in "A Caregiver's Voice," Box 3.1) and monitoring chronic illnesses.

BOX 3.1: A Caregiver's Voice

Bridget L Ryan

My daughter, Sarah, 3 years old, has been referred to Dr Connor, a pediatric ENT, for chronic ear infections. She is used to having her ears examined by our family physician who is very kind and respectful to her. He has taught her that the instrument he uses is an otoscope and always asks permission to look in her ears. When she sees him with the otoscope, she now automatically turns her head and offers her ear.

Dr Connor's fellow enters the examining room and speaks to my daughter. "Hi Sarah, how are you today?" he says warmly. She smiles warily as is her nature with strangers. He takes a bit of history and says Dr Connor should be in shortly. After a long wait, Dr Connor arrives. He goes immediately to the examination table, grabs and turns Sarah's head, preparing to use the otoscope. Sarah is taken aback and afraid; she screams. Dr Connor says, "Oh don't worry – they all cry like that." I think to myself, "I hope that young physician manages to maintain his patient-centered manner in this hostile environment."

I call my family physician's office and tell my nurse that I cannot take Sarah back to this person. We are referred to another pediatric ENT. We are fortunate to live in a city where it is possible to find more than one pediatric ENT.

At our first visit with Dr Singh, he introduces himself to Sarah. He shows her a little finger puppet and asks her if she would like to wear it. He asks if he can use his otoscope to examine her ears. She says he can; he gently asks her to turn her head. The appointment is no longer than the one with Dr Connors. There is no crying, and Sarah leaves thrilled with her finger puppet and tells me that she liked this doctor.

The physical examination is carried out, as much as circumstances allow, in a private setting. Care is taken to seek permission from the patient before examining any part of the body. "May I examine more closely your swollen ankles?" Proper draping is done to maintain modesty, and for some examinations, a chaperone may be necessary. It is important that the clinician ask the patient if they would be more comfortable with a chaperone in the room, rather than expecting the patient to request one.

A skillfully done examination blends the necessary gathering of objective signs while also reassuring and comforting the patient and keeping the clinician grounded.

The increasing use of virtual care through telephone or video as well as portable technologies such as ultrasound have raised alarm about the decline in the frequency of physical examinations and clinician competence and confidence in carrying out this traditional aspect of clinical care[16, 17] (see Chapter 9 for a discussion of some technologies and patient-centered care).

In the example of Rex, presented earlier in this chapter, his presentation with symptoms of an acute MI would have been dealt with using chiefly a biomedical approach. His disease, however, had begun years before this life-threatening event. At that time, he occupied the left side of the Disease circle in Figure 3.3. He had a disease but no symptoms. When he presented with chest pain, breathlessness and diaphoresis, he had moved to the center of the overlapping circles-symptomatic disease with diminished health. Now that he is 8 months post-MI, his clinician is focusing on his illness and health while also monitoring the underlying disease. See the left-hand column of Figure 3.3, which summarizes that the clinician began the visit with the follow-up of Rex's coronary artery disease and progress on the plan that included watching his weight and cholesterol. The conversation about the exercise program, which had been going well, revealed symptoms of sadness and possible depression. A physical examination was not conducted at this visit.

EXPLORING DIMENSIONS OF HEALTH

We propose that clinicians keep in mind the definition of health as being unique to each patient and encompassing not only absence of disease but also the meaning of health to the patient and the patient's ability to realize aspirations and purpose in their lives. For one person, health may mean being able to run in the next marathon; for another, health is when the back pain is brought under control.

Assuming the importance of the role of health promotion in all of health care, we recommend that clinicians listen for cues to the meaning of health for the patient and to patients' aspirations for health. Some of these possible cues have been identified by rich literature on health promotion, such as patients' perceived susceptibility[18]; their perceived health status and sense of well-being[19]; their attitudes toward health consciousness and health behaviors[20]; the degree to which patients feel they can create their own health, often called "self-efficacy"[21]; and things that help people get through tough times, often called "resiliency".[22]

As well, clinicians may ask persons coming to the clinic for periodic health examinations[23] or minor ailments: "What does the term 'health' mean to you in your life?" Such questions adapted

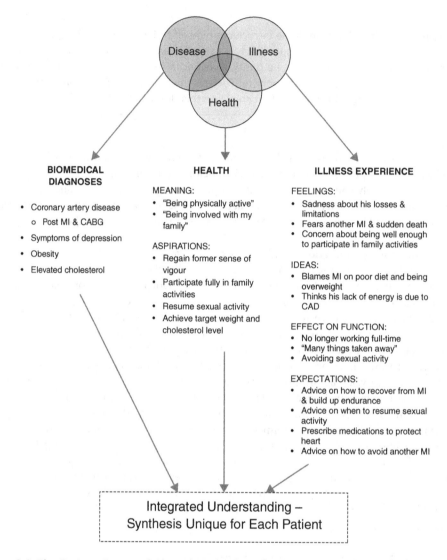

BIOMEDICAL DIAGNOSES

- Coronary artery disease
  - o Post MI & CABG
- Symptoms of depression
- Obesity
- Elevated cholesterol

HEALTH

MEANING:
- "Being physically active"
- "Being involved with my family"

ASPIRATIONS:
- Regain former sense of vigour
- Participate fully in family activities
- Resume sexual activity
- Achieve target weight and cholesterol level

ILLNESS EXPERIENCE

FEELINGS:
- Sadness about his losses & limitations
- Fears another MI & sudden death
- Concern about being well enough to participate in family activities

IDEAS:
- Blames MI on poor diet and being overweight
- Thinks his lack of energy is due to CAD

EFFECT ON FUNCTION:
- No longer working full-time
- "Many things taken away"
- Avoiding sexual activity

EXPECTATIONS:
- Advice on how to recover from MI & build up endurance
- Advice on when to resume sexual activity
- Prescribe medications to protect heart
- Advice on how to avoid another MI

Integrated Understanding –
Synthesis Unique for Each Patient

Figure 3.3 The Patient-Centered Clinical Method Applied

to the culture and individuality of each patient will serve two purposes clinically: first, the questions will reveal to the clinician previously unknown dimensions in the patient's life; second, the questions will "develop the patients' knowledge", as Cassell[24] says, a health-promoting act, in itself.

When patients are very sick, perhaps with multiple conditions and experiencing hospitalizations, the clinician can explore the aspirations and purposes using the following types of questions taken from Cassell: "What is really bothering you about all this? . . . Are there things that you feel are very important that you want to do now . . . things that, if you got those done or started . . . you would have a better sense of well-being?"[24]

Rex, the patient who was recovering from a previous myocardial infarction in the case study presented earlier in this chapter, saw himself as "no longer a healthy man". We see in Figure 3.3, in the center column, the meaning of health to Rex and his aspirations for a fully healthy life. The clinician seeks an understanding of the meanings and aspirations as well as the individual's self-perceived health, susceptibility and seriousness of disease, ideas about health promotion, and the perceived benefits and barriers to health promotion and prevention.

It might be said that Rex sees his "not healthy" state as the losing end of an all-or-nothing continuum. Engaging Rex in considering his health, as his ability to pursue his own aspirations, can support Rex to regain a sense of health in his new context; this could be described as health-promoting patient-centered care.

EXPLORING THE PATIENTS' ILLNESS EXPERIENCES

To examine patients' illness experiences, we suggest that practitioners should attentively and actively listen for patients' *cues* and explore these four dimensions: (1) patients' feelings, especially their fears, about their problems; (2) their ideas about what is wrong; (3) the effect of the illness on their functioning; and (4) their expectations of their clinician (look again at Figure 3.2).

What are the patient's feelings? Does the patient fear that the symptoms they present may be the precursor of a more serious problem such as cancer? Some patients may feel a sense of relief and view the illness as a reprieve from demands or responsibilities. Patients often feel irritated or culpable about being ill.

What are patients' ideas about their illnesses? On one level, the patient's ideas may be straightforward – for example, "I wonder if these headaches could be migraine headaches". However, at a deeper level, patients may struggle to make sense of their illness experience. Many people face illness as an irreparable loss; others may view it as an opportunity to gain valuable insight into their life experience. Is the illness seen as a form of punishment, or, perhaps, as an opportunity for dependency? Whatever the illness, knowing the patients' explanation is significant for understanding the patient.

What are the effects of the illness on function? Does it limit patient's daily activities? Does it impair their family relationships? Does it require a change in lifestyle? Does it compromise the patient's quality of life by preventing them from achieving important goals or purposes?

What are the patient's expectations of the clinician? Does the presentation of a sore throat carry with it an expectation of an antibiotic? Does the patient want the clinician to do something or just listen? In a review and synthesis of the literature on patient expectations of the consultation, Thorsen et al. provide a further conceptualization of patients' expectations of the visit. They suggest that patients may come to a visit with their practitioner with "a priori wishes and hopes for specific process and outcome".[25] At times, these expectations may not be explicit, and, in fact, patients may modify or change their expectations during the course of the consultation.

Figure 3.3 describes, in its right-hand column, Rex's illness experience elicited by the clinician following Rex's cues to his sadness.

The following examples of patient–practitioner dialogue contain broad questions that clinicians might ask to elicit the four dimensions of the patient's illness experience.

- To the clinician's question, "What brings you in today?" a patient responds, "I've had these severe headaches for the last few weeks. I'm wondering if there is something that I can do about them".
- The patient's feelings about the headaches can be elicited by questions such as, "What concerns you most about the headache? Is there something worrisome for you about the headaches?"

- To explore the patient's ideas about the headaches, the clinician might ask questions such as, "What do you think is causing the headaches? Have you any ideas or theories about why you might be having them? Do you think there is any relationship between the headaches and current events in your life? Do you see any connection between your headaches and the guilty feelings you have been struggling with?"
- To determine how the headaches may be impeding the patient's function, the clinician might ask, "How are your headaches affecting your day-to-day living? Are they stopping you from participating in any activities? Is there any connection between the headaches and the way your life is going?" Mold suggests a useful question: "How is your symptom affecting your ability to do things you want to do?"[26]

"A Patient's Voice" (see Box 3.2) provides an example of a patient's reaction to the clinician exploring function, simultaneously assisting the patient to adjust, cope, and heal.

Eric Cassell challenges physicians to broaden their concept of their role to include a careful assessment of how disease impairs the patient's function:

> The focus is wider. Knowing the disease, the healer is concerned with establishing the functional status of the patient – what the patient can and cannot do. What is interfering with the accomplishment of the patient's goals? How does the patient attempt to surmount these impairments?[24]

BOX 3.2: A Patient's Voice

Moira Stewart

Falling at the age of 71 is no joke. It is traumatic, painful, and scary. I was alone, flat on my back, immobile in a snow-bank at dusk for maybe 6 minutes before a jogger came by to help me. At that moment, I lost my independence, my ability to take care of myself, my ability to play music, and most importantly my confidence in my body. Could I walk outside again? Could I keep my balance? Was it all over for me?

After my husband came quickly home and took me to the urgent care center for assessment of the humerus (arm) broken near the shoulder, it was a week before I had a visit with the orthopedic surgeon at the outpatient clinic and the orthopedic fellow. After a week of pain, ebbing confidence, and feeling that life-as-I-had-known-it was at an end, their approach was a godsend.

The orthopedic fellow took the lead. "Tell me about yourself." "I am a professor, and I do research". "OK so what does your day look like?" "Oops but I should tell you that I am retired". "OK so what do you do each day now that you are retired?" "Well I play music". "What kind of music?" "Percussion in big concert bands". "Well what does that mean? I have never done that myself. Show me with your good arm, what the motions are that you do on your drums?" Pause, while I mimic playing a drum with my left hand. "I can tell you that, with your injury, seeing the X-ray, you will be drumming again within months". Within 10–20 seconds, she had taken a huge weight off me and my broken arm/shoulder!

He, too, suggests expanding the scope of questions: "Fatigue (or dyspnea, heartburn, or abdominal pain)?" "Does that get in your way?" or "Does that interfere in your life?" "How?" "Tell me about it".[24]

Finally, to identify the patient's expectations of the practitioner at this visit, the clinician might ask, "What do you think would help you to deal with these headaches? Is there some specific management that you want for your headaches? In what way may I help you? What do you think would reassure you about these headaches?"

As the following case illustrates, listening to the patient's story and exploring the disease and illness experience are essential aspects of patient-centered care.

CASE EXAMPLE

At 3 a.m., Jenna Jamieson was awakened by a sharp pain in her right lower quadrant. She dismissed it as bothersome menstrual pain and tried to get back to sleep. However, sleep was not an option, as the pain became unremitting.

Jenna was a 31-year-old single woman who lived alone. A committed teacher of special needs children, she had just begun working at a new school. She was also an accomplished rower who had led her team to several national victories. At 3:30 a.m., Jenna, feeling feverish and nauseated, staggered to the bathroom. In her stupor of pain she was thankful on two counts: it was Saturday – at least she would have a couple of days to recover from whatever this was before returning to school – and being winter there was no rowing practice.

By 6 a.m., the pain had reached the point that Jenna could hardly get her breath. She felt weak, sweaty, and nauseated. In desperation Jenna called a close friend to take her to the hospital.

Three hours later, after undergoing numerous tests and examinations, the surgeon on call diagnosed acute appendicitis. Jenna was promptly taken to the operating room for surgery. While medication had alleviated Jenna's pain, her anxiety and fear had intensified. In a few brief hours, she had gone from feeling healthy and vital to someone who was very ill.

In the recovery room, Jenna felt groggy and disoriented. She sighed and then blinked to see her surgeon standing over her. "Well, Jenna" he said, "It was not your appendix after all. In fact it was a bit more serious". Jenna had a Meckel's diverticulitis requiring a partial bowel resection. Because it had ruptured and she developed peritonitis, she would be in hospital for several days for intravenous antibiotics. Her recovery would require at least 4–6 weeks. The diagnosis was a shock, and the surgery had been intrusive. Jenna found it hard to comprehend how all this had transpired, and to some extent she denied her current reality.

Daily, her surgeon came to see her and offer support. On one occasion, sensing her irritability, he asked Jenna if she was angry. While initially surprised by his question, upon reflection Jenna realized that she was angry and also felt as if her once healthy body had betrayed her. She was struggling to make sense of why this had happened. Her life had been turned upside down, and the things that were important to her were now even more precious. She missed her students and her work and wondered if she would have the physical stamina to return to work. She was also fearful that her other passion, rowing, would have to be forsaken – at the pinnacle of her career. Her team was so close to an international victory – an event she might now miss. Jenna's surgeon listened and understood her anger and fears. He did not dismiss them or render them superfluous. Rather, he validated Jenna's concerns and reassured her that she would be able to enjoy all her activities and zest for living. These actions on the part of the doctor were central to Jenna's recovery. The doctor's acknowledgment of her present anger and future fears assisted in Jenna's own self-knowledge and belief in becoming well again. Had the surgeon only focused on her disease, her emotional recovery could have been delayed. Exploring Jenna's unique illness experience and supporting her through the recovery period to regain her health was as essential to her care as the surgical intervention.

Certain illnesses or events in the lives of individuals may cause them embarrassment or emotional discomfort. As a result, patients may not always feel at ease with themselves or their clinician and may cloak their primary concerns in multiple symptoms. The doctor must, on occasion, respond to each of these symptoms to create an environment in which patients may feel more trusting and comfortable about exposing their concerns. Often, the doctor will provide them with an avenue to express their feelings by commenting: "I sense that there is something troubling you or something more going on. How can I help you with that?"

Identifying how to ask key questions ought not to be taken lightly. Malterud has described a method for clinicians to formulate and evaluate the most effective wording of key questions. By trying out different wording, the physician was able to discover key questions with wording that facilitated patients answering questions that they had previously avoided. For example:

By including . . . 'let me hear' . . . or . . . 'I would like to know' . . . , I heard myself signalling an explicit interest towards the patient's thoughts
. . . When asking the women directly about their expectations, they often responded – somewhat embarrassed: . . . 'I thought that was up to the doctor to decide . . .' The response became more abundant when I hinted that she surely had been imagining what might happen (. . . 'of course you have imagined' . . .).[27]

Key questions were usually open-ended, signaled the doctor's interest, invited the patient to use her imagination, and conveyed that the doctor would not withdraw from medical responsibility.

The remaining two sections in this chapter amplify some of the important concepts of Component 1: common responses to illness and patients' cues and prompts.

COMMON RESPONSES TO ILLNESS

The reasons patients present themselves to their practitioners when they do are often as important as the diagnosis. Frequently the diagnosis is obvious, or it is already known from previous contacts; often there is no biomedical label to explain the patient's problem. Thus, it is helpful to answer the question "Why now?" In chronic illness, for example, a change in a social situation, or a change in the internal sense of health agency/control, are more common reasons for presenting than a change in the disease or the symptoms.

Illness is often a painful crisis that will overwhelm the coping abilities of some patients and challenge others to increased personal growth.[28–31]

Stein describes four common feelings that accompany serious illness: terror, loss, loneliness, and betrayal. Understanding these predictable responses to illness can help prepare both patients and clinicians for the struggles that patients may experience in attempting to come to terms with the impact of disease on their bodies and their lives. "Terror is the beginning of the end of the illusion that illness isn't that bad".[32] Losses associated with illness come one after another and sometimes feel endless. "Disfigurement offers the most literal understanding of loss, of change, of the fragility and vulnerability of the body".[32] Stein refers to the unbearable loneliness of serious illness, how patients conceal their struggles with pain or chemotherapy without revealing the fears and many inconveniences illness brings. Betrayal refers to the feeling that the body has let the patient down – it can no longer be trusted or counted on to let the patient do what matters to them. Stein describes betrayal this way:

> Health is familiar, predictable, reliable, and, we hope enduring. It provides a sense of orientation. Illness is a break in the established, continuous sameness and comfort of health. Betrayal arrives without arrangement, unpredictably, spontaneously, carrying danger. It is a threat, and we are vulnerable. It has revealed a secret about us. Personal worth and value are undermined. All of us idealize our own bodies (even if not every piece of them) so we are deeply disappointed by illness. We are strong and vigorous one moment, helpless the next; we have power one moment and are without it the next. We take account of our assets and resources, but when betrayed, we feel useless.[32]

PATIENTS' CUES AND PROMPTS

Patients often provide clinicians with cues and prompts about the reason they are coming to the clinician that day. These may be verbal or non-verbal signals. The patients may look tearful, sigh deeply, or be breathless. They may say directly, "I feel awful, Doctor. I think this flu is going to kill me". Or, indirectly, they may present a variety of vague symptoms that are masking a more serious problem such as depression. Other authors have described patients' cues and prompts using different terminology, such as clues[7, 33] or offers,[34] but regardless of the name assigned, the patient behaviors are the same. Lang et al.[7] describe a useful taxonomy of clues revealed in patients' utterances and behaviors reflecting their underlying ideas, concerns, and/ or expectations:

- Expression of feelings (especially concern, fear, or worry)
- Attempts to understand or explain symptoms
- Speech clues that underscore particular concerns of the patient
- Personal stories that link the patient with medical conditions or risks
- Behaviors suggestive of unresolved concerns or expectations (e.g., reluctance to accept recommendations, seeking a second opinion, early return visit).

In contrast to Lang et al., Levinson et al. (2000) define a clue as:

> a direct or indirect comment that provides information about any aspect of a patient's life circumstances or feelings. These clues offer a glimpse into the inner world of patients and create an opportunity for empathy and personal connection . . . [thus] physicians can deepen the therapeutic relationship.[33]

In order to assess how primary care physicians and surgeons respond to patient clues they assessed 116 patient–physician encounters (54 of primary care physicians and 62 of surgeons).

Through their qualitative analysis, Levinson and colleagues found that most clues were emotional in nature. The physicians frequently missed opportunities to adequately acknowledge patients' feelings, and as a result some patients repeatedly brought up the clue only to have it ignored again and again.

Thus, as doctors sit down with patients and ask them, "What brings you in today?" they must ask themselves, "What has precipitated this visit?" They need to listen attentively to patients' cues not only of their diseases but also of their experience of illness and their perceptions of their health. Of equal importance to hearing patients' cues and prompts are empathic responses that help patients feel understood and recognized.

Chapter 12 in this book deals with the importance of teaching about cues.

CONCLUSION

In this chapter, we have described the first component of the patient-centered clinical method, exploring disease, health, and the patient's illness experience. Prior research has demonstrated how clinicians have concentrated mostly on disease and failed to acknowledge the patient's personal and unique experiences of health and illness. Also the authors note that patient-centeredness has been mistakenly associated with an absence of consideration of disease. Our emphasis in this chapter has been on the synthesis of disease, health, and illness in the clinical method. Caring for patients in a way that promotes health and attends to the illness experience requires a broad definition of the goals of practice. The importance of exploring the dimensions of health (through thoughtful questions) and illness experience (particularly the four dimensions of the patient's illness experience: feelings, ideas, function, and expectations) has been described and demonstrated through case examples. The bridge between health promotion and patient-centered care has been elucidated; a person's perception of health and the practitioner's openness to that person's perceptions create opportunities for enhanced patient-centered healing. The balance among the three elements of Component 1 has been redressed.

The final two cases that follow bring to life the synthesis, the integrated approach, weaving among health, disease, and illness, leading to the clinician and the patient achieving a healing integrated understanding.

In the next case, this family physician working in a walk-in clinic enacts Component 1 by eliciting the patient's feelings, fears, and struggles, as well as supporting her decisions.

EMPOWERING A TEEN'S DECISION

Melad Marbeen

As I began another interesting day at the walk-in clinic, I grabbed the first patient's chart: Joan, 15-year-old female, here to follow-up on her pregnancy. Her last visit to the clinic was a week ago when another physician saw her and the encounter note conveyed: unplanned 7 weeks pregnancy, poor social support, declines to have any prenatal care or smoking cessation counseling. I headed to the examination room and met a young woman, sitting on the examination table, looking down, wearing a long-sleeved brown top over black pants.

"I know smoking is bad for my child, but I'm not quitting", Joan said flatly. Then I inquired why she didn't want to do any prenatal tests. "I don't care; everybody tells me get rid of this pregnancy, but I don't want to!" her eyes welling with tears. I asked who those people were. The following spilled out, "When my boyfriend knew that I was pregnant, he wanted to have nothing to do with this. He left me. My mother tells me to have abortion so I won't repeat her mistake, which I was the product of, unfortunately! My friend tells me to have abortion like she did, and I want to tell you that I'm not carrying this child for 9 months then give it up for adoption!" Her voice was soft; the sentences punctuated by sobs in her throat. I wondered if she was considering an abortion.

After pausing for a few seconds I gently approached her asking, "Joan, do you want to keep this pregnancy or not?" Her down cast eyes started overflowing with tears "I don't want to hate myself forever if I kill my baby", Joan continued, "being a teen mom is terrifying, but I'd like to have a baby". I asked why she considered it terrifying. "I'm all alone and everybody is against me. I don't know how I will be responsible for another person when I can barely take care of myself!"

I still could not fully understand what Joan wanted to do and which direction to go. She seemed overwhelmed by the despair with her present life. A few moments of silence passed as vivid thoughts coursed through my brain about her being a mother in the future, so I calmly asked her, "Joan, could you tell me where you see yourself in few years from now?" Joan surprisingly lifted her eyes from the ground and through her tears, she smiled and said, "busy mom, picking my child from kindergarten, buying Christmas gifts for him". I felt her answer reflected her inner desire of mothering this baby and how much she may have thought and dreamed about it during the past week.

"So Joan, it sounds to me that you want to keep this pregnancy if you get enough support, am I correct?" She nodded her head without saying anything. I acknowledged her fears and frustrations, reassuring her that I would support whatever decision she made. If she wanted to continue with the pregnancy there were community services that support single teen moms like her with finances, housing, schooling, and childcare. I offered to refer her to a social worker who could connect her with such services. Joan seemed receptive and relieved; she maintained eye contact, and her tears were drying up.

I informed her that in a walk-in-clinic I can't assume her full prenatal care, however, I would be happy to support her new journey with pregnancy and motherhood, I could see her regularly and listen to her concerns, whether medical or psychosocial. Whenever Joan felt ready, we could talk about smoking. For her antenatal care, I offered to refer her to the family medicine obstetrical clinic in the city that provides prenatal care for women without a family doctor.

Joan agreed with the plan and uttered "In the past week I was feeling frozen, lost, and having no sense of direction, but now I can find myself and see hope, thank you!" Joan was able to see the world with a new perspective and recognize that she would have the support that most women at her age need to deal with such a challenging life-altering event.

Providing a safe environment, nonjudgmental caring presence, and open discussion was what this vulnerable young woman needed to build the courage to express her wishes, face life challenges, and make important decisions. This case illustrates that identifying patients' feelings, fears, and struggles in finding the meaning of their problems are keys to exploring their illness experience. This story also demonstrates how validating patients' concerns, defining their life goals, enlisting support, and empowering their voice and role in decision-making when facing uncertainty facilitates the process of finding common ground.

This next case is written by family physicians in Nigeria. It represents the first component – exploring the disease (including prevention), health (including health promotion), and illness experiences of the patient and her husband. It also represents the second component – following the family; the third component – finding common ground; and the fourth component – continuity of care over time (in this case, four visits over 6 months).

INDECISION AROUND CONTRACEPTIVE USE

IkeOluwapo O Ajayi and Omolara Lewechi-Uke

Aduke is a 41-year-old nursing mother who had presented with blood pressure (BP) readings (146/88 mmHg and 140/90 mmHg) measured 2 days apart in her neighbourhood by a nurse. Since she was not previously known to have high BP, she attributed this finding to inadequate sleep and the stress of caring for her newborn. She was scared it could lead to a stroke. Aduke had just given birth to her sixth child 6 weeks before the presentation. This pregnancy was unplanned, and despite not having the financial resources to raise another child, she did not consider terminating the pregnancy due to her religious beliefs. She was a housewife, married to a pathology technician in a monogamous setting with six children (three males and three females). Their first child was 15 years old, while the last was a 6-week-old infant.

The physician explored awareness of contraceptives with Aduke, and she responded in the affirmative – "I am aware and even used Implanon and Cu-T intrauterine contraceptive device (IUCD) in the past, but I discontinued it because of the belief that Implanon could cause cancer. Cu-T made me gain weight too". The physician thereafter sought objective evidence of any weight gain, but there was none. The physician also enquired about the source of the idea that Implanon could cause cancer, and Aduke mentioned that a friend had told her.

The physician then checked Aduke's BP, which was 130/84 mmHg and 126/88 mmHg, on two occasions, 30 minutes apart. Her body mass index (BMI) was 24.82 kg/m², which was normal. Aduke was glad to hear that the BP readings were normal and that she was not at risk of stroke. However, the physician was quick to tell her she needed to do other things to prevent hypertension and stroke. Aduke then asked what these things could be. The physician asked Aduke her preferred diet and if she engaged in exercise habitually, to which Aduke responded that she works hard with much physical movement within the house, which could equate to exercise. "I do not have a dedicated time for exercise, but the amount of movement in the house doing house chores is even more than doing exercise." The physician educated her on healthy lifestyle practices such as salt reduction, regular intake of fruits and vegetables, and regular exercise (which will also help with weight control). The physician added that a healthy lifestyle would help to prevent the onset of hypertension. Aduke was asked if she understood, and she indicated her understanding by recapping her learnings. She was asked if she had any questions, and her response was no.

The physician asked Aduke, "What is your plan to prevent unwanted pregnancy in the future?" Aduke indicated that she had exceeded her desired family size and was confused about which contraceptive method to use, considering her fears about some contraceptive techniques she had earlier expressed. The physician counselled and educated her about the various contraceptive methods. The perception that Cu-T caused undesired weight gain was addressed by informing her about the common side effects of each contraceptive method and that weight gain was not a documented side effect of Cu-T. She was also told that cancer was not a known side effect of Implanon. Aduke was asked if she understood or still had any concerns. Despite affirming her understanding of the various forms of contraceptives, she was hesitant about the best method to use and said she would need her husband's opinion and approval.

The physician saw Aduke and her husband on her second visit, and the various methods of contraception were explained to them. The physician counselled that bilateral tubal ligation (BTL) or vasectomy was the most appropriate method for them, considering their family size. This suggestion was followed by silence from the couple. Aduke sighed and said, "Uhmm, God forbid for my tubes to be tied; if anything should happen to my children, how will I bear children to replace the loss? Nobody knows tomorrow". The husband was quick to dismiss the option of vasectomy. They both opted for IUCD insertion. The couple was given a leaflet on contraceptives to peruse at home.

The physician reminded the couple about the reason for the encounter and the idea that stress could have been the cause of the "hypertension". The physician asked the couple how they could reduce the stress of caring for the baby and the house chores. Aduke mentioned that the baby's siblings had been of help, but this was inadequate. The physician suggested that the couple consider employing paid helpers or an extended family member, which the husband agreed to.

IUCD insertion was done at her third clinic visit after obtaining informed consent, and the procedure was well tolerated. Aduke's BP was 130/86 mmHg at this visit. The husband was asked what he knew about hypertension and if he had checked his BP recently. He had not, and the physician asked for his consent to check his BP. The BP was 136/88 mmHg. The physician reiterated the need to adopt a healthy lifestyle to prevent hypertension. Aduke was followed up for 6 months post-IUCD insertion with no side effects or complaints of weight gain.

Discussion of the case: This case uniquely showcases different components of patient-centered clinical method. Component 1 (exploring the disease and the patient's health and illness experience) and Component 4 (enhancing the patient–practitioner relationship) were vividly utilized by eliciting the patient's fear and ideas, and prescribing lifestyle modification for Aduke and her husband to delay the onset of hypertension. The cultural milieu of Aduke influenced her management by involving the partner in reaching a common ground. In the African culture (Nigeria inclusive), the married woman does not exclusively own the right to reproductive and sexual choices. The male (husband) culturally must consent to such decisions as contraceptive use. Otherwise, the woman is seen as disobedient or rebellious. Bilateral tubal ligation and vasectomy are not widely chosen in Nigeria. Using the second component of patient-centered clinical method, we understood the whole person and her context and offered the appropriate care acceptable to her and her partner. Component 3 was employed in assisting the couple with finding common ground regarding the proper contraceptive method to use.

REFERENCES

1. World Health Organization. *Health Promotion: Concepts and Principles in Action – A Policy Framework*. London: WHO; 1986.
2. Green LA, Fryer Jr GE, Yawn BP et al. The ecology of medical care revisited. *N Eng J Med*. 2001;344(26):2021–2025.
3. Frostholm L, Fink P, Christensen KS et al. The patients' illness perceptions and the use of primary health care. *Psychosom Med*. 2005;67:997–1005.
4. Hatcher S, Arroll B. Assessment and management of medically unexplained symptoms. *BMJ*. 2008;336:1124–1128.
5. McWhinney IR, Freeman TR. *McWhinney's Textbook of Family Medicine*. 4th ed. New York, NY: Oxford University Press; 2016: 36.
6. Rosenberg CE. The tyranny of diagnosis: Specific entities and individual experience. *Milbank Q*. 2002;80(2):237–260. Doi: 10.1111/1468-0009.t01-1-00003.
7. Lang F, Floyd MR, Beine KL. Clues to patients' explanations and concerns about their illness. A call for active listening. *Arch Fam Med*. 2000;65(7):1351–1354.
8. Launer J. *Narrative-Based Practice in Health and Social Care: Conversations Inviting Change*. New York, NY: Routledge; 2018: 19–23.
9. Beckman HB, Frankel RM. The effect of physician behavior on the collection of data. *Ann Int Med*. 1984;101(5):692–696.
10. Charon R, DasGupta S, Hermann N. *The Principles and Practice of Narrative Medicine*. New York, NY: Oxford University Press; 2017.
11. Launer J. *Reflective Practice in Medicine and Multi-Professional Healthcare*. Boca Raton, FL; CRC Press; 2022: 121–122, 128.
12. Tinetti ME, Fried T. The end of the disease era. *Am J Med*. 2004 Feb 1;116(3):179–185. Doi: 10.1016/j.amjmed.2003.09.031.
13. Rosenberg CE. The tyranny of diagnosis: Specific entities and individual experience. *Milbank Q*. 2002;80(2):237–260. Doi: 10.1111/1468-0009.t01-1-00003.
14. Kelly M, Svrcek C, King N, Scherpbier A, Dornan T. Embodying empathy: A phenomenological study of physician touch. *Med Educ*. 2020 May;54(5):400–407. Doi: 10.1111/medu.14040.
15. Kelly MA, Freeman LK, Dornan T. Family physicians' experiences of physical examination. *Ann Fam Med*. 2019 Jul;17(4):304–310. Doi: 10.1370/afm.2420.
16. Hyman SL, Levy SE, Myers SM. Council on Children with Disabilities, Section on Developmental and Bahavioral Pediatrics. Identification, evaluation, and management of children with autism spectrum disorder. *Pediatrics*. 2020 Jan;145(1):e20193447. Doi: 10.1542/peds.2019-3447.
17. Kelly MA, Gormley GJ. In, but out of touch: Connecting with patients during the virtual visit. *Ann Fam Med*. 2020 Sep 1;18(5):461–462.
18. Boudreau JD, Cassell E, Fuks A. *Physicianship and the Rebirth of Medical Education*. Oxford, UK: Oxford University Press; 2018.
19. Gillis AJ. Determinants of a health-promoting lifestyle: An integrative review. *J Adv Nurs*. 1993;18(3):345–353.
20. Reifman A, Barnes GM, Dintcheff BA et al. Health values buffer social-environmental risks for adolescent alcohol misuse. *Psychol Addict Behav*. 2001;15(3):249–251.
21. Bandura A. *Social Foundations of Thought and Action: A Social Cognitive Theory*. Englewood Cliffs, NJ: Prentice Hall; 1986.

22. Leppin AL, Bora PR, Tilburt JC, Gionfriddo MR, Zeballos-Palacios C, Dulohery MM, Sood A, Erwin PJ, Brito JP, Boehmer KR, Montori VM. The efficacy of resiliency training programs: A systematic review and meta-analysis of randomized trials. *PloS One*. 2014 Oct 27;9(10):e111420. Doi: 10.1371/journal.pone.0111420.

23. Birtwhistle R, Bell NR, Thombs BD, Grad R, Dickinson JA. Periodic preventive health visits: A more appropriate approach to delivering preventive services: From the Canadian Task Force on Preventive Health Care. *Can Fam Phys*. 2017 Nov 1;63(11):824–826.

24. Cassell EJ. *The Nature of Healing: The Modern Practice of Medicine*. New York, NY: Oxford University Press; 2013: 89, 126, 128.

25. Thorsen H, Witt K, Hollnagel H, Malterud K. The purpose of the general practice consultation from the patient's perspective – Theoretical aspects. *Family Practice*. 2001 Dec 1;18(6):638–643.

26. Mold JW. *Goal-Oriented Medical Care: Helping Patients Achieve Their Personal Health Goals*. Chapel Hill, NC: Full Court Press; 2020: 42–43.

27. Malterud K. Key questions – A strategy for modifying clinical communication. Transforming tacit skills into a clinical method. *Scand J Prim Health Care*. 1994;12(2):121–127.

28. Sidell J. Adult adjustment to chronic illness: A review of the literature. *Health and Soc Work*. 2001;22(1):5–12.

29. Wainwright D (ed). *A Sociology of Health*. Thousand Oaks, CA: Sage; 2008.

30. Marini I, Stebnicki M. *The Psychological and Social Impact of Illness and Disability*. New York: Springer; 2012.

31. Lubkin IM, Larsen PD. *Chronic Illness – Impact and Intervention*. 8th ed. Burlington MA: James and Bartlett Learning; 2013.

32. Stein M. *The Lonely Patient – How We Experience Illness*. New York: HarperCollins; 2007: 61, 95, 165.

33. Levinson W, Gorawara-Bhat R, Lamb J. A study of patient clues and physician responses in primary care and surgical settings. *JAMA*. 2000;284(8):1021–1027.

34. Balint M. *The Doctor, His Patient, and the Illness*. 2nd ed. New York, NY: International Universities Press; 1964.

4

The Second Component: Understanding the Whole Person, Section 1 – Individual and Family

JUDITH BELLE BROWN AND W WAYNE WESTON

It is impossible to practice effective primary medical care without attention to the range of psychological and social issues embedded in the lives of all human beings.[1]

We all face the many challenges and demands presented at each stage of human development. The ascendancy to independence in adolescence, the creation of intimate partnerships in adulthood, and the realignment of roles and tasks that transpire in the senior years are all examples of expected life cycle changes. How we traverse each stage will be influenced by prior life experience. For many individuals, the successful achievement of the tasks and expectations of each developmental phase steers them through life relatively unscathed. However, for others, each ensuing life phase may be marred by past failures, previous losses, and lack of supportive relationships. For them, life's challenges are experienced as overwhelming and often unachievable.

The second component of the patient-centered clinical method is the integration of the concepts of health, disease, and illness with an understanding of the whole person, including an awareness of the patient's position in the life cycle and their life context. The patient's position in the life cycle takes into consideration the individual's own personality development, whereas the patient's context includes both their proximal (e.g., familial) and their distal (e.g., cultural) contexts. Distal context will be addressed in Chapter 5.

THE PERSON: INDIVIDUAL DEVELOPMENT

There are multiple theoretical frameworks that can help clinicians understand patients' individual development and provide both explanation and prediction about patient behavior and responses to illness. For example, they include psychoanalytic theory (i.e., ego psychology, object relations, and self-psychology); feminist theory; and cognitive theory. A comprehensive overview of these various theoretical frameworks has been provided by numerous authors[2-12] including Piaget, Erikson, and many others. The intent of this section of the chapter is to highlight understanding individual development and to demonstrate how its exploration can be achieved in the practice of patient-centered care.

DOI: 10.1201/9781003394679-6

Healthy individual development is reflected by a solid sense of self, positive self-esteem, a position of independence, and autonomy, coupled with the capacity for connectedness and intimacy. The motives, attachments, ideals, and expectations that shape each individual's personality evolve as they traverse each developmental phase. Each person's life is profoundly influenced by each stage of development, which may be isolated and lonely for an elderly widow or vast and complex for a middle-aged woman with multiple responsibilities as wife, mother, daughter, and worker. Thus, their position in the life cycle, the tasks they assume, and the roles they ascribe to will influence the care that patients seek. As an illustration of the impact of illness on human development, consider the teenager grappling with the demands of peer acceptance who is ostracized because of their acne or the elderly person whose multiple health issues remind them of their limited ability for independence.

Understanding the patient's current stage of development and the relevant developmental tasks that need to be accomplished assists clinicians in several ways. First, knowledge of expected life cycle crises that occur in individual development helps the clinician recognize the patient's problems as more than isolated, episodic phenomena. Second, it can increase the clinician's sensitivity to the multiple factors that influence the patient's problems and broaden awareness of the impact of the patient's life history. For example, the onset of a chronic illness at an early age may interfere with negotiation of age-specific tasks. Such is the case with type 1 diabetes, which may create difficulty for an adolescent attempting to negotiate the turbulent process of becoming independent. Third, understanding the whole person may also expand the clinician's level of comfort with caring as well as curing.

Patient stories depict how disease not only affects organs and organ systems of the body but also diminishes patients' ability to achieve goals and aspirations that give meaning to their lives. Often the patients presenting before us bear no resemblance to their former selves. We view them in their present context and fail to understand their past. Sometimes we make assumptions about these patients that cause us to exclude them from conversations about their health care as in "A Caregiver's Voice," Box 4.1.

BOX 4.1: A Caregiver's Voice

Bridget L Ryan

My mother, 89 years old and in good health physically and cognitively, was admitted to cardiology for newly diagnosed atrial fibrillation, where she stayed for 4 days.

Each day, a different person enters her room. None of them introduce themselves, but we assume from their officious and hurried nature that they are cardiologists.

Each day, I stand by Mom's side and the physicians speak only to me – in soft voices. I direct them to my Mom, sharing that she is cognitively competent but has trouble hearing – could they please speak up so that she can hear them? Day 1 – I ask; they continue to speak only to me and will not speak louder. Day 2 – I ask; they continue as if not hearing my request. Day 3 – again I ask – nothing. After the third visit, Mom comments to me that they seem competent but she guesses that they are too busy to be kind. Day 4 – my energy flags as yet a fourth new physician enters the room, and I steel myself to try again. The physician greets us warmly. He introduces himself to Mom and to me in a volume that she can hear. He sits down next to Mom; he calls her by name and gently takes her hand to be sure he has her attention. He tells her he has good news; she is going home today. I can tell he is genuinely happy to share this news. He explains atrial fibrillation to her and describes her treatment and asks if she or I have any questions. Afterwards, Mom expresses to me how lovely he was. I was grateful that someone finally took the time to speak directly to my mother, to respect her, and to show both of us simple courtesy and compassion.

Regardless of age and the presence of a family member, every patient deserves to be addressed directly and respectfully and in keeping with their own capacities. The fourth physician was as efficient and clinically thorough as the other three – perhaps more so. The difference was that he treated my mother as a whole person and not just as a body containing a heart in need of treatment. Though our interaction was less than 10 minutes long, he established a compassionate, trusting patient-caregiver-clinician relationship that allowed both my mother and me to leave the hospital reassured about how to handle this new condition.

In the following two case examples, we witness the loss of independence and its devastating impact on patients in their later years.

CASE EXAMPLE

As the nurse cleaned up another soiled diaper of her patient in Bed C, Room 557, all she saw was a frail old man, eyes at half-mast, bent over in his wheelchair, unable to speak. What she failed to capture was Allen, the Renaissance man.

Allen had been diagnosed with Parkinson's disease at the age of 68 – shortly after the death of his wife, Maria, following a protracted course of breast cancer. While her death had been devastating, Allen had adapted stoically. Together they had raised three children who had gone on to lead successful and happy lives – of this he was proud and content. Initially the diagnosis of Parkinson's had not fazed him, but as the symptoms of the disease rapidly progressed, he was suddenly projected into a place he had never imagined. The family home was sold, and Allen was placed in a long-term facility. At a frightening rate, Allen experienced a loss of multiple functions – he could no longer walk and was now confined to a wheelchair, and he was unable to dress or feed himself without some catastrophic incident such as a serious fall. Ultimately, he lost the ability to communicate – while his internal voice remained strong and his cognition intact, Allen's ability to speak was gone. Allen the Renaissance man had vanished, with only his children remembering the history of this amazing man.

In particular, his one daughter, Jordan, tried vehemently to retain her father's spirit and zest for life. She reminisced with him about his passion for classical music and their times together at the opera. Allen had been an avid sailor, and with care and devotion he had refitted an ancient teak sailboat that was the envy of his yacht club. Jordan and her father could now see the humor in his disastrous finish in the Boston Marathon when he was aged 60 – Allen had come in as the 300th runner, but at least he had finished! As a successful entrepreneur in the sale of "used but not abused" clothing he had done well, but more important was the commitment Allen had made to the betterment of his community – not just financially but also through active participation in campaigns to make it safer, cleaner, and viable for all who lived there.

Allen was a remarkable man in his time, but as his time began to diminish and slip away Jordan took note. She reflected on his life and grieved the inevitable loss of her beloved father, the Renaissance man – but at the same time she took hold of the moment to be with him as he, with her care and love, moved toward the end of his life.

Imagine how the health care professional's care of Allen may have changed if she had shown interest and taken the time to know the man he had been.

CASE EXAMPLE

At the age of 88, Thompson felt very satisfied with his life as he reflected on his loving marriage of 58 years with Victoria, his two successful children, Clarice and Gibson, and a very fulfilling career in the technology industry. After being a widower for 3 years, Thompson had made the decision to sell the family home with the blessing of his children, and he now resided in a retirement home. Thompson had gradually adjusted to this new lifestyle at the retirement home – although with some reluctance. He was still very independent, and in fact still remained, although peripherally, engaged with the technology industry.

Thompson's health had been remarkable for his age – high blood pressure controlled by medications and some intermittent arthritis. He viewed the latter as part of aging. But in the winter of his 88th year his health status and quality of life was dramatically altered. After an episode of shortness of breath, ankle edema, and general malaise, the nursing staff at the retirement home had Thompson transferred by ambulance to the local emergency department. Thompson was admitted to hospital, and the next 10 days were uncertain and dispiriting for Thompson. It took the wind out of his sails. He felt unsteady and confused, and he lacked interest in common routines such as the daily news.

The cardiology team assessed him as being severely compromised with a 20% ejection fraction of his left ventricle. Thompson's life as he knew it was about to change. Because of his compromised cardiac status, he was abruptly informed that his driver's license would be revoked. Thompson was shocked. He felt as though his independence had been violently stripped away. How would he manage to go out for lunch, get his hair cut, or just run a few errands? While perhaps viewed as mundane activities to many, these outings framed the passing of Thompson's days. The thought of being dependent on others was hard to grasp, let alone his loss of freedom to go when and where he pleased. Also, the thought of "giving up" his beloved car was inconceivable. While the cardiologist's decision was based on sound guidelines, it underestimated the psychological and social ramifications for the patient. In the weeks following Thompson's discharge from hospital he slowly recovered physically, but his emotional health suffered as he deeply grieved his loss of independence.

In addition to managing his heart failure, the clinician needed to provide Thompson with an opportunity to discuss the increasing loss of his independence and his increased risk of depression.

Understanding the patient's personality structure, in particular the defense mechanisms they use to ward off anxiety, both internal and external, can enhance clinicians' understanding of patients' varied responses to disease and illness. Defense mechanisms, which are automatic and unconscious, serve an important function in protecting the self or the ego from real or perceived danger.[13-16] Patients use a variety of defense mechanisms, including more primitive or immature defenses such as denial and projection. Higher-level or more mature defenses such as rationalization and sublimation are used to ward off toxic threats to the ego and thus help patients to cope. The defenses are used to prevent ego disintegration and as such need to be respected. As Broom observes:

> The patient defends himself against the 'intolerable' by setting in place structures that are not ideal but are actually adaptive within the patient's total economy, and we should expect resistance to any change in this. I may be imprisoned and long for freedom, but also be terrified of venturing out into a wider world. There may also be some comforts in the prison cell that those of us outside may scorn as objects to be clung to, but this may be very understandable within the patient's perspective.[17]

The following case serves as an example of a patient's use of defense mechanisms and takes place in the context of what is normally a happy event, the birth of a child.

CASE EXAMPLE

When the delivery room nurse announced to 28-year-old Isabella that her baby was a healthy 8-pound boy the patient cried out, "I didn't want a boy!" She refused to hold the baby, and the shocked nurse handed the baby over to his father.

A few days later, when the visiting nurse made a home visit, she found Isabella stiffly holding her infant. She denied that there were any problems and rationalized her outburst in the delivery room as a result of exhaustion from a long labor. Over the next several weeks as the nurse continued to visit Isabella, she observed that mother and child were bonding well. Isabella's initial displeasure about the baby's sex seemed to have disappeared. Her anger was now being displaced onto her husband, Lucio, whom she described as never being around or helping out with young Antonio. The source of the marital discord was apparently Lucio's "obsession with work." From Isabella's perspective, Lucio was "hell-bent" on proving he could successfully operate the pizza business inherited from his father – a legacy she deeply resented. Her husband was just like her father, who had never been physically or emotionally available during her childhood. "All men are the same," concluded Isabella, "never there when you need them most."

The nurse's attempts to explore Isabella's feelings during subsequent visits were met with denial and rationalization. Because mother and child were doing well, the nurse's role had been fulfilled; yet, as she closed the case she had a nagging feeling that Isabella's defenses were protecting her from some deeper distress. We will return later in this chapter to Isabella's story.

An understanding of the whole person enhances the clinician's interaction with the patient and may be particularly helpful when signs or symptoms do not point to a clearly defined disease process or when the patient's response to an illness appears exaggerated or out of character. On these occasions, it is often helpful to explore how the patient is dealing with the common issues related to their stage in the life cycle. Knowing that a patient has minimal family interaction or limited social supports alerts the practitioner to an individual at risk. Also, being aware of prior losses or developmental crises assists the clinician to identify vulnerable junctures in the patient's life.

The genesis of our mental and physical health has its origins in early childhood and adolescent experiences. The groundbreaking work of Felitti and colleagues[18] over 25 years ago provided strong evidence of the link between adverse childhood experiences (ACEs) and both mental and physical health across the lifespan. ACEs are defined as exposure, between infancy to 18 years of age, to one or more of the following: physical, emotional, and sexual abuse; a family member attempting or dying by suicide; experiencing family dysfunction including mental illness, substance abuse, violence, parental separation or divorce; and incarceration of a family member.[19] ACEs have been associated with poor health status later in life and the cumulative nature and intensity of exposure has been noted.[20, 21] In particular, ACEs have been found to be associated with increase in health risk behaviors including high consumption of alcohol and nicotine and with poor health outcomes in adulthood such as coronary heart disease, stroke, diabetes, obesity, depressive disorder, cancer, and chronic obstructive pulmonary disease.[22-24] Research has identified that the prevalence of ACEs is substantial. A study by Joshi et al.[25] reported exposure to at least one ACE among adults in Canada aged 45 to 85 years with physical abuse, intimate partner violence, and emotional abuse being the most prevalent.

The work of ACE researchers can guide clinicians in using the empirical evidence to create primary care and public health interventions. Several authors have highlighted the importance of clinicians developing and promoting trauma-informed care to address the needs of patients across the lifespan who have suffered ACEs.[23, 25] Primary care clinicians can play a significant role in the prevention of ACEs through screening for women abuse or being alert to abuse during well-child exams. When treating a sexually transmitted infection, the potential of sexual assault should be considered. Obtaining a family history of exposure to ACEs in the past can potentially alter the cycle of ACEs in the family system, replacing it with preventative and protective factors.[23] Furthermore, clinicians' exploration and evolving understanding of their patients as whole persons can assist them in ameliorating the harm associated with ACEs – ranging from an adolescent engaging in high-risk behaviors[26] to the impact on physical activity in adulthood.[22]

Being knowledgeable about ACE exposure and comfortable in exploring these issues with patients is at the core of understanding the whole person. This comes with training (see Chapter 11) and experience, complemented by the attributes of the patient–clinician relationship articulated in Chapter 7 such as the capacity for compassion, creating a trusting and safe therapeutic relationship, and being a healer.

The following case serves as an illustration of the impact of exposure to ACEs at an early age and how this reverberates throughout an individual's life. The case entitled "About Christine" in Chapter 7 is also an excellent example of the influence of ACE exposure across the life span.

CASE EXAMPLE

Dr Wang was perplexed. This was the sixth time he had seen his 23-year-old patient, Petra, and her daughter, Mica, in the last 2 months. At each visit, Petra had expressed concern about her 5-year-old daughter's health, but from the clinician's perspective, Mica's, or rather her mother's, complaints were minor, such as a sore throat or a stomach ache. On each occasion, Dr Wang reassured Petra that her daughter's problem was self-limiting and would resolve quickly. Yet Petra continued to bring her daughter to see the doctor.

Petra and her daughter had joined the practice a year ago, and, upon reflection, Dr Wang realized he knew little of Petra's life and experiences. At the end of the next visit, he asked Petra if she would be interested in coming back alone to talk to him regarding her concerns about Mica. She agreed and when she returned, the following story was revealed.

Petra, a single parent on welfare, was finding it difficult to cope with the demands of her active daughter. She had become increasingly more physical with Mica in her attempts to control her behavior. She was concerned that she might unintentionally harm Mica when her anger got "out of control." In order to cope with the pressure and calm herself down, she had started to drink "the odd shot of vodka," which at times had led to consuming the whole bottle.

Petra described her feelings of guilt after having struck Mica and how these feelings added to her sense of helplessness and growing reliance on alcohol. She often ruminated about "what could have been" if her boyfriend had not "got her pregnant and taken off." Her goal had been to go to university and train as a physiotherapist; her above-average high school grades would have ensured admission into the program. Petra was angry with herself for "wasting" her life. She felt extremely lonely and confused. Finally, she questioned her ability to be a "good" mother and in turn demanded near-perfection in her mothering skills (e.g., hygiene and child nutrition).

Dr Wang then asked about her early years and learned important information about Petra's past that illuminated her current problems and concerns. Petra, the eldest of three daughters, was raised in a rural community. Her father had held an executive position with a nearby food processing and distributing company for 30 years. He was an alcoholic who controlled his binge drinking in such a way that it did not interfere with the demands of his job. However, when intoxicated he would emotionally and physically abuse his wife. Often, Petra and her younger sisters "got in the way" and would also suffer physical and emotional abuse from their father.

Her pregnancy had been a shameful experience for the family and became a well-kept family secret. Forced to leave the family home and small, close-knit community where she had been raised, all Petra's supports and connections had been severed. Furthermore, her father had forbidden her to have contact with her mother and sisters. Consequently, Petra was raising Mica on her own, with no family support and limited social supports.

In listening to Petra's story, the doctor gained a greater understanding and deeper appreciation of the influence of the patient's past on her current behavior. Her frequent visits to the doctor and her "over concern" about her daughter's health were being fueled by multiple factors, both present and historical. A pattern of multigenerational behaviors and responses was now evident. Dr Wang was no longer perplexed by his patient's actions but, rather, was informed by her difficult and tragic history of abuse and alcoholism. The patient's disclosure of this important information would assist the patient and doctor in their work together – helping Petra remain a loving and responsible mom.

Individuals' pasts can haunt them, immobilizing their ability to act in the present and preventing their movement toward future goals and aspirations. As Fraiberg et al.[27] so aptly wrote, there are "ghosts in the nursery" – demons of the past that can be dissipated by the clinician's careful and attentive listening to the patient's life story, not just their disease.

The normal achievement of developmental milestones by a child can often serve as triggers for the parent of unresolved issues from their past. Returning to the case of Isabella serves as an illustration.

CASE EXAMPLE

When Isabella's son, Antonio, was 2 years of age, she began presenting to her family doctor with a variety of complaints including headaches, dizziness, leg weakness, and buzzing in her ears. Each round of investigations failed to uncover a cause for her symptoms. Reassurance from her doctor that "nothing was wrong" did not alleviate her distress; rather, her symptoms intensified and the frequency of her visits increased. Finally, during one of her many visits, Isabella burst into tears, crying out, "I think I'm dying." The doctor was initially baffled by the intensity of her response since none of her symptoms were life threatening. She appeared to have a happy home life with a healthy and active toddler and a loving husband. However, clearly Isabella's ongoing presentation of multiple and unexplained physical symptoms was a signal of some deeper distress in her life.

What unfolded was a complex multigenerational story activated by the normal developmental progression of her toddler. As Antonio began to assert his autonomy and independence, Isabella felt anxious and abandoned. The root of these powerful emotions rested in the patient's own childhood and her family of origin.

Isabella was the eldest of five children, all of whom had been born in rapid succession, thus propelling her from the maternal nest. By the age of seven, she had become her mother's "little helper," assisting in the care of her younger siblings. Unconsciously, she had assumed this role in an attempt to have her own needs addressed. When this failed, Isabella turned in desperation to her father, but he was self-absorbed with his failing business and his physical problems, including chronic leg weakness as a result of having polio in his youth. Isabella's father frequently complained how the burden of providing for his family was "killing him."

Isabella's early years had been filled with abandonment and uncertainty. Now in her late twenties, these feelings had resurfaced as her son, in whom she had invested all her love and attention, was asserting his own independence. Unable to understand or describe her inexplicable sense of loss, she had voiced her feelings through bodily symptoms.

This is a difficult and multifaceted case. The patient's story was uncovered during many visits with the family doctor, and this was assisted by the expert skills of a therapist. It highlights the intricate relationship between mind and body, past and present.[17, 28, 29] While not all patients' stories are this complex, this case demonstrates how clinicians can use their understanding of the whole person to enhance patient-centered care. Learning about the patient's developmental journey helps clinicians realize that patients are more than just their diseases. As Broom observes:

> The patient's story is, amongst many other things, a woven tapestry – of events, of perceptions of events, and of highly idiosyncratic responses to events. Many of the very significant events have to do with the vicissitudes of the patient's relationships with the world, and with other significant persons. Therefore, when a patient and a doctor collaborate together to look for the meaning of an illness, they are usually looking for the story of a person in relationship.[17]

CONTEXT

There are multiple contextual factors that influence patients' health, disease, and illness experience; many of which are elaborated in Chapter 5. Here we focus on two: (1) the role and significance of a patient's spirituality and (2) the individual's unique position in the family life cycle as well as the role of families in promoting health, living with chronic diseases, and traversing the multitude of challenges they must overcome.

Spiritual Issues

Religion can play an important role in some adults' lives, while for others it serves little or no function.[11] Nonetheless, different religious faiths bring with them various traditions and doctrines that may influence a person's daily living and source of support. Spirituality is a broad concept, conveying an individual's search for meaning in life through connection to a greater entity than themselves and more recently includes an appreciation for Indigenous spirituality.[11] Spirituality can be defined as the many ways individuals seek to find purpose, meaning, and connection "to the moment, to self, to others, to nature and to the significant or sacred."[30] Spirituality can be a source of transcendence and hope.[11, 30, 31]

Exploring patients' spiritual needs is often viewed as being exclusive to palliative care or end of life scenarios.[32] But patients' spiritual issues, in particular spiritual distress in the face of acute or chronic illness and subsequent suffering, also need to be considered. Spiritual care is an integral dimension of whole person care.

Until recently, physicians have abdicated issues of patient spirituality to the clergy or other spiritual care providers.[33] Physicians are hesitant to discuss religious or spiritual issues with their patients, perhaps because they feel such inquiry is outside their area of expertise or perhaps from fear of offending patients.[30, 32, 34] However, research has revealed patients' desire for their physicians' involvement in the spiritual aspects of their personhood.[35, 36] Selman and colleagues, in their international qualitative study across nine countries examining patient and caregiver spiritual care issues, found that offering human connection was fundamental to addressing their spiritual care needs.[35]

Furthermore, physicians have expressed an interest in engaging their patients in discussions about spirituality, recognizing that this must be approached with an appreciation of the uniqueness of each patient.[30, 32, 35] While physicians recognize the relationship between spirituality and patient overall well-being, barriers to assessing patients' spiritual resources include lack of time, inadequate training, and a belief that discussion of spiritual issues is beyond the proper boundaries of patient care and not part of the conventional medical culture.[24-32, 30, 37] In Lee-Poy's study, physicians' beliefs about the importance of religion and spirituality and their comfort level were significantly associated with asking about patients' beliefs.[36] A survey of U.S. physicians reported that the majority of respondents agreed with having a limited role in providing spiritual care to their patients; however, variability in their perspectives was associated with the physicians' religious characteristics.[32]

Appleby, Wilson, and Swinton conducted an integrated review of the qualitative literature from nine studies representing six countries on family physicians' views about spirituality and their role in addressing patients' spiritual needs. From their analysis, they derived four categories of providing spiritual care. These were (1) family physicians who "embraced" the role of providing their patients' spiritual care viewing it as caring for the whole person; (2) family physicians who assumed a "pragmatic" stance seeing this role as appropriate if helpful and desired by the patient; (3) family physicians who were "guarded" about offering spiritual care and would only do so in certain situations; and (4) family physicians who unequivocally rejected this role viewing spiritual care as not their responsibility.[38] They questioned whether these categories were "fixed or fluid" and could be influenced by training, hence requiring further future research.

Serious illness raises questions about meaning: why has this happened, why me, what did I do to deserve this, what will become of me, what will become of my family? Such questions (which reflect our desire to make sense of our lives and our experience of illness) may have no easy answers and are unique to each person. These questions may lead to a deepening of patients' spiritual lives or, conversely, to a loss of faith based on a feeling of being abandoned or a sense that life has no meaning. Thus, these questions are intensely important. Yet because they are so personal, they may not be discussed with anyone, not even family or close friends. This may leave the patient alone with these fundamental doubts and concerns at a time when they most need to share them and regain meaning, purpose, and hope in the midst of illness and suffering.[39]

In summarizing the findings of their narrative synthesis, López-Tarrida et al. state:

> Patients ask their doctors to address their spiritual needs because they need to feel that someone has listened to them and cares about their problems, worries, and concerns when they are faced with the challenge of a serious illness or even the end of their life. This attention strengthens the patient–doctor relationship and, from an ethical point of view, favours joint clinical decision-making, as well as respecting the patient's autonomy and dignity, and ensure that the care given in the clinical practice is both holistic and humanized.[40]

De Diego-Cordero et al., in their integrated literature review conclude that "addressing spiritual needs of individuals leads to a reduction in stress, anxiety, depression and an increase in resilience and hope among patients."[41]

Several authors[32, 35, 39] describe the qualities of effective dialogue about spiritual issues which include offering a safe space to share, quiet listening, and being fully present and nonjudgmental. The goal is not to provide answers but to offer existential support at a difficult time in a patient's life and can extend caring to the family as well. The attributes of compassion and being a healer described in Chapter 7 are very salient to spiritual care and contribute to establishing human connection.

The following case examines the role of spirituality in a couple's attempt to deal with a devastating health event. How the case evolves highlights, also, the importance of teamwork described in Chapter 8.

CASE EXAMPLE

Together they had carefully mapped out their early retirement plan. Over the years, Constance and Mert had been diligent in their financial planning to ensure a solid 10 years of travel to exotic venues – adventures they had always dreamed of. Suddenly, Constance's and Mert's life together was irrevocably altered and their careful plans shattered. At 60 years of age, Mert had suffered a debilitating stroke, rendering him hemiplegic. In the early days, Constance explained, "of course our way of life has changed and his world is only what he can reach. But I'm so glad he's here." But as much as they attempted to work together in confronting and adjusting to their present situation, both Constance and Mert also described grieving the dramatic change in their relationship.

Mert felt guilt and self-loathing for the burden he placed on Constance. "If I wasn't here, Constance could go on with her life. I'm pulling her down." Over time, Mert became more uncommunicative and withdrawn. For Constance, the ongoing demands of constant caregiving gave rise to negative reactions that were also damaging to the couple's relationship. An accumulation of feelings – vulnerability, irritability, fatigue, loss, and guilt – began to surface, undermining Constance's attempt to pull her husband back into their relationship.

Constance, who, throughout their 30-year marriage, had devoted herself to Mert, experienced his withdrawal as abandonment and rejection. While distraught because of Mert's profound disability, Constance could not quiet her anger – not at their situation but at Mert. They had been so close, so connected, such kindred spirits. How could he withdraw from her at this moment! She was disappointed that he had also turned his back on God. Their religion had been so important to both of them, and now, when they most needed it, he would not discuss his feelings about his situation. When, together, they met with their family doctor to discuss Mert's management options they were sad, angry, confused, and in conflict. The doctor was overwhelmed by their powerful display of emotions. In previous contacts with this couple, he had observed their very measured and clear decision-making. Yet now they were in serious distress. Recognizing that they needed more time and expertise than he could offer, the doctor referred them to the social worker affiliated with the clinic.

Several sessions with the social worker, and then with a pastoral counselor, were needed to help Mert and Constance overcome the conflict-laden behaviors they were expressing. Conversations about their shared joy of exotic travel brought them back into conflict and disappointment because such opportunities were no longer possible. However, exploration of other shared interests led them to express their common belief in the healing power of their spiritual values. Their sense of connectedness increased as together they regained their shared sense of faith. Recognizing and reaffirming their shared religious commitments helped them continue to share together what gave their lives meaning, even in the face of Mert's chronic illness.

The Person and the Family Life Cycle

Patients may be parents, partners, and sons or daughters; they all have a past, a present, and a future. We are all connected on some level to a family, which in turn shapes who we are as people and as patients. Healthy relationships and kinships bind us to one another, making us feel needed, loved, and connected. Illness can enhance or sever these essential ties in human relationships, leaving both the sick and the well feeling alone and rudderless. The journey to recovery or, at best, attainment of the status quo can be experienced as an extreme effort, and for some this is beyond the realm of possibility.

Similar to individual development, a vast literature on family theory exists to explain and understand the intricacies and dynamics of family systems. Again, it is not the purpose of this chapter to provide a comprehensive overview of this area but, rather, to highlight the important role of the family in understanding the whole person. The reader is directed to texts that provide clear and thoughtful presentations of the family life cycle and family systems.[42, 43] Additional works link family systems and primary care as well as medical family therapy.[44-47]

How the concept of family is defined has in recent years become more diverse, encompassing, and inclusive. As Kane states:

The family is a social group created and maintained by the goal of nurturing the well-being of all family members and the family unit as a whole. When it is recognized that we are all in need of care, and when our desire for caring relationships makes clear how much we value care in our day-to-day lives, we seek to form, maintain, or enhance caring relations with others who also recognize and value caring relations. Since families are not often newly created, but are groups that have expanding and contracting memberships over time, families are maintained by joint activity that works toward the shared goal of mutual well-being over the long term.[48]

While Kane maintains that families should not be defined by biological similarities she, as well as other authors, endorse the critical role of screening for family history of chronic disease for prevention and risk reduction.[49, 50] The conceptualization of family extends beyond the traditional notion of the family (of being biologically or legally connected) to encompassing unions such as gay and lesbian couples, common-law relationships, single-parent families, couples without children, and households composed of friends. While the composition and roles of the family have changed and expanded, the function of the family has remained constant – to provide a nurturing and safe environment that promotes the physical, psychological, and social well-being of its members.

In today's society creating and sustaining a healthy and caring family environment is a daunting task. The family is being buffeted by internal and external forces. The increase in single-parent households, changes in traditional sex-role relationships, and both parents often working outside the home all challenge the function of the family. The health and well-being of families is assaulted by problems such as child and woman abuse, suicide, and substance abuse. Families must also face the enormous strain imposed by unemployment, poverty, serious illness, and being homeless. Around the world, families are being torn apart, both literately and figuratively. Seeking asylum from war-torn countries or untenable living conditions, families are being tragically separated with no knowledge of the safety or survival of their family members. Children are suddenly becoming "orphans," and the elderly are left behind to die.

In March 2020, the world was irrevocably changed by the COVID-19 pandemic, often pitting family members against one another over issues of masks and vaccination to mitigate the severity of the disease. Those living in long-term care facilities or admitted to hospital due to infection with the COVID-19 virus suffered intense isolation and loss of family support. Family members on the "outside" experienced the pain and profound grief of not being in attendance with their dying family member and were unable to find closure in saying goodbye.

The additional burden of illness, either acute or chronic, may cause severe disruption to an already overtaxed family system.[51-54] Illness, either acute or chronic, is a powerful agent of change. The impact of illness on the family ranges from the devastating loss of the breadwinner role caused by a cardiovascular accident to the riveting effect on a family when a child is diagnosed with cerebral palsy. Jack Medalie, as a young family physician practicing on a kibbutz in Israel, experienced a powerful example of the impact of illness of one member of the family resulting in illness in the caregiver – what he referred to as the "hidden patient."[55] Medalie had been making regular home visits to an elderly man recovering from a myocardial infarction, and he observed the attentive care provided by the man's wife. Late one night, Medalie was called to the home for an emergency. Expecting his patient may have suffered another heart attack, Medalie was surprised to see he had improved. Instead, Medalie learned that the patient's wife had committed suicide by jumping off a cliff. This is a dramatic example of the great stress that illness in the family can place on caregivers.

When chronic illness strikes, each partner must accept the new role of either caregiver or care receiver, and each must subsequently reconcile how this role change affects their role as a partner in a couple relationship. This necessitates revising their own, as well as their partner's, understanding and interpretation of their respective roles. When the illness is chronic and deteriorating, with no hope for improvement, couples need assistance in understanding and accepting the changes brought about by the chronic illness. They need guidance and new skills to help express and realize both their individual and their shared needs, wants, and expectations.

Healthcare professionals can help couples maintain and build on their strengths of reciprocity, mutuality, and concern. Supporting couples to discuss and work through feelings of guilt, anger, and frustration may alleviate negative experiences and facilitate positive, reciprocal exchanges. Specific interventions, such as providing more in-home care, increasing utilization of respite services, or giving the well spouse "permission" for time out for themselves, may assist couples in shifting from instrumental needs to relationship needs.

For all couples living with a chronic illness, an intervention directed at improved communication would include dialogue between the partners that is sensitive, open, and always patient-centered, acknowledging that both partners in the dyad are patients. This will result in a more positive balance of roles and function within their relationship and strengthen the clinician's relationship with both members of the dyad, recognizing them both as a couple and as individuals.

The following case illustrates how the family's response to illness can have a ripple effect among its members.

CASE EXAMPLE

The possibility of breast cancer had been a foreboding presence in Jocinda's mind since her mother died of breast cancer when Jocinda was in her first year of law school. In the passing years, Jocinda had appropriately grieved the loss of her mother and became a mother herself to three sons and a daughter. Jocinda shared a law practice with Nicolas, her husband of 20 years, and together they had built successful careers and a happy, albeit busy, home.

While Jocinda's diagnosis of breast cancer 1 year ago had not been completely unexpected, the news was devastating for the entire family. However, the family quickly rallied around Jocinda to support her in her battle against cancer. The exception was 14-year-old Alexandria – her mother's cancer rocked the foundations of her being.

Jocinda faced her breast cancer with her usual strong will and determination. In character with her life view, she was positive and proactive, making the necessary lifestyle changes required to tackle her cancer. Jocinda knew and believed that cancer research had made significant strides since her mother succumbed to the disease over 22 years ago. Treatments were much more successful and survival rates for her type of breast cancer had improved significantly. All this Jocinda had conveyed to her family and most pointedly to her fearful daughter.

Always a somewhat anxious child, prone to abdominal pain, Alexandria's symptoms of anxiety were exacerbated by her mother's diagnosis. In the early months, during which her mother underwent a lumpectomy and radiotherapy, Alexandria kept her growing anxiety hidden from her family. Now that her mother had returned to work part-time, Alexandria could no longer keep her symptoms at bay. Alexandria began complaining of heart palpitations and dizziness, and she was biting her nails down to the quick. On a few occasions, Jocinda had discovered her daughter plucking at her eyelashes. In Jocinda's mind, this was the last straw. Pushing aside her guilt for being the source of Alexandria's mounting anxiety, Jocinda took action. Now was the time to wrap the family's love and energy around Alexandria. With her husband Nicolas's support, and the wholehearted encouragement of her sons, the family stepped forward to eradicate Alexandria's debilitating anxiety. Together they attended family therapy, and together they learned more about one another – and themselves. In particular, Jocinda came to understand how her sometimes overly enthusiastic approach to attacking her cancer may have preempted her daughter's ability to voice her concerns and fears of losing her mother – just as she had lost her own mother to cancer. In addition, Jocinda recognized how denying the possibility of a recurrence of her cancer would only serve as false reassurance for the already anxious Alexandria.

Together, the family gained insight into how their "fighting stance" toward Jocinda's breast cancer had squelched the opportunity for all of them to share their fears and worries about their future together. This was a new healing experience for Jocinda and her family. This family's story illuminates their journey from time of diagnosis to cancer survivorship emphasizing how a family's response can be adaptive and functional versus employing non-adaptive family coping mechanisms.[56]

Illness in the family causes a major disruption, altering how families relate, and it may ultimately impede their ability to overcome the ramifications of the illness experience. Illness may demand a change in the family role structure and task allocation. Changes in routine may be required, such as childcare responsibilities or visits to the hospital. Major alterations may be needed, such as substantial home renovations to accommodate a wheelchair-bound family member or a return to the workforce to provide for the financial needs of the family.

The disequilibrium in the family resulting from illness can also alter the established rules and expectations of the family, transform their methods of communication, and substantially alter the family structure. For example, after a disabling stroke, a mother transferred her responsibilities for the care of her five children to her eldest daughter, aged 18. The daughter, in turn, quit school, assumed the full caregiver role for her siblings, and became her father's confidant as he watched his wife resign herself to her disability. The changes imposed on families by illness are limitless and are accompanied by a host of feelings: loss, fear, anger, resignation, anxiety, sadness, resentment, and dependency.

Involving the family is also important, given that over one-third of patients are accompanied by one or more family members during a visit to their doctor.[57, 58] Family members may be as concerned as the patient about the problem or potential treatments.[59] They can also provide important information about the patient and be an invaluable resource in the patient's recovery or the management of their chronic disease.[59] However, as Lang et al.[60] observed, involving family members in an office visit can present specific challenges, such as maintaining confidentiality and addressing family conflict. The particular needs of the patient and knowledge of the family's dynamics will assist clinicians in deciding who to involve within the family and when to approach them. The use of a genogram may help simplify a complex family structure by displaying relationships and patterns.

How families have coped previously will influence how they negotiate the impact of the illness on their family roles, rules, patterns of communication, and structures. Therefore, in understanding the impact of the illness on the family some key questions can guide the clinician's inquiry: At what point in the family life cycle is the family (e.g., starting a family, launching pad, or retirement)? Where is each member in the life cycle (e.g., adolescence or middle age)? What are the developmental tasks for each individual and for the family as a whole? How does the illness affect the achievement of these multiple tasks? What kinds of illnesses have the family experienced? What kinds of support have they mobilized in the past to help them cope with illness? Is there currently an established support network? How has the family dealt with illness in the past? Have they responded with functional or dysfunctional patterns of behavior? For example, has the family demonstrated potential maladaptive responses, such as rejection of the sick person or overprotection that stifles responsibility for self-care?

These latter questions are important because they elicit how families may contribute to or perpetuate illness behavior in their members.[61] The family may represent a safe refuge for the ill person or, conversely, the family may aggravate the illness through maladaptive responses.

The impact of the diagnosis on the patient and family will depend on the juncture in the life cycle when it occurs. For example, an adult male with a preexisting history of diabetes mellitus may find his disease has less impact on his role (as a husband and father) than a teenager who is diagnosed at the point when he and his family are struggling with adolescent issues of independence and identity. Similarly, the preoccupations and struggles of families in each stage may be vastly different – for example, how does the diagnosis of multiple sclerosis impact on the childrearing responsibilities of the family system; what meaning does the death of an adult child have on aging parents who were relying on that child for support; and, conversely, how do aging parents plan and prepare for the care of their adult child with an intellectual disability?

Families caring for a child with a chronic illness such as diabetes, asthma, chronic pain, muscular dystrophy, or a traumatic brain injury face multiple challenges.[62, 63] Parents may experience feelings of sadness, anger, or guilt and struggle to negotiate multiple demands and responsibilities. Relationship discord may ensue as parenting styles clash, and siblings may experience survivor guilt. Family conflict can push the entire family constellation into a state of disequilibrium. At the epicenter is the child with the lifelong illness. For clinicians, establishing a caring and trusting relationship with all the members of the affected family is paramount.[62] Primary care providers are well positioned to serve as the "quarterback" helping families navigate all the various specialists, treatments and transitions of care. They also provide continuity of care, which is extremely important as families and their individual members traverse each phase in the life cycle.

Finally, while the illness of an individual family member reverberates throughout the family system,[64] the family also plays a powerful role in modifying the illness experience of the individual. There is now a strong body of research demonstrating how families affect health, ranging from maternal-infant bonding[65, 66] to the consequences of bereavement.[67, 68] Both McWhinney & Freeman[69] and McDaniel and colleagues[45] provide excellent reviews of the empirical evidence documenting the significant influence of the family on the health and disease of its members.

CONCLUSION

Clinicians develop an evolving understanding of the social and developmental context in which their patients live their lives. Usually, this information is not gathered in a single encounter as part of a formal social history but rather is accumulated over many visits that can span months or years. As the patient and clinician have shared life experiences, this understanding becomes richer and more detailed. With certain patients, this information may help the clinician understand the patient's complex dynamics and idiosyncratic responses to illness or demands for care.[70] Specific aspects of the patient's family dynamics or developmental difficulties may not necessarily be shared with the patient but guide the practitioner in the management and care of the patient. In other instances, facilitating patients' awareness of the origin of their conflicts or distress may help patients make sense of their struggles and pain. Finally, understanding the whole person can deepen the clinician's knowledge of the human condition, especially the nature of suffering and the responses of persons to sickness.[71-73]

The following story reveals the impact of a chronic illness and its implications on the individual's personal growth and future goals.

NOW I KNOW WHAT IT'S LIKE

Britta Laslo

"OK, who wants to try?" the diabetes nurse educator looks at us earnestly. Her display table is filled with models of the kidney, insulin vials, injection devices, needles, and various information sheets. We just finished a paper-based exercise to practice titrating insulin doses. I can tell she is very excited to be working with six young medical students on their nephrology clerkship rotation. A few of us raise our hands, myself included.

The nurse educator is referring to checking our capillary blood sugars to "see what it's like" to be someone who has diabetes. We are all eager try the exercise. It's not every day that we have hands-on teaching on ourselves! My classmates get up and get pricked by the lancet device. Turn by turn they read out their normal values with a sense of pride – "4.7," "5.1," "4.8" they bolster. My turn! I'm excited to follow suit.

The nurse educator lances my right index finger and I flinch – "Geez, patients aren't kidding, this does sting!" I joke with the others. A few seconds pass before the reading appears on the little black screen. I don't think I will ever forget those flashing red numbers on the small hand-held meter or her smile suddenly fleeing from her expression. She pauses for seemingly an eternity.

"19.8," she says as her shock silences the room while I shuffle quietly in my chair. Again, a pause.

"That can't be right," she says. "What did you eat for lunch? What time did you eat? Do you have anything sticky on your hands?" The questions flew at me – bang, bang, bang – my classmates are looking on.

I answer as best as I can, "I had some pasta and a small salad and a clementine. I ate over 2 hours ago at noon. I've definitely washed my hands since then."

She quickly mulls over these answers, seeking desperately for an explanation. "You must have some clementine juice on your hands – go wash them, thoroughly, and we will try again," she insists.

I get up and wash my hands, not knowing what else to do. A feeling settles so deep into the pit of my stomach I do not know how to tell her I don't want to check my sugar again, especially in front of my classmates. Nevertheless, I am a good student and want to please this well-intentioned woman; I hold out my finger a second time for the sharp prick. Again, that same pause.

"20.3," she states aloud. "Are you feeling okay? Any troubles with urinating or weight loss? Any headaches? Anyone with type 1 diabetes in your family?" – Bang, bang, bang, bang – round two of questions.

"I feel fine. No symptoms. My maternal grandmother has type 2 diabetes but that's it," I find myself telling her. I feel like I am on television with the audience intently watching on.

"You should go see your family doctor, just to make sure everything is okay and to get some blood work done," she instructs me, now trying to hide the elephant in the room – I have diabetes.

My family doctor, Dr Wright, ushers me into her office. She has kind and gentle eyes. We sit in privacy and she asks me what has brought me in today. I recount my story of the capillary blood sugar exercise and tell her without prompting that I feel fine and have none of the classical symptoms, or any symptoms for that matter, of diabetes. I guess this could be deemed my denial phase. Dr Wright is soft-spoken and agrees that the whole scenario seems atypical but nonetheless we agree to pursue some confirmatory bloodwork. I am calm and collected, but as I gather my bag to leave she places her hand on my arm and says, "I am off the rest of the week and I don't typically call patients during my off-time but would it be okay if I called your cellphone once I receive the results? I'll check for them. I know you must be worried." I thank her and tell her I would appreciate the phone call.

Friday morning, I am rounding with the nephrology fellow, two junior residents, and a fellow classmate. We are in a large teaching center and seeing patients with whom the complications of diabetes have taken their toll – amputated limbs, blindness, and chronic kidney disease requiring dialysis – when my phone vibrates indicating an incoming call. I quietly excuse myself to go to the dictation room.

"Hello."

"Hi, is this Britta?" I hear Dr Wright's voice. Her tone is shaky.

"Yes, hi Dr Wright."

"Hi Britta. I wanted to call you because I got your results back and I'm sorry. Your hemoglobin A1c was 8.9 and your fasting sugar was 10.1 and random sugar was 13.5. I'm so sorry."

I process these values. All three of them indicate a diagnosis of diabetes. I have diabetes. There is no doubt, I think to myself. I suddenly feel the heaviness of the phone in my hand and tears silently streaming down my cheeks.

"I've already called Endocrinology Clinic and they have an opening this afternoon if you can make it. I think it would be best to see them as soon as possible because they have a great team of specialists there, and, to be honest, I only have one patient with type 1 diabetes in my practice, so this is a bit beyond my scope. I want to see you in a week or two though if you're willing to come back in just to talk about all of this." Dr Wright finishes and pauses. I can tell she feels guilty for some reason and I want to make her feel better.

"Thanks so much for calling, Dr Wright. I guess I knew this was coming, so it's not as much of a surprise, just kind of hard to hear out loud. I will definitely go to the appointment this afternoon and would be happy to see you again in a couple of weeks."

As I put my phone back in my lab coat pocket, I fall into the chair. I am still crying, more loudly now, and I try my best to get a grip as my supervisors and countless students are about 10 feet away. I can't help but picture myself as one of the patients we had just reviewed as a team; a 34-year-old woman, legally blind from the complications of her poorly controlled diabetes, one leg amputated, the other at risk of being cut off as we, her medical team, are unable to treat the infection creeping from her skin into her bones. Just a few days ago I felt like I was thriving and healthy. Part of me no longer feels whole.

I move numbly in to the endocrinologist's office that afternoon. On the outside I am a composed, young, bright medical student. On the inside, I am a confused and angry 23 year old. My new doctor and his team are beyond kind. His handshake is warm and I feel my anger dissipating already. We go through my history and the physical examination.

We discuss the diagnosis of type 1 diabetes. We discuss its management and the need to start insulin right away. The nurse practitioner reviews injection technique and they state that they have great faith in me considering how much I know about the disease and how quickly I am learning the injection skills.

It's Friday afternoon and I am the last patient in clinic. My endocrinologist has excused himself to finish some dictations in another room and tells me he looks forward to seeing me in follow-up. Once the nurse practitioner has completed the necessary paperwork, she loads me up with my new glucometer, test strips, a patient information booklet, injection pens, and a prescription for insulin. We say our goodbyes for now and I head out to the waiting room to rebook in three months time.

"Britta, wait!" my endocrinologist hurries towards me and places his hands on mine squeezing ever so slightly.

"I wanted to tell you . . ." he pauses, his eyes focus and he squeezes my hands just a little tighter, "it's not your fault that any of this happened. I know it's a lot to take in, but we will be with you in this. I do not anticipate any reason that you won't be able to live a long and healthy life and that you will be a great doctor and have a healthy family of your own one day. If you only remember one thing when you leave here, though, just remember that it's not your fault." My eyes start to fill with tears as I listen. My fears had been heard, even without voicing them. Knowing all of the possible complications of type 1 diabetes, he knew I was not only suffering and grieving the loss of my health, but also the threatened loss of my future as a physician and as a mother. I take a deep breath, my confusion lifts, and most of my anger feels more manageable. Starting to accept this diagnosis, its prognosis, its complications, scares me, there is no doubt, but I also believe that, with support, I will be able to manage what has come my way.

"Now I know what it's like." I thought to myself; to have a diagnosis, to be confused, to be angry, to be in denial, to be scared and to begin to accept my journey. This diagnosis will now be part of my personhood for the rest of my life but it won't be everything.

Postscript: I saw Dr Terry four years later after having finished my family medicine residency training in another city. He was so happy to hear how well I had been doing. He still had those warm, kind eyes, and his handshake still brought with it the same calmness, hope, and sense of healing that I experienced 4 years ago.

This last case in this chapter illustrates the whole person in the context of her family and the role of culture in health.

FINDING A VOICE

Nisanthini Ravichandiran

I looked across the examining room at Salima, feeling as if a large gulf stood between us, and I was not sure how I could cross it. Salima was a woman in her forties, an immigrant to Canada from a rural village, who could not speak any English. Many of my patients had limited English fluency, but through a combination of unofficial and official translators, and perseverance by both patient and physician, we usually managed to cross the language barrier to some extent. However, Salima was different. She had not only a language barrier, but also an undiagnosed intellectual disability. She came to her appointment with her aunt Fatima, a kind but somewhat preoccupied woman who seemed eager to get this appointment over with and move on with her day.

A few seconds into the appointment, Fatima let me know that what Salima needed was to be on birth control. She gestured at Salima and said, "Look at her; she can't take care of a baby." I learned that Salima was married and had a young daughter. Salima had her still undiagnosed intellectual disability since she was a young child, although it was not clear whether it was congenital or acquired. Her family members, including her aunt, had formed a tightly-knit support network around Salima, making sure that her needs and those of her young child were met. Her husband had little involvement in childcare but worked hard at multiple jobs to provide for his family. They all agreed that Salima's daughter was well cared for, but that Salima could not care for another baby.

As I looked over again at Salima, I wished that I could bridge the language barrier and speak to her directly, as I was used to doing in almost every other patient–physician interaction. My training had not prepared me for this unique, complex, unpredictable scenario. I understood that her aunt had Salima's best interests in mind, but I also knew that prescribing contraception without Salima's consent was a violation of her personhood and autonomy. When I tried to explain my concerns to Fatima, she shook her head, looking perplexed, and just repeated the words, "she can't take care of a baby." Feeling at a loss, I scheduled a follow-up visit, hoping in the meantime to gain a better understanding of Salima's competence and identify resources for translation.

My search for a translator gave me a glimpse into the reality of practising family medicine in an urban, multicultural setting. Except in limited settings, there is no funding for translators, and many patients who would require translation cannot afford to pay. The cost of a translator typically far exceeds the cost of a publically funded medical visit. I heard that the local community health centre provided translation services for their family doctors, but this family had neither the interest nor the ability to travel halfway across the city for this purpose. Phone translation was an option, but in the context of Salima's intellectual disability and the complex conversations that needed to happen about birth control, I felt that phone translation would hardly bridge the language barrier. Fatima was well intentioned, but she was too concerned about Salima's well-being to act as an impartial translator and tended to provide her own answer to every question I asked. Translation by a family member also raised concerns about confidentiality and conflict of interest. At the end of the day, I felt that Salima was left without a voice.

At the next visit, Salima came with a different family member, her niece Aisha. Aisha was a young adult who formed part of Salima's support network. Fortunately, for me, Aisha was more passive in her role as a translator. She translated my words to Salima, and Salima's responses to me. I had always taken for granted this passivity in a translator, but now I realized that this was actually a difficult task for an untrained family member. It was a task at which Aisha was adept. This was an imperfect solution – the concerns about confidentiality, particularly in discussing the sensitive topic of birth control, remained. However, this seemed to be the best option available, and both Aisha and Salima agreed to proceed with Aisha as the translator. Finally, I felt that I was hearing Salima's voice – and I learned that she had a lot to say!

Through Aisha, I heard that Salima wished she could have another baby. Salima looked at me as she mimed what it would be like to hold a baby, and her face blossomed into a smile. However, Salima also understood that she could not care for a baby because her daughter already required much love and care. She agreed that she wanted to be on birth control so she would not have another baby. In fact, she said, another doctor had already put something inside her a long time ago, so she would not have babies. How long ago? Many, many years – just after her 10-year-old daughter was born. None of her family members knew about it. Not because it was a secret, but because no one had thought to ask her, and Salima had never thought to mention it. When I examined her, sure enough, I found an intrauterine device – which, if Salima's memory was accurate, must have been present for almost 10 years. Grateful that I had not missed this key piece of information, I removed the intrauterine device, and we formed a new plan for her birth control.

There was more to Salima's story, however. When I asked Salima what she knew about her intellectual disability, she said something in her own language that caused Aisha to laugh uncomfortably and hesitate. I asked what she had said, and Aisha translated that Salima believed that her intellectual disability was a curse that she had acquired because she had walked through a haunted graveyard when she was younger. This was a belief shared by many of her family members and had been engrained in her mind and self-concept as she grew up.

As I got to know Salima over the subsequent months, along with her daughter and other family members, I realized that the gulf between us still existed but was beginning to shrink. I was finally beginning to know my patient as a person: a person at the centre of a tapestry of relationships that formed a supportive network around her; a person whose beliefs, roles, and ability to communicate were shaped not only by her intellectual disability but also by the culture in which she grew up and the culture into which she had migrated; a person who did have a voice and was able to make that voice heard under the right circumstances.

REFERENCES

1. Pincus H. Alcohol, Drug and mental disorders, psychosocial problems, and behavioural intervention in primary care. In Showstack J, Rothman AA, Hassmiller SB (eds). *The Future of Primary Care*. San Francisco, CA: Jossey-Bass; 2004: 243.
2. Piaget J. *The Psychology of Intelligence*. San Diego, CA: Harcourt; 1950.
3. Erikson EH. *Childhood and Society*. New York, NY: Norton; 1950.
4. Erikson EH. *The Life Cycle Completed: A Review*. New York, NY: Norton; 1982.
5. Kohut H. *The Analysis of the Self*. New York, NY: International Universities Press; 1971.
6. Kohut H. *The Restoration of the Self*. New York, NY: International Universities Press; 1977.

7. Bowlby J. *Attachment and Loss: Vol. 2, Separation: Anxiety and Anger.* New York, NY: Basic Books; 1973.

8. Bowlby J. *Attachment and Loss: Vol. 1, Attachment.* 2nd edition. New York, NY: Basic Books; 1982.

9. Gilligan C. *In a Different Voice: Psychological Theory and Women's Development.* Cambridge: Harvard University Press; 1982.

10. Berzoff J, Melano Flanagan L, Hertz P. *Inside Out and Outside In: Psychodynamic Theory and Practice in Multicultural Settings.* Northvale, NJ: Jason Aronson; 1996.

11. Santrock JW, Mondloch C, Mackenzie A. *Essentials of Life-Span Development.* Toronto, ON: McGraw-Hill; 2020.

12. Broderick P, Blewitt P. *The Life Span: Human Development for Helping Professionals.* 3rd edition. Hoboken, NJ: Merrill-Prentice Hall; 2010.

13. Shamess G. Ego psychology. In Berzoff J, Melano Flanzagn I, Hertz P (eds). *Inside Out and Outside In: Pschodynamic Clinical Theory and Practice in Contemporary Multicultural Contexts.* London, UK: Jason Aronson; 1996.

14. Cramer P. Understanding defense mechanisms. *Psychodyn Psychiatry.* 2015 Dec;43(4):523–552. Doi: 10.1521/pdps.2015.43.4.523.

15. Bond M, Perry JC. Long-term changes in defense styles with psychodynamic psychotherapy for depressive, anxiety, and personality disorders. *Am J Psychiatry.* 2004 Sep 1;161(9):1665–1671.

16. Larsen A, Boggild H, Mortensen JT, et al. Psychology, defense mechanisms, and the psychosocial work environment. *Int J Soc Psychiatry.* 2010;56(6):563–577.

17. Broom B. *Somatic Illness and the Patient's Other Story: A Practical Integrative Mind/Body Approach to Disease for Doctors and Psychotherapists.* London, UK: Free Assn Books; 1997: 1–2, 66–67.

18. Felitti VJ, Anda RF, Nordenberg D, Williamson DF, Spitz AM, Edwards V, Koss MP, Marks JS. Relationship of childhood abuse and household dysfunction to many of the leading causes of death in adults: The adverse childhood experiences (ACE) study. *Am J Prev Med.* 1998;14(4):245–258. Doi: 10.1016/S0749-3797(98)00017-8.

19. Jones CM, Merrick MT, Houry DE. Identifying and preventing adverse childhood experiences: Implications for clinical practice. *JAMA.* 2020 Jan 7;323(1):25–26. Doi: 10.1001/jama.2019.18499.

20. Chang X, Jiang X, Mkandarwire T, Shen M. Associations between adverse childhood experiences and health outcomes in adults aged 18–59 years. *PloS One.* 2019 Feb 7;14(2):e0211850. Doi: 10.1371/journal.pone.0211850.

21. Krinner LM, Warren-Findlow J, Bowling J, Issel LM, Reeve CL. The dimensionality of adverse childhood experiences: A scoping review of ACE dimensions measurement. *Child Abuse Negl.* 2021 Nov;121:105270. Doi: 10.1016/j.chiabu.2021.105270.

22. Hadwen B, Pila E, Thornton J. The associations between adverse childhood experiences, physical and mental health, and physical activity: A scoping review. *J Phys Act Health.* 2022 Nov 1;1(aop):1–8.

23. Jones CM, Merrick MT, Houry DE. Identifying and preventing adverse childhood experiences: Implications for clinical practice. *JAMA.* 2020 Jan 7;323(1):25–26. Doi: 10.1001/jama.2019.18499.

24. Chang X, Jiang X, Mkandarwire T, Shen M. Associations between adverse childhood experiences and health outcomes in adults aged 18–59 years. *PloS One.* 2019 Feb 7;14(2):e0211850. Doi: 10.1371/journal.pone.0211850.

25. Joshi D, Raina P, Tonmyr L, MacMillan HL, Gonzalez A. Prevalence of adverse childhood experiences among individuals aged 45 to 85 years: A cross-sectional analysis of the

Canadian Longitudinal Study on Aging. *CMAJ Open*. 2021 Mar 2;9(1):E158–E166. Doi: 10.9778/cmajo.20200064.

26. Garrido EF, Weiler LM, Taussig HN. Adverse childhood experiences and health-risk behaviors in vulnerable early adolescents. *J Early Adolesc*. 2018 May;38(5):661–680. Doi: 10.1177/0272431616687671.

27. Fraiberg A, Adelson E, Shapiro V. Ghosts in the nursery: A psychoanalytic approach to the problems of impaired infant-mother relationships. *J Am Acad Child Psychiatry*. 1975;14:387–421. 1975:389.

28. Broom BC. Medicine and story: A novel clinical panorama arising from a unitary mind/body approach to physical illness. *Adv Mind Body Med*. 2000;16(3):161–177.

29. Broom B. *Meaning-Full Disease – How Personal Experience and Meanings Cause and Maintain Physical Illness*. London: Karnac; 2007.

30. Appleby A, Wilson P, Swinton J. Spiritual care in general practice: Rushing in or fearing to tread? An integrative review of qualitative literature. *J Relig Health*. 2018 Jun;57(3):1108–1124. 2018:1109. Doi: 10.1007/s10943-018-0581-7.

31. Koenig H, Koenig HG, King D, Carson VB. *Handbook of Religion and Health*. Oxford, UK: OUP; 2012 Feb 29.

32. Smyre CL, Tak HJ, Dang AP, Curlin FA, Yoon JD. Physicians' opinions on engaging patients' religious and spiritual concerns: A national survey. *J Pain Symptom Manag*. 2018 Mar 1;55(3):897–905.

33. Selby D, Seccaraccia D, Huth J, Kurrpa K, Fitch M. A qualitative analysis of a health-care professional's understanding and approach to management of spiritual distress in an acute care setting. *J Palliat Med*. 2016 Nov;19(11):1197–1204. Doi: 10.1089/jpm.2016.0135.

34. López-Tarrida ÁD, de Diego-Cordero R, Lima-Rodríguez JS. Spirituality in a Doctor's practice: What are the issues? *J Clin Med*. 2021 Jan;10(23):5612.

35. Selman LE, Brighton LJ, Sinclair S, Karvinen I, Egan R, Speck P, Powell RA, Deskur-Smielecka E, Glajchen M, Adler S, Puchalski C, Hunter J, Gikaara N, Hope J; InSpirit Collaborative. Patients' and caregivers' needs, experiences, preferences and research priorities in spiritual care: A focus group study across nine countries. *Palliat Med*. 2018 Jan;32(1):216–230. Doi: 10.1177/0269216317734954.

36. Lee-Poy M. *The Role of Religion and Spirituality in the Care of Patients in Family Medicine*. Masters Thesis; 2012.

37. de Diego-Cordero R, Ávila-Mantilla A, Vega-Escaño J, Lucchetti G, Badanta B. The role of spirituality and religiosity in healthcare during the COVID-19 pandemic: An integrative review of the scientific literature. *J Relig Health*. 2022 Jun;61(3):2168–2197. Doi: 10.1007/s10943-022-01549-x.

38. Appleby A, Wilson P, Swinton J. Spiritual care in general practice: Rushing in or fearing to tread? An integrative review of qualitative literature. *J Relig Health*. 2018 Jun;57(3):1108–1124. 2018:1120. Doi: 10.1007/s10943-018-0581-7.

39. Rogers M, Hargreaves J, Wattis J. Spiritual dimensions of nurse practitioner consultations in family practice. *J Holist Nurs*. 2020 Mar;38(1):8–18. Doi: 10.1177/0898010119838952.

40. López-Tarrida ÁD, de Diego-Cordero R, Lima-Rodríguez JS. Spirituality in a doctor's practice: What are the issues? *J Clin Med*. 2021 Jan;10(23):5612. 2021:8–9.

41. de Diego-Cordero R, Ávila-Mantilla A, Vega-Escaño J, Lucchetti G, Badanta B. The role of spirituality and religiosity in healthcare during the COVID-19 pandemic: An integrative review of the scientific literature. *J Relig Health*. 2022 Jun;61(3):2168–2197. Doi: 10.1007/s10943-022-01549-x.

42. Walsh R. *Strengthening Family Resilience*. 3rd edition. New York: Guilford Press; 2017.
43. McGoldrick M, Hardy KV, editors. Revisioning *Family Therapy: Addressing Diversity in Clinical Practice*. 3rd edition. New York: Guilford Press; 2019.
44. Doherty WJ, Baird MA. Developmental levels in family-centered medical care. *Fam Med*. 1986 May–Jun;18(3):153–156.
45. McDaniel SH, Campbell TL, Hepworth J, et al. *Family-Oriented Primary Care*. 2nd edition. New York: Springer; 2005.
46. Doherty WJ, McDaniel SH. *Family Therapy*. Washington: American Psychological Association; 2010.
47. Falke SI, D'Arrigo-Patrick E. Medical family therapists in action: Embracing multiple roles. *J Marital Fam Ther*. 2015 Oct;41(4):428–442. Doi: 10.1111/jmft.12104.
48. Kane LW. What is a family? Considerations on purpose, biology, and sociality. *Public Aff Q*. 2019;33(1):65–88.
49. Carroll JC, Campbell-Scherer D, Permaul JA, Myers J, Manca DP, Meaney C, Moineddin R, Grunfeld E. Assessing family history of chronic disease in primary care: Prevalence, documentation, and appropriate screening. *Can Fam Phys*. 2017 Jan;63(1):e58–e67. Erratum in: *Can Fam Phys*. 2017 Oct;63(10):754–755.
50. Ginsburg GS, Wu RR, Orlando LA. Family health history: Underused for actionable risk assessment. *Lancet*. 2019 Aug 17;394(10198):596–603. Doi: 10.1016/S0140-6736(19)31275-9.
51. Medalie JH, Cole-Kelly K. The clinical importance of defining family. *Am Fam Physician*. 2002;65(7):1277–1279.
52. Newman D. *Families: A Sociological Perspective*. New York: McGraw-Hill; 2008.
53. Gorman E. Chronic degenerative conditions, disability and loss. In Harris DL (ed). *Counting Our Losses: Reflecting on Change, Loss and Transition in Everyday Life*. New York, NY: Routledge; 2011.
54. Chambers D. *A Sociology of Family Life – Change and Diversity in Intimate Relations*. Cambridge, UK: Polity Press; 2012.
55. Medalie, J, Borkan J, Reis S, Steinmetz D, et al. *Patients and Doctors: Life Changing Stories from Primary Care*. Madison, WI: University of Wisconsin Press; 1999.
56. Rubin G, Berendsen A, Crawford SM, Dommett R, Earle C, Emery J, Fahey T, Grassi L, Grunfeld E, Gupta S, Hamilton W, Hiom S, Hunter D, Lyratzopoulos G, Macleod U, Mason R, Mitchell G, Neal RD, Peake M, Roland M, Seifert B, Sisler J, Sussman J, Taplin S, Vedsted P, Voruganti T, Walter F, Wardle J, Watson E, Weller D, Wender R, Whelan J, Whitlock J, Wilkinson C, de Wit N, Zimmermann C. The expanding role of primary care in cancer control. *Lancet Oncol*. 2015 Sep;16(12):1231–1272. Doi: 10.1016/S1470-2045(15)00205-3.
57. Brown JB, Brett P, Stewart M, Marshall JN. Roles and influence of people who accompany patients on visits to the doctor. *Can Fam Phys*. 1998 Aug;44:1644–1650.
58. Marvel MK, Epstein RM, Flowers K, et al. Soliciting the patient's agenda: Have we improved? *JAMA*. 1999;281(3):283–287.
59. Zisman-Ilani Y, Khaikin S, Savoy ML, Paranjape A, Rubin DJ, Jacob R, Wieringa TH, Suarez J, Liu J, Gardiner H, Bass SB, Montori VM, Siminoff LA. Disparities in shared decision-making research and practice: The case for black American patients. *Ann Fam Med*. 2023 Mar–Apr;21(2):112–118. Doi: 10.1370/afm.2943.
60. Lang F, Marvel K, Sanders D, et al. Interviewing when family members are present. *Am Fam Physician*. 2002;65(7):1351–1354.

61. Davidson JE, Jones C, Bienvenu OJ. Family response to critical illness: Postintensive care syndrome – Family. *Crit Care Med.* 2012;40(2):618–624.

62. Birnkrant DJ, Bushby K, Bann CM, Apkon SD, Blackwell A, Colvin MK, Cripe L, Herron AR, Kennedy A, Kinnett K, Naprawa J, Noritz G, Poysky J, Street N, Trout CJ, Weber DR, Ward LM; DMD Care Considerations Working Group. Diagnosis and management of Duchenne muscular dystrophy, part 3: Primary care, emergency management, psychosocial care, and transitions of care across the lifespan. *Lancet Neurol.* 2018 May;17(5):445–455. Doi: 10.1016/S1474-4422(18)30026-7.

63. Law E, Fisher E, Eccleston C, Palermo TM. Psychological interventions for parents of children and adolescents with chronic illness. *Cochrane Database Syst Rev.* 2019 Mar 18;3(3):CD009660. Doi: 10.1002/14651858.CD009660.pub4.

64. Saunders JC. Families living with severe mental illness: A literature review. *Issues in Mental Health Nursing.* 2003;24:175–198.

65. Klaus MH, Kennell JH, Klaus PH. *Bonding: Building the Foundation of Secure Attachment and Independence.* Cambridge, MA: De Capo Press; 1996.

66. Mooney CG. *Theories of Attachment: An Introduction to Bowlby, Ainsworth Gerber, Brazelton, Kennell, and Kraus.* St Paul, MN: Redleaf Press; 2010.

67. Schulz R, Mendelsohn AB, Haley WE, et al. End-of-life care and the effects of bereavement on family caregivers of persons with dementia. *N Engl J Med.* 2003;349:1936–1942.

68. Stroebe M, Schut H, Stroebe W. Health outcomes of bereavement. *Lancet.* 2007;370:1960–1973.

69. McWhinney IR, Freeman TR. *McWhinney's Textbook of Family Medicine.* 4th edition. London, UK: Oxford University Press; 2016: 36.

70. Hani MA, Keller H, Vandenesch J, Sönnichsen AC, Griffiths F, Donner-Banzhoff N. Different from what the textbooks say: How GPs diagnose coronary heart disease. *Fam Pract.* 2007 Dec 1;24(6):622–627.

71. Cassell EJ. *The Nature of Suffering and the Goals of Medicine.* 2nd edition. Oxford: Oxford University Press; 2004.

72. Cassell EJ. *The Nature of Healing – The Modern Practice of Medicine.* Oxford: Oxford University Press; 2013.

73. Schleifer R, Vannatta JB. *The Chief Concern of Medicine – The Integration of the Medical Humanities and Narrative Knowledge into Medical Practices.* Ann Arbor: University of Michigan Press; 2013.

5

The Second Component: Understanding the Whole Person, Section 2 – Context

THOMAS R FREEMAN AND JUDITH BELLE BROWN

Hippocrates said:

> Whoever would study medicine aright must learn of the following subjects. First he must consider the effect of each of the seasons of the year and the differences between them. Secondly . . . the warm and the cold winds . . . the effect of water on the health must not be forgotten. . . . Then think of the soil. . . . Lastly consider the life of the inhabitants themselves.[1]

"Understanding context is as much precision medicine as it should be practiced by physicians as anything molecular and maybe more so. To truly appreciate context requires heart as well as head".[2]

INTRODUCTION

Consideration of contextual factors in clinical practice is a hallmark of the patient-centered clinician.[3] The meaning of both illness and health varies with the surrounding circumstances just as the meaning of a word depends on the sentence in which it resides. In the clinical world, information only becomes useful knowledge when it is placed in the context of a particular patient's world. To ignore context will lead to errors in both the interpretation of findings and the therapies recommended.[4, 5] A clinician will want to remember that just as the body is made up of a number of interlocking systems, the individual, too, exists within larger systems, including family, community, and ecology.

Central to the patient-centered clinical approach is finding common ground (Chapter 6 in this book) between the patient and the clinician, and this requires knowledge of the context of the patient's life and current circumstances. Focusing only on the presenting symptom or behavior with no regard for the health history or life situation is called "context stripping" and considered a form of medical error.[4] Taking into account contextual variables in arriving at an understanding

DOI: 10.1201/9781003394679-7

of the patient reflects the dynamic tension between two notions of ill health that have existed since antiquity.[6-8] The ontological or structuralist viewpoint is that diseases are specific entities that have an existence separate from the sufferer. The task of the clinician is to correctly categorize the disease that is afflicting the patient, based on the symptoms, signs, and investigations. Therapeutics will, naturally, be directed at eliminating or mitigating the disease entity. The organismic or holistic or ecological view, on the other hand, sees ill health as the outcome of an imbalance or failure of the organism to adapt to the environment understood as the psychological and social and economic realm as well as the physical. Genetic, epigenetic, and early childhood experience all play a role in the adaptability of the organism to its environment.[9] In this approach, diagnosis involves arriving at an understanding of these many factors and their interplay with respect to the patient's propensity for health and illness. One arrives at a diagnosis of the *person* rather than a *disease* category. Therapeutics, then, in the organismic approach, is multifactorial and interdisciplinary in nature.

> Even when caused by a toxin, by a microbe, or by the dysfunction of an organ, illness is a fluid process that changes as we change – enigmatic, insubordinate, subjective. It captures bodies, minds, and emotions; remains at its deepest level inaccessible to language; and alters under the influence of non-medical events from divorce to climate change. What biomedicine finds hard to recognize or to accept is that different observers – patient, spouse, doctor, pastor, insurance provider, hospital administrator, epidemiologist, to name a few – examining the same illness from their separate perspectives will observe different aspects of its truth.[10]

In the 20th century, these views – the structuralist and the organismic – assumed separate pathways. The structuralist view dominates allopathic medicine and focuses on the individual patient using powerful, and increasingly, technical diagnostic and therapeutic methods. The organismic view became the arena of public health focusing on whole populations,[8] but this view also continued *sub rosa* in clinical medicine, being incorporated into whole person medicine. Whole person medicine uses both these concepts, structuralist and organismic, recognizing that each describes an element of the truth providing a broader array of therapeutic approaches and understanding. In this way, the fruits of biomedicine are used as tools placed in the greater service of providing individualized, humanistic medicine. It seeks a synthesis of the universal and the particular. Using this approach, Candib[11] has reframed the obesity and diabetes epidemics as involving several complex factors including genetics, physiology, psychology, family, social, economic, and political issues. It takes into account "fetal life, maternal physiology and life context, the thrifty genotype, the nutritional transition, health impact of urbanization and immigration, social attributions and cultural perceptions of increased weight and changes in food costs and availability resulting from globalization".[11]

Neuroscientific research has made great progress in defining the biological pathways involved in adaptation to stressful life challenges, such as those contextual factors that activate the neural, neuroendocrine, and neuroendocrine-immune mechanisms to maintain homeostasis through change.[12] They also suggest that chronic stress can have a cumulative effect or allostatic load[13] that ultimately overtaxes the body's adaptive capacity, predisposing one to disease processes[14] and accelerated cellular aging.[15]

A life course perspective assesses the influence of changing context on an illness trajectory.[16] Astute clinicians will try to take into account contextual issues in helping patients to arrive at a meaning for the symptoms. Similarly, practitioners will attend to contextual issues in contemplating health promotion and disease prevention strategies recognizing, for example, for some patients food insecurity and shelter may be of more immediate concern than disease screening programs. The patient's context includes not only the physical, interpersonal, and immediate environment of the person but also, increasingly, global factors affecting health and health care such as the recent COVID-19 pandemic and climate change.[17]

Health promotion and disease prevention require that the "whole person" be understood with a wider lens, encompassing "community" and the larger societal context. As knowledge of the broader social determinants of health has evolved, the paradigm of individualized responsibility for and focus on health, health promotion, and disease prevention no longer suffice. Thus, healthcare professionals will question whether society at large, the healthcare system in general, and the local community provide individual patients with the options they need for optimal health. When appropriate, practitioners will explore these larger contextual components with patients. For example, are the foods that constitute a healthy diet available and affordable? Does their community context enable them to exercise safely? Does air or water pollution place their health at risk? Do their living accommodations and work circumstances undermine their health?

Contextual circumstances that potentially jeopardize individuals' health are of concern to the entire healthcare community, not just to the public health sector.

CONTEXT IN HEALTH AND ILLNESS

Research from various fields continues to contribute to our knowledge of contextual factors that influence people's health and propensity for illness. Some of the chief ones follow:[18]

Family

As Scarf so eloquently states, the family unit can be viewed as

> a great emotional foundry, the passion-filled forge in which our deepest realities – our sense of who we are as persons, and of the world around us – first begins to form and take shape. It is within the enclave of the early family that we learn those patterns of being, both of a healthy and a pathological nature, which will gradually be assimilated into, and become a fundamental part of, our own inner experience.[19]

The interaction of family in health and illness is covered in Chapter 4.

Financial Security

The inverse relationship between household income and all-cause mortality is well established.[20-25] Lower income is associated with poorer health overall and lower life expectancy.

Education

The number of years of schooling is positively associated with better diet, lower obesity, and lower mortality. Education and household income, though related, have been found to be independent predictors of health.[26-28]

Employment

Burnout is recognized as a risk of chronic stress at work and is associated with hyperlipidemia, type 2 diabetes, coronary heart disease, musculoskeletal pain, fatigue, headaches, gastrointestinal issues, respiratory problems, and mortality.[29-32] Unemployment has long been recognized as deleterious for health, though the effects may differ for different subgroups.[33]

Occupation

"To know someone's occupation is to learn something about their social status, education, specialized knowledge, responsibilities, hours worked, income, muscular development, skills, perspective on life, politics, housing, and so much more".[34]

Housing

Housing insecurity is associated with negative effects on both mental and physical health.[35] Being homeless increases the risk of disease, disability, and early death.[36] The neighborhood has effects on health through such factors as walkability, safety, pollution (both air and noise),[37] access to social resources, and social cohesion. The inclusion of home visits provides immediate appreciation of context including family, household, neighborhood, and values.

Leisure

Leisure activities that also satisfy social needs prevent isolation and loneliness and improves physical and mental health in the elderly.[38, 39]

Social Support

Meaningful social support networks aid in overcoming adversity and barriers to accessing aid but may also inhibit upward mobility.[40] Social isolation is associated with mortality rates similar to common clinical risk factors.[41, 42]

Culture

Culture is understood to be the "language and accumulated knowledge, beliefs, practices, assumptions and values that are passed between individuals, groups and generations."[43] Cultural differences are not only about ethnicity but include subcultures defined by age, social status, sex, sexual preference, education, occupation, religion, and some diseases or disabilities (e.g. deafness).[44] Cultural differences influence how individuals perceive and respond to illness. A move from one culture to another is a major upheaval that can have negative effects on self-esteem, self-coherence, and health.[45]

Macroeconomics

There is a complex relationship between microeconomics and individual health and macroeconomics and population health.[46] In places where income inequality is greater, overall population health is poorer,[47] though this effect is mitigated by a strong primary care system.[48]

HealthCare System

The system of health care itself is a component of the illness experience and may have both positive and negative effects. Compassionate care requires smooth communication between team members and across the sectors of the system. There is a need for strong leadership and support at all levels of the system to achieve patient-centered care.[49] The rapid transition to virtual healthcare due to the COVID-19 pandemic is one of many technological challenges to the patient–physician relationship; these challenges have become significant factors in context.

Sociohistorical

Advances in epigenetics are providing an understanding of how historical and social circumstances influence health across generations by influencing the biological response to environmental stressors and may lead to chronic patterns of poverty, poor health, and early mortality.[50, 51]

Ecosystem

Climate change has been associated with increases in respiratory, cardiovascular, infectious, immune, metabolic, and neoplastic diseases as well as negative effects on mental health.[52] Anxiety may arise from the direct effects of storms, floods, and wildfires but range up to an existential dread that has been identified as significant in younger people. This has led to a sharp increase in research on the influence of climate change on population health.[53-55]

Media

Mass media in its various forms (print, visual, digital) help to shape our worldview and influence our behavior in both positive and negative ways.[56] Media can be an effective tool in health promotion and health education, but it can also be the source of misinformation leading to higher morbidity and mortality.[57, 58] Social media has been associated with negative effects on mental health and academic work[59] but may also be a source of important peer support.[60]

Taxonomy of Contextual Factors

Knowledge of contextual factors that influence health and disease continues to rapidly expand leading to a variety of methods to categorize that knowledge, and there are several taxonomies to organize thinking in this field.

A widely used categorization of contextual influences on health is *proximal* and *distal*, with proximal factors conceived as those closest to the individual such as family, financial security, education, employment, leisure, social support, and occupation; distal factors are thought to be more remote such as neighborhood, community, culture, and country. The proximal/distal categorization became incorporated into the thinking of social scientists in the late 19th century and adopted into public health thinking in the mid-20th century to accommodate the recognition of multicausal chains of disease causation. Inherent in proximal/distal thinking is the idea of a nested hierarchy of influences on health with clinicians focusing on proximal variables and public health on the distal ones. This way of thinking has been criticized for confusing time, distance, and power in the relationship of contextual variables known to influence health.[61] For example, in a particular situation, distal influences may have more impact on health than proximal ones. Proximal/distal categorization of context invites thinking in causal chains with distal factors influencing proximal factors through intermediaries, ignoring that effects on one level can directly influence non-adjacent levels rapidly with no intermediaries as when a change at the policy level bears directly on personal health. Given current understandings of genetics/epigenetics and the ways in which the environment influences genetic expression, even something so proximal as one's chromosomes are closely and directly connected to context. A gene carried by an individual since conception may not be expressed until environmental changes trigger it, as in many cases of adult onset celiac. The proximal/distal categorization of contextual variables has the consequence of laying the responsibility for addressing risk factors, sometimes described as lifestyle choices, with the individual and their physician rather than examining the social and economic forces that determine how those factors are distributed in a population.

Whether one conceives of risk as either individual or social determines where accountability is thought to lie – with the individual or with society and social/economic forces.

Another common taxonomy of contextual influences on health is micro- (family, working conditions, home, social networks), meso- (institutions and institutional structures), and macro-(historical time, changing cultural representations, economic cycles, income distribution, national wealth),[62] but this adds little and overcomes none of the criticisms of the binary one of proximal/distal.

Any of these methods of categorization are most useful for purposes of summarizing the results of research on the social determinants of health usually using populations as the unit of analysis. They do not lend themselves easily to the reasoning of clinicians for whom the individual patient is the unit of analysis, which requires an interpretive, inductive approach.[63] To put it another way, listing all the social variables that have been shown to have an impact on health does not inform the clinician about which ones pertain to *this* patient at *this* time. Nor do they answer the question of *how much* contextual knowledge is enough in a clinical situation?

The method of Hinds et al.[64] sees context as four nested, interactive layers: (1) the *immediate context* focused on the individual, in the present time, where rapid changes may happen or be effected; (2) the *specific context* oriented to the individual, including consideration of the immediate past as well as the relevant present, and again change can be rapid; (3) the *general context*, including both the personal and the cultural dimensions and past as well as current variables, and change, while possible, is slower to effect; and (4) the *metacontext*, which is generally shared, although rarely articulated in a clinical encounter unless explicitly sought. It is socially constructed and predominately past-oriented. Only very slow change is possible in the metacontext. These layers are distinguished by three characteristics: (1) the degree to which meaning is shared, whether individual or universal; (2) the dominant time focus: past, present, or future; and (3) the speed with which change can occur within the layer. The clinician's task is to help the patient arrive at a shared meaning of the events, a finding of common ground, or understanding that is mutually agreed upon. Meaning comes from a purposeful interaction with various layers of the context. Each layer can act as a source of prediction and explanation, but, generally speaking, the immediate and specific layers of context tend to be more predictive while the general and metacontext are more explanatory in nature. However, either of these layers can affect a patient's health and/or perception of health.

ELAINE

Immediate Context: Thirty-year-old nurse's aide presenting with sudden onset of painful shoulder.

Specific Context: Shoulder pain onset following a work mishap in which, while transferring a patient from wheelchair to bed, the patient's legs gave out causing excessive strain on Elaine's left arm in her efforts to avoid the patient falling. Examination was consistent with strained rotator cuff muscle on the left side. Treatment was started with rest, an urgent physiotherapy appointment, and cautious use of analgesics. Application for benefits for work-related injury was initiated.

General Context: She is a single mother with a daughter age 13. Her family physician (FP) had treated her for fibromyalgia and anxiety. He was aware that she had been sexually abused by a family member when in her teens, about the same age as her daughter is at present. Her ancestry is that of a racialized group. He is also aware that what should have been a two-person transfer was made by one, due to staff shortages and under-funding of homecare programs. Worker's compensation benefits ended after 4 weeks based on the average time to recovery stipulated by the compensation board, but she continued to have pain and functional limitation.

Metacontext: The effect of adverse child experiences on the developing nervous system and central sensitization[65] helped her physician to understand why her recovery would be expected to be longer. Knowing the general and metacontext enabled her FP to advocate successfully for extension of benefits. He shared this information with the patient who was able to understand that her prolonged recovery was not a personal failure but part of her larger life narrative.

Another useful way for clinicians to think about context is found in ecosocial theory.[61, 66, 67] The concept of *embodiment* views our bodies as the literal biological repositories of our physical and social lives. It is a process resulting in the ongoing transformation of the body interacting with the biological, psychological, social, and material environment. Bodies tell stories about our past from pre-conception (the genomic and epigenomic markers of our immediate and remote ancestry) to the present (biological, psychological, and social experiences). All of the contextual issues listed earlier, and more, leave marks, often not visible, on the body. The relevant patient context is embodied. This way of thinking reframes considerations of health and illness arising from individual lifestyle choices to being a result of social inequities with deep historical and contemporary roots.[67] For example the observation that hypertension is more prevalent among African Americans is not seen to be solely due to inherited biological tendencies and lifestyle but, rather, due to a complex interaction of a history of slavery, lack of access to healthy foods, unsafe neighborhoods in which to exercise isn't possible, and systemic racism. Recognizing that embodiment is a process raises the potential for mitigating negative consequences by changing the context at whatever level of interaction that an efficacious intervention is available.

ELAINE – AN ECOSOCIAL VIEW

Viewing Elaine through the lens of embodiment reminds us that her painful shoulder is more than a strained trapezius muscle (though it is that), but it also includes the circumstances that led to her needing to undertake alone what should have been a two-person transfer. Underfunding of homecare services is a political determination, as well as a business decision with personal consequences. Her body's response to the injury is influenced by the comorbidity of fibromyalgia which, in turn, is related to the associated central nervous system sensitivity[65] likely associated with the experience of physical abuse in childhood. Being a single mother living close to the poverty line and in need of employment adds to her anxiety, which in turn affects her experience of a painful shoulder. These factors occur concurrently and across time. She is not one day a member of racialized historically abused minority, another day the victim of sexual abuse as a child, another day a single mother struggling to keep her job, and another day a woman with a shoulder injury. She is all of these together seen as whole, and the clinician seeks the most direct and efficacious way to intercede in the process of recovery.

Cues to the Need to Explore Context

There are patient cues that alert the astute clinician to the need to explore more of the patient's context. During the course of a continuous patient–doctor relationship this knowledge is accumulated over multiple encounters enabling the clinician to develop a deeper understanding of the patient and strengthening the relationship. Table 5.1 shows cues to the need to examine context more deeply.

Table 5.1 Cues to the Need to Examine Context More Deeply

1. Verbal (e.g. "It's been tough since the plant closed") and non-verbal (e.g. change in patient's demeanor or clinician intuitive sense that something isn't).[74]
2. Inability to adhere to recommended treatment, e.g. inability to continue a prescribed medication or therapy due to lack of insurance coverage or the needed financial resources.
3. Multiple symptoms involving multiple systems presenting frequently or repeatedly.[75]
4. Absence of a diagnosis despite adequate investigation, e.g. medically unexplained symptoms.
5. Exacerbation of a previously controlled chronic condition, e.g. reemergence of symptoms in previously controlled major psychiatric illness.
6. All chronic illnesses.
7. Prolonged recovery from illness, injury, or surgery.
8. Frequent visits by a parent with a child with minor problems.
9. An adult patient accompanied by a relative.
10. First visit with a problem that has been present for a long time.

Clinicians too are part of and affected by the context and community in which they practice.

This is one of the essential things about rural practice, the fact that you are part of a community . . . caring for people was about listening to them, understanding them, trying to put yourself in their shoes, accepting each person for who they are, recognizing them as a person. Because that's important to people and it's part of the broader context of good health.[68]

Existing and new technologies can help make the patient's context more visible to the clinician at the time of the encounter. The concept of "community vital signs"[69, 70] offers a way for visualizing patients' neighborhoods using publicly available sociodemographic, economic, and health data to populate the EMR and can be combined with readily available street view photos of the place of residence. The addition of social determinants of health modules into the patient's chart provides a visual reminder to the clinician at point of contact of important elements of context[71, 72] and facilitates interventions and referrals for necessary support.[73]

CASE: FREDA

Dr S had attended to Freda for over 10 years during which time she treated her for frequent migraines, diabetes, anxiety, depression, and fibromyalgia. Now age 66, and due to increasing weakness, Freda required a motorized device to assist in mobility on the sidewalk near her home. On this visit Freda mentioned her new apartment on the second floor of her son's home. Knowing the neighborhood in which she lived lacked resources and was marginalized, Dr S wondered about the accessibility of the streets and sidewalks for someone with Freda's disabilities. After asking Freda's permission to see her new home, Dr S turned to her computer and brought up a street view of the son's home and found that the access to the second floor was by way of a wooden staircase on the outside of the building. She turned back to her patient and asked, "Freda, how do you get up those stairs?" Her patient's answer startled her. "Doctor, I leave my scooter at the bottom and crawl up them. I keep a walker in my apartment to get around there". This view into the neighborhood and house in which her patient lived gave Dr S her first insight into what her patient had to cope with on a daily basis and provided the impetus to initiate a referral to find something more suitable.

CONCLUSION

Being patient-centered involves being aware of the many layers of contextual nuance in which both patient and clinician reside. In arriving at a shared understanding or common ground, meaning can only occur within a particular set of circumstances or context.

THE POWER OF CONTEXT AND CONTINUITY*

Peter Lucassen and Juul Houwen

Together with biomedical knowledge, knowledge of the context and the quality of the doctor–patient relation are essential. Knowledge of the context, personal continuity and the gradual development of the 'gut feeling' reduce diagnostic uncertainty, as the following case shows. In this rendering of the case, we focus mostly on the context.

Case: Atypical Complaints

The 61-year-old Froukje Ypma comes to my office (JH) with a burning sensation in the stomach and chest region that has existed for five days without radiation in the arms or back, does not worsen with exertion or after meals, but does worsen when lying on the left side. She is not short of breath and does not suffer from vegetative symptoms. These complaints are new to her. She is known to have hypertension and she smokes. On physical examination I find no abnormalities and the blood pressure is good. I am unsure if there is a cardiac problem behind the atypical presentation. The ECG machine at the practice has just been gone for repair for two days, so I request a troponin test, something I hardly ever do. At the end of the afternoon the serum troponin appears to be elevated. After consultation with the cardiologist I refer her. She is seen that evening at the ER and after ECG and chest X-ray she is sent home with a diagnosis of atypical complaints. She does have an appointment for a transthoracic ultrasound.

I know Froukje Ypma well. She divorced two years ago. Contact with her ex is good. Together they have two sons, one of whom died unexpectedly last year at the age of 39 from a myocardial infarction. The other son lives in Bulgaria. Froukje has had no contact with her daughter-in-law and grandchildren since the death of her son. She is very sad about that. After the unexpected death, I have had regular contact with her and her ex. The consultations were usually about the loss, grief and processing, almost never about physical complaints. I know her as someone who does not often come to consultations on her own initiative and tends to minimize complaints ('It must be nothing'). It is special that she visits me with physical complaints. I also see Froukje's sadness during this consultation. I mention the situation of her deceased son and ask if she is also afraid that something is wrong with her heart. Froukje denies that, and that fits her pattern.

Knowledge of the Context

Important in a patient's context is knowledge of their socioeconomic status, important relations, life events and how the patient deals with illness. This knowledge (the patient does not often come by herself and tends to deny complaints) can make the General Practitioner (GP) alert, but also led astray (mourning period after death of son). After all, a mourning period is often accompanied by non-specific complaints. This makes the GP's work complex, but attention to these aspects is the only way to apply evidence-based knowledge to the individual patient.

Two days later, Froukje Ypma becomes unwell at work and is taken to hospital by ambulance with a diagnosis of suspected myocardial infarction. That suspicion is confirmed in the hospital. After discharge I visited her at home. She is very shocked and also angry because nothing was found at the ER at first.

Conclusion

Personal contact and knowledge of living conditions, way of responding and important events in the patient's life can lead to a sharpening of the GP's intuition. This gradually sharpened intuition gives the GP an extra diagnostic tool – the gut feeling – that removes some of the inherent uncertainty and actually enables the GP to provide individualized care. In the case described here, knowledge of the patient's response contributed to the troponin determination and referral to the cardiologist. But this knowledge could also have led to the thought 'It must be complaints as a result of the mental state'. The GP himself also had doubts, but decided on the troponin determination on the basis of intuition, caution and familiarity with the patient.

---

* This case was published by Lucassen PL and Houwen J. Reprinted with permission of Medisch Contact.

REFERENCES

1. Hippocrates. *Airs, Waters, Places: An Essay on the Influence of Climate, Water Supply and Situation on Health. Hippocratic Writings.* Hammondsworth: Penguin Books; 1986.
2. Aron DC. *Complex Systems in Medicine: A Hedgehog's Tale of Complexity in Clinical Practice, Research, Education and Management.* Gewerbestrasse 11, Cham, Switzerland: Springer Nature; 2020.
3. McWhinney IR, Freeman T. *McWhinney's Textbook of Family Medicine.* 4th Ed. Oxford, New York: Oxford University Press; 2016: 18.

4. Weiner S, Schwartz A. *Listening for What Matters: Avoiding Contextual Errors in Health Care*. New York, NY, Oxford, UK: Oxford University Press; 2015 Dec 17.
5. Konopasky A, Durning SJ, Artino AR, Ramani D, Battista A. The linguistic effects of context specificity: Exploring affect, cognitive processing, and agency in physicians' think-aloud reflections. *Diagnosis*. 2020 Sep 1;7(3):273–280.
6. Aronowitz RA. *Making Sense of Illness: Science, Society and Disease*. Cambridge, UK: Cambridge University Press; 1998.
7. Crookshank FG. The theory of diagnosis. *Lancet*. 1926;2:934–942, 995–999.
8. Reiser SJ. *Technological Medicine: The Changing World of Doctors and Patients*. Cambridge, New York: Cambridge University Press; 2009: 132–134, 151.
9. Karr-Morse R, Wiley MS. *Scared Sick: The Role of Childhood Trauma in Adult Disease*. New York, NY: Basic Books; 2012.
10. Morris A. *Illness and Culture in the Postmodern Age*. Berkeley: University of California Press; 1998: 5.
11. Candib L. Obesity and diabetes in vulnerable populations: Reflection on proximal and distal causes. *Annals of Family Medicine*. 2007;5(6):547–555.
12. McEwen B. A life course, epigenetic perspective on resilience in brain and body, chapter 1. In *Stress, Resilience: Molecular and Behavioral Aspects*. A Chen (ed.). San Diego, CA, Cambridge, MA, Oxford, UK: Elsevier Science and Technology, Academic Press; 2020.
13. Guidi J, Lucente M, Sonino N, Fava GA. Allostatic load and its impact on health: A systematic review. *Psychotherapy and Psychosomatics*. 2020 Dec 15;90(1):11–27.
14. McEwen BS. Stress, adaptation, and disease. Allostasis and allostatic load. *Annals of the New York Academy of Sciences*. 1998 May 1;840:33–44. Doi: 10.1111/j.1749-6632.1998.tb09546.x.
15. Zalli A, Carvalho LA, Lin J, Hamer M, Erusalimsky JD, Blackburn EH, Steptoe A. Shorter telomeres with high telomerase activity are associated with raised allostatic load and impoverished psychosocial resources. *Proceedings of the National Academy of Sciences*. 2014 Mar 25;111(12):4519–4524.
16. Daaleman TP, Preisser JS. *The Life Course: Chronic Illness Care: Principles and Practice*. Gewerbestrasse 11, Cham, Switzerland: Springer Nature; 2018: 469–478.
17. Ebi KL, Boyer C, Ogden N, Paz S, Berry P, Campbell-Lendrum D, Hess JJ, Woodward A. Burning embers: Synthesis of the health risks of climate change. *Environmental Research Letters*. 2021 Mar 30;16(4):044042.
18. Braveman P, Gottlieb L. The social determinants of health: It's time to consider the causes of the causes. *Public Health Reports*. 2014;129(1_suppl 2):19–31.
19. Scarf M. *Intimate Worlds: Life Inside the Family*. New York, NY: Random House; 1995: xxii.
20. Kitigawa EM, Hauser PM. *Differential Mortality in the United States: A Study in Socio-Economic Epidemiology*. Cambridge, MA: Harvard University Press; 1973.
21. Pappas G, Queen S, Hadden W, et al. The increasing disparity in mortality between socioeconomic groups in the United States, 1960 and 1986. *The New England Journal of Medicine*. 1993;329(2):103–109.
22. Kaplan GA, Neil JE. Socioeconomic factors and cardiovascular disease: A review of the literature. *Circulation*. 1993;88(4):1973–1998.
23. Khullar D, Chokshi DA. Health, income and poverty: Where we are and what could help. *Health Affairs, Health Policy Brief*, October 4, 2018. www.healthaffairs.org/do/10.1377/hpb20180817.901935/.
24. Martikainen P, Mäkelä P, Koskinen S, Valkonen T. Income differences in mortality: A register-based follow-up study of three million men and women. *International Journal of Epidemiology*. 2001 Dec 1;30(6):1397–1405.

25. Report from StatCan Sociodemographic and Socioeconomic Factors Linked to COVID-19 Mortality Rates, 2020–2021. *Stats Canada; The Daily*. https://www150.statcan.gc.ca/n1/daily-quotidien/220308/dq220308d-eng.htm.

26. Veenstra G, Vanzella-Yang A. Does household income mediate the association between education and health in Canada? *Scandinavian Journal of Public Health*. 2021;49(8):857–864. Doi: 10.1177/1403494820917534.

27. Takashi Y, Kunkel SR. An international comparison of the association among literacy, education, and health across the United States, Canada, Switzerland, Italy, Norway, and Bermuda: Implications for health disparities. *Journal of Health Communication*. 2015;20(4):406–415. Doi: 10.1080/10810730.2014.977469.

28. Zajacova A, Lawrence EM. The relationship between education and health: Reducing disparities through a contextual approach. *Annual Review of Public Health*. 2018 Apr 1;39:273–289. Doi: 10.1146/annurev-publhealth-01816-044628.

29. Salvagioni DAJ, Melanda FN, Mesas AE, GonzaÂlez AD, Gabani FL, Andrade SMD. Physical, psychological and occupational consequences of job burnout: A systematic review of prospective studies. *PloS One*. 2017;12(10):e0185781. Doi: 10.1371/journal.pone.0185781.

30. McKee-Ryan FM, Song ZL, Wanberg CR, Kinicki AJ. Psychological and physical well-being during unemployment: A meta-analytic study. *Journal of Applied Psychology*. 2005;90(1):53–76.

31. Paul KI, Moser K. Unemployment impairs mental health: Meta-analyses. *Journal of Vocational Behavior*. 2009;74(3):264–282.

32. Murphy GC, Athanasou JA. The effect of unemployment on mental health. *Journal of Occupational and Organizational Psychology*. 1999;72:83–99.

33. Norström F, Virtanen P, Hammarström A, et al. How does unemployment affect self-assessed health? A systematic review focusing on subgroup effects. *BMC Public Health*. 2014;14:1310.

34. Cassell EJ. *The Nature of Suffering and the Goals of Medicine*. New York, NY, Oxford, UK: Oxford University Press; 2004: 164.

35. Vasquez-Vera H, Palencia L, Magna I, Mena C, Neira J, Borrell C. The threat of home eviction and its effects on health through the equity lens: A systematic review. *Social Science & Medicine*. 2017;175:199–208.

36. Kushel MB, Vittinghoff E, Haas JS. Factors associated with the health care utilization of homeless persons. *JAMA*. 2001;285(2):200–206.

37. Wheaton B, Nisenbaum R, Glazier RH, Dunn JR, Chambers C. The neighbourhood effects on health and well-being (NEHW) study. *Health & Place*. 2015 Jan 1;31:65–74.

38. Ten Bruggencate TI, Luijkx KG, Sturm J. Social needs of older people: A systematic literature review. *Ageing & Society*. 2018 Sep;38(9):1745–1770.

39. Paggi ME, Jopp D, Hertzog C. The importance of leisure activities in the relationship between physical health and well-being in a life span sample. *Gerontology*. 2016;62(4):450–458.

40. Lubbers MJ, Small ML, García HV. Do networks help people to manage poverty? Perspectives from the field. *The ANNALS of the American Academy of Political and Social Science*. 2020;689(1):7–25, 340.

41. Pantell M, Rehkopf D, Jutte D, Syme SL, Balmes J, Adler N. Social isolation: A predictor of mortality comparable to traditional clinical risk factors. *American Journal of Public Health*. 2013;103(11):2056–2062.

42. Leigh-Hunt N, Bagguley D, Bash K, Turner V, Turnbull S, Valtorta N, Caan W. An overview of systematic reviews on the public health consequences of social isolation and loneliness. *Public Health*. 2017 Nov 1;152:157–171.

43. Boyden (2004) as cited by Eckersley RM, Chapter 9. In *Macrosocial Determinants of Population Health*. S Galea (ed.). New York: Springer; 2007: 194.

44. Sacks O. *Seeing Voices: A Journey into the World of the Deaf.* Berkeley: University of California Press; 1989.

45. George U, Thomson MS, Chaze F, Guruge S. Immigrant mental health, a public health issue: Looking back and moving forward. *International Journal of Environmental Research and Public Health.* 2015 Oct;12(10):13624–13648.

46. Bishai DM, Kung Y-T. Macroeconomics, chapter 8. In *Macrosocial Determinants of Health*. S Galea (ed.). New York: Springer; 2007.

47. Pickett KE, Wilkinson RG. Income inequality and health: A causal review. *Social Science & Medicine.* 2015 Mar 1;128:316–326.

48. Detollenaere J, Desmarest AS, Boeckxstaens P, Willems S. The link between income inequality and health in Europe, adding strength dimensions of primary care to the equation. *Social Science & Medicine.* 2018 Mar 1;201:103–110.

49. Tehranineshat B, Rakhshan M, Torabizadeh C, Fararouei M. Compassionate care in healthcare systems: A systematic review. *Journal of the National Medical Association.* 2019;111(5):546–554. Doi: 10.1016/j.jnma.2019.04.002.

50. Shantz E, Elliott SJ. From social determinants to social epigenetics: Health geographies of chronic disease. *Health & Place.* 2021 May 1;69:102561.

51. Vick AD, Burris HH. Epigenetics and health disparities. *Current Epidemiology Reports.* 2017 Mar;4:31–37.

52. Panu P. Anxiety and the ecological crisis: An analysis of eco-anxiety and climate anxiety. *Sustainability.* 2020 Sep 23;12(19):7836.

53. Crane K, Li L, Subramanian P, Rovit E, Liu J. Climate change and mental health: A review of empirical evidence, mechanisms and implications. *Atmosphere.* 2022 Dec 13;13(12):2096.

54. Harper SL, Cunsolo A, Babujee A, Coggins S, de Jongh E, Rusnak T, Wright CJ, Domínguez Aguilar M. Trends and gaps in climate change and health research in North America. *Environmental Research.* 2021;199. Doi: 10.1016/j.envres.2021.111205.

55. Rocque RJ, Beaudoin C, Ndjaboue R, et al. Health effects of climate change: An overview of systematic reviews. *BMJ Open [Internet].* 2021 Jun 9;11(6).

56. Viswanath K, Ramanadhan S, Kontos EZ. Mass media, chapter 13. In *Macrosocial Determinants of Health*. S Galea (ed.). New York: Springer; 2007.

57. Bagherpour A, Nouri A. COVID misinformation is killing people. *Scientific American*, October 11, 2020. https://www.scientificamerican.com/article/covid-misinformation-is-killing-people1/.

58. Rocha YM, de Moura GA, Desidério GA, de Oliveira CH, Lourenço FD, de Figueiredo Nicolete LD. The impact of fake news on social media and its influence on health during the COVID-19 pandemic: A systematic review. *Journal of Public Health.* 2021 Oct 9:1–10.

59. Braghieri L, Levy R, Makarin A. Social media and mental health. *American Economic Review.* 2022;112(11):3660–3693.

60. Berkanish P, Pan S, Viola A, Rademaker Q, Devine KA. Technology-based peer support interventions for adolescents with chronic illness: A systematic review. *Journal of Clinical Psychology in Medical Settings.* 2022 Dec;29(4):911–942.

61. Krieger N. Proximal, distal, and the politics of causation: What's level got to do with it? *American Journal of Public Health.* 2008 Feb;98(2):221–230.

62. Richter M, Dragano N. Micro, macro, but what about meso? The institutional context of health inequalities. *International Journal of Public Health*. 2018 Mar;63:163–164.

63. Montgomery K. *How Doctors Think: Clinical Judgment and the Practice of Medicine.* Oxford, New York: Oxford University Press; 2006: 125, 130.

64. Hinds PS, Chaves DE, Cypress SM. Context as a source of meaning and understanding. In *Qualitative Health Research.* JM Morse (ed.). Newbury Park, CA: Sage Publications; 1992.

65. Yunus MB. Editorial review: An update on central sensitivity syndromes and the issues of nosology and psychobiology. *Current Rheumatology.* 2015;11(2):70–85.

66. Krieger N. *Ecosocial Theory, Embodied Truths, and the People's Health.* New York, NY, Oxford, UK: Oxford University Press; 2021 Sep 17.

67. Krieger N. Embodiment: A conceptual glossary for epidemiology. *Journal of Epidemiology and Community Health.* 2005 May;59(5):350–355. Doi: 10.1136/jech.2004.024562.

68. Morland P. *A Fortunate Woman: A Country Doctor's Story.* Dublin, UK: Pan Macmillan; 2022: 68.

69. Bazemore AW, Cottrell EK, Gold R, Hughes LS, Phillips RL, Angier H, Burdick TE, Carrozza MA, DeVoe JE. "Community vital signs": Incorporating geocoded social determinants into electronic records to promote patient and population health. *Journal of the American Medical Informatics Association.* 2016 Mar;23(2):407–412. Doi: 10.1093/jamia/ocv088.

70. Angier H, Jacobs EA, Huguet N, Likumahuwa-Ackman S, Robert S, DeVoe JE. Progress towards using community context with clinical data in primary care. *Family Medicine and Community Health.* 2019;7(1).

71. Greene JA. *The Doctor Who Wasn't There: Technology, History and the Limits of Telehealth.* Chicago and London: University of Chicago Press; 2022.

72. Pinto AD, Bondy M, Rucchetti A, Ihnat J, Kaufman A. Screening for poverty and intervening in a primary care setting: An acceptability and feasibility study. *Family Practice.* 2019;36:364–368.

73. Moscop A, Ziebland S, Bloch G, Iraola JR. If social determinants of health are so important, shouldn't we be asking about them? *BMJ.* 2020;371:m150. Doi: 10.1136/bmj.m4150bs.

74. Campbell L, Angeli EL. Embodied healthcare intuition: A taxonomy of sensory cues used by healthcare providers. *Rhetoric of Health & Medicine.* 2019;2(4):353–383.

75. Rosendal M, Olde Hartman TC, Aamland A, van der Horst H, Lucassen P, Budtz-Lilly A, Burton C. "Medically unexplained" symptoms and symptom disorders in primary care: Prognosis-based recognition and classification. *BMC Family Practice.* 2017 Feb 7;18(1):18. Doi: 10.1186/s12875-017-0592-6.

6

The Third Component: Finding Common Ground

JUDITH BELLE BROWN, W WAYNE WESTON, CAROL L MCWILLIAM,
THOMAS R FREEMAN, AND MOIRA STEWART

> It is less technique than a manner of communication that seeks to spring clients from the trap of indecision. For the patient facing a choice, as doctors see it, other options compete. Only the patient can resolve his ambivalence by choosing among them. And resolution takes time.[1]
>
> Change takes time and is meted out in the mutuality of human relationship – where the doctor and patient cling to a common log on the rising river.[1]

A central goal of the patient-centered clinical method is finding common ground with patients about their health problems – achieving a consensus with patients on a plan for addressing their medical problems and health goals that reflects their needs, values, and preferences and is informed by evidence and guidelines. This goal is realized by first exploring the patient's experience of health and illness and, at the same time, the signs and symptoms implying disease. This evolving understanding is placed in the context of the patient's personhood, family, other significant relationships, and the environment in which they live. This complex process is accomplished through collaboration between clinician and patient based on trust, caring, and mutual respect.

Finding common ground is often mistakenly understood as the final step in the clinical method, only occurring after all the information about the patient's problems is obtained and sorted out by the clinician. However, we suggest that finding common ground must begin at the beginning. It is a process based on a relationship in which patients are treated as partners in exploring their health and health problems and deciding on treatment. As described by Tuckett et al.,[2] it is a meeting between experts – physicians are the expert in the biomedical aspects of the problems, and patients are the expert in their experience of health and illness and how illness is interfering with the achievement of their aspirations in life. While a skilled and often detailed collection of biomedical data is obviously essential for understanding the patient's medical problems, it is incomplete without an equally detailed understanding of the person who is suffering from the problems. A "checklist" approach emphasizing biomedical data or a perfunctory review of the patient's ideas or concerns will give a clear message that the doctor is preoccupied with the biomedical task of diagnosis. Trying to switch gears at the end of the interview, by

DOI: 10.1201/9781003394679-8

inviting the patient's perspective on a menu of treatment options offered by the physician, will be challenging. Having spent most of the interaction as a passive source of medical information, it is difficult for patients to engage in a conversation in which their ideas, values, and preferences occupy center stage.

In this chapter we will examine the third interactive component of the patient-centered method, finding common ground. This will include a brief review of the research demonstrating the importance of patients and clinicians finding common ground; a description of finding common ground; and strategies to assist the clinician in finding common ground, such as motivational interviewing and shared decision-making. Finding common ground is the process through which the patient and clinician reach a mutual understanding and mutual agreement in three key areas: (1) defining the problem, (2) establishing the goals and priorities of treatment, and (3) identifying the roles to be assumed by both the patient and the clinician. Achieving common ground often requires that two potentially divergent viewpoints be brought together in a reasonable plan. Once agreement is reached on the nature of the problems, the patient and clinician must determine the goals and priorities of treatment. What will be the patient's involvement in the treatment plan? How realistic is the plan in terms of the patient's perceptions of their health, disease, and illness experience? Does the plan address all the impediments to pursuing the life goals and purposes that really matter to the patient? What are the patient's wishes and their ability to cope? Finally, how do each of the parties – patients and clinicians – define their roles in this interaction?

THE IMPORTANCE OF FINDING COMMON GROUND

As noted in Chapter 1, a recent movement toward focusing care on patients' goals has gained momentum. It is called goal-oriented care, and it holds much similarity to finding common ground. It stresses the crucial importance of the process itself, i.e. the mutual discussion of patients and clinicians. "The process . . . when patient and clinician collaborate to clarify goals and priorities, develop and attempt to carry out agreed upon strategies, is of, by for, and with patients, an end in itself".[3]

In a paternalistic model, healthcare professionals are in charge – they make decisions on behalf of their patients that they believe are in the patient's best interests without involving them. Over the past 50 years paternalism has gradually lost ground as patients' rights have gained support.[4-6] Although there is general agreement in the literature that patients should be better informed regarding their medical condition, offered choices, and asked their opinions about all decisions concerning their health care,[7] clinicians still fall short of this ideal. "Not being properly informed about their condition and the options for treating is a very common source of patient dissatisfaction worldwide".[8] For over 50 years research has documented how doctors have failed to find common ground.[9-13] In a seminal study of primary care physicians and surgeons, Braddock et al.[14] reviewed audiotapes of informed decision-making and found that discussion of alternatives occurred in 5.5%–29.5% of interactions, discussion of pros and cons in 2.3%–26.3%, and discussion of uncertainties associated with the decision in 1.1%–16.6%. Physicians rarely explored whether patients understood the decision (0.9%–6.9%).

Almost 22 years later, building on Braddock and colleagues work, Long and her team[15] examined informed consent and informed decision-making in relation to high-risk surgery. Similar to Braddock's and colleagues' results, the surgeons rarely explored the patients' understanding of the decision during informed consent conversations; however when using an informed decision-making approach almost 60% assessed the patient's level of understanding.

Studies exploring physician prescribing behaviors and patients' use of medication also report a paucity of finding common ground.[16-19] For example, a qualitative study by Britten et al.[17] revealed that an essential precursor to finding common ground was an exploration of the patient's illness experience (described in Chapter 3). However, Dowell et al.[18] found that when a consultation process included an exploration of their illness experience and finding common ground, previously nonadherent patients were assisted in following their medication regimen.

Another study highlighting the centrality of finding common ground is Stewart et al.,[20] who found that the most important association with good outcomes was the patient's perception that the physician and patient had found common ground.

Healthcare providers in the community are recognized as reliable sources of information related to health promotion and disease prevention. At the level of the individual, it is first important to understand their *personal* meaning of health, which will vary from time to time and over the life course. In this sense, health promotion is the development of a person's general resistance resources.[21] Health is then seen as attainable "a healthy environment, balanced diet, and physical fitness, as well as the fostering of coping skills, self-confidence, and self-control".[22] The threshold between health and illness is often defined as whether a person can carry out those physical, social, and mental functions that are important to their self-identity. To the extent that these become impaired, a person begins to experience illness, an encroachment on their identity and aspirations in life. An important element in a person's approach to prevention is their health beliefs: perceived severity of the problem, susceptibility, efficacy of prevention, benefits of taking action, and perceived barriers.[23] However, when Street and Haidet[24] studied physicians' awareness of their patients' health beliefs they found that physicians had a relatively poor understanding, generally underestimating how much patients perceived value in natural remedies or preferred being a partner in their care. "Such understanding forms the foundation for formulating therapeutic plans that patients are more likely to follow, since such plans take into account the patient's perspective on how the illness works and what therapies are feasible, given their unique circumstances".[25]

In summary, research indicates how physicians still fail to find common ground with patients, but at the same time it also reveals how finding common ground is important for both patients and physicians – it is the lynchpin of the patient-centered clinical method.

DEFINING THE PROBLEM

Seeking an understanding or explanation of worrisome symptoms is a fundamental human response to illness. Most patients want a "name" or label for their disease to help them gain some sense of control over what is happening to them,[26–28] "adding meaning to the patient's experience".[29] When patients can assign a label to their problems it helps them understand the cause, what to expect in terms of the course or timeline of the problem, and what will be the outcome. It also assists them in regaining some degree of mastery over what may have been a frightening symptom. Some patients may develop quite magical notions of what is happening to them when they become ill. It may seem better to have an irrational explanation of the problem than no explanation at all. Other patients will blame themselves for the problem rather than see the disease as something beyond their control.

To have a diagnosis is to have a vision of what one is up against, no matter how terrible the possible future: "Better the devil you know than a devil you don't know". Enduring a long period when one's diagnosis is uncertain can be a painful and frustrating experience. Even when a doctor only "suspects" something, patients and families want to know what it is.[30]

Patients have usually formed some ideas about their problems before presenting to the doctor. They have commonly consulted family, friends, and the Internet to gain some understanding of what is happening to them. Failure to elicit the patient's perspective may jeopardize agreement on the nature of the problem(s). Without some agreement about what is wrong, it is difficult for a patient and a clinician to agree on a treatment protocol or plan of management that is acceptable to both. It is not essential that the practitioner fully agrees with the patient's formulation of the problem, but the practitioner's explanation and recommended treatment must at least be consistent with the patient's point of view and make sense in the patient's world.

Problems develop when patient and doctor have quite different ideas of the cause of the problems. For example

- The patient dismisses her back pain as aging and osteoarthritis, yet the doctor is concerned that it may represent metastases from her breast cancer.
- The practitioner has diagnosed hypertension, but the patient insists that his blood pressure is probably only elevated because he is working overtime on a big assignment at work and refuses to see his blood pressure as a problem.
- The parent of a 6-year-old child thinks there is something seriously wrong because the child has frequent colds: six a year. The clinician thinks this number is within normal limits, and that the parent is overly protective of the child.

In defining and describing the problem it is essential that practitioners give the information in language patients can understand; thus complex medical terms and clinical language should be avoided. If patients are intimidated by medical jargon, it may limit their ability to express their ideas and concerns or to even raise important questions. Failure to elicit these patients' expressions may result in a failure to find common ground. Gill and Maynard[31] suggest that the "canonical organization" of the medical interview powerfully structures the interaction, thus making it hard for patients to insert their ideas or for physicians to even hear them. Doctors are so busy collecting information to sort out the diagnosis that they resist being "sidetracked" by the patient's ideas.

Although in some cases doctors do evaluate patients' explanations immediately in information-gathering contexts, they typically stay on course when this option is provided and continue to collect data from patients without outwardly indicating that they heard patients insert their analyses into the conversation. Thus, as in previous research, we find that physicians may leave patients' explanations unassessed or even unacknowledged. However, this is at least partly due to both participants' orientation to the overall organization of the medical interview.[31]

To counter this unspoken rule about what and how information is to be collected in medical interviews, patients need to be encouraged to ask questions and not fear being ridiculed or embarrassed for not knowing or not understanding technical terms and procedures. Just as active listening is key to exploring patients' health and illness experiences, it is also central to finding common ground. Thus it is important to understand and acknowledge patients' perspectives on their problem. The format in which the patient's history of their illness is collected determines what information is gathered and also shapes the nature of the relationship between patient and physician and the role of the patient. If the history is simply the result of answers to a series of questions – an interrogation – the patient's role is to be a source of information in response to the physician's lead. However, if the history is acquired by listening intently to the patient's story of their illness, the information is rich with personal details and values, and the patient has a more important role in constructing their medical history. But it's not that simple. Patients are often uncertain about their story and sometimes fearful of what it might mean; they may need assistance in putting it into words. Howard Brody refers to the "joint construction of narrative" in which physicians assist in writing the story:

> The physician who takes stories seriously will . . . adopt as a working hypothesis that the patient is asking a question like the following: "Something is happening to me that seems abnormal, and either I cannot think of a story that will explain it, or the only story I can think of is very frightening. Can you help me to tell a better story, one that will cause me less distress, about this experience?" If this formulation seems overly wordy, a shorter form of the patient's possible plea to the physician might be, "My story is broken; can you help me fix it?"[32]

From this perspective, taking the patient's history is more like a conversation in which the history is co-created. The clinician's role is to be curious, asking questions for clarification, following the patient's lead, and sometimes suggesting another viewpoint.[33] Often the patient's story will reveal the diagnosis. Osler's oft-quoted aphorism reminds us: "Listen to the patient, he is telling you the diagnosis".[34] Also, a narrative approach usually provides insights into the patient's experience of their illness – how it is affecting the patient's life; how the patient has made sense of it; the patient's feelings, especially their fears about the illness; and the role the patient hopes the physician will play. However, sometimes physicians must ask questions to fill in gaps in the patient's story to explore cues to possible diagnoses and to clarify aspects of the patient's illness experience. It is also important to attend to the relational aspects of the interaction:

> Patients value positive relationships with health professionals not only (or not mainly) because of the benefits of task-related information exchange and choice but also because it matters to them that they feel cared for as individuals and respected as part of the care team.[35]

A special, but not uncommon, challenge in finding common ground occurs when, after examination and investigation, symptoms are not classifiable into a known diagnostic category. Patients with symptoms that lack a diagnosis (medically unexplained symptoms [MUS]; somatic symptom disorder) constitute up to one third of common symptoms in primary care and, of these, 20–25% become chronic or recurring.[36] They are one reason for excessive investigations. Approaches to patients with MUS that have been tried and failed include simple reassurance ("Nothing is wrong. Everything is normal") and attributing their symptoms to psychological origins (reattribution).[37, 38] These strategies lead to dissatisfaction, anger, and loss of trust on the part of patients and feelings of frustration and helplessness in clinicians.[39, 40] Approaches that result in more satisfied patients and less stressed physicians and greater trust in the relationship begin with first listening, carefully seeking to understand all aspects of the problem including context; recognizing the patient's own ideas, their fears, and how the symptoms affect their function; careful physical examination as indicated; and acknowledging and validating the person's suffering. Patient-centered clinicians engage their patients in co-creating an explanation for the symptoms even if that account is at variance with their own understanding.[38] The use of "explanatory fragments" drawing on the patient's particular circumstances and biomedical, psychological, and social frameworks can be used to achieve concordance between patient and physician while recognizing that this may be revised as new information becomes available.[41] This is followed by specific recommendations to alleviate symptoms, such as diet, exercise, and counseling.[42]

In the care of patients with chronic diseases, once the diagnosis has been established, follow-up visits concentrate on therapy. History taking will focus on how the treatment is changing the story – has the patient been able to follow through on the therapeutic plans, are the symptoms improving, are there any side effects of treatment, are there any new problems, and, most important, are the impediments to the achievement of important life goals and purposes addressed adequately? In addition, effective care of patients with chronic diseases is dependent on skilled self-management.[43-46] The following case example demonstrates the value of collaboration between patient and physician. By acknowledging and respecting the patient's perspective, the doctor encouraged the patient to contribute to a shared understanding of her problem and take an active role in developing a more effective approach to the treatment of her depression.

CASE EXAMPLE

Zoya struggled. Some days felt interminable, while others were barely within Zoya's meager control. Zoya struggled to mother her 7-year-old son, Arun, as a single parent; she struggled to keep a roof over their heads and food on the table; she struggled to maintain her quota as a sales representative for a local flower distributor – a loss of income would be catastrophic. However, Zoya's greatest struggle was her depression. Her depression was a demon Zoya could not conquer. It swept over her, delivering Zoya to a fearful and uncertain place she could not manage alone.

Dr Adria was more than familiar with his 28-year-old patient Zoya. He knew and empathized with her multiple struggles – how each day was a monumental effort to take a step forward – to merely survive. Yet there was some underlying frustration, given his many failed attempts to find common ground with Zoya. Various antidepressant medications had been prescribed, but each one had resulted in an undesired outcome – drowsiness, weight gain, agitation. From a pharmacological perspective Dr Adria was at a loss how best to treat Zoya. Nothing seemed to address her overwhelming depressive symptoms without some negative consequence or adverse reaction. Dr Adria was uncertain about how to proceed with Zoya's care. At the same time, he too struggled to address all the other complex dimensions of Zoya's life – often unspoken but evident in her haggard profile.

The chaotic presentation in the office with her son, Arun, was particularly worrisome. Did this little boy's "hyperactivity" warrant an official diagnosis and intervention or was it rather a reflection of his mother's chaos – both internal and external? These questions sat suspended before Dr Adria.

On a few rare occasions Zoya had shared her frustrations in caring for Arun – how when his behavior would escalate, so too would hers. The resulting yelling match left Zoya feeling depleted and guilty about her poor parenting skills. As a consequence she often avoided disciplining Arun for fear that such confrontations would lead to more angry outbursts from both of them. Zoya blamed her inability to parent on her persistent fatigue, indecision, and irritability – all part of her depression.

With some further probing, Dr Adria discovered that Zoya despised being on medication and the stigma associated with depression. Zoya believed she should be able to cope on her own, and her inability to do so led to further frustration and self-loathing. Zoya revealed how, on several occasions, she had decreased or increased her medication – in the absence of consultation with her doctor. This new information opened the door for Dr Adria to seek common ground with his patient.

Zoya's goals were to decrease her depressive symptoms and to gain an understanding of how to better approach parenting and discipline of her son. Dr Adria shared his patient's goals but realized simply telling her to be more "compliant" with the antidepressant medication had failed before and would fail again. He needed to engage Zoya in tackling the problem together. He suggested that they brainstorm possible approaches to her problems. Zoya realized that she had been fighting to avoid acknowledging her depression and that her "on-again, off-again" approach to the medication was not working. When she had maintained a regular dose, she had felt better, so it made sense to try this again and stick to it. Also, she had read about parenting self-help groups on the Internet and asked Dr Adria if there was a similar program that he would recommend in her community. Dr Adria supported Zoya's suggestion and provided a referral. Dr Adria also wondered aloud if Zoya was interested in resuming journaling, as in the past she had found this to be helpful in sorting out her many struggles; Zoya agreed that this would be a good idea. Zoya suggested that it might be helpful to maintain regularly scheduled visits with Dr Adria in order to monitor her progress with their agreed-upon plan. Zoya's struggles were not over yet – but they both felt more confident. They had reached common ground and together they could move forward.

Every contact between patients and clinicians is an opportunity to consider health promotion and prevention. In the four components of the patient-centered clinical method, the exploration of health-promoting values and beliefs is considered as part of Component 1, found in Chapter 3 of this book. Statistics from the United States[47] revealed that six risk factors each individually accounted for more than 5% of risk-attributable, disability adjusted life years (DALYs): tobacco use, high body mass index (BMI), poor diet, alcohol and drug use, high fasting glucose, and high blood pressure. All of these risk factors represent the potential for prevention and health promotion in the clinical setting. At first glance disease prevention wouldn't seem to be a source of problems. After all, wanting to avoid ill health is normally taken for granted. However, the behaviors and practices known to support good physical and mental health, such as healthy diet, exercise, meaningful work, and good relationships are sometimes difficult to attain and sustain. Moreover, some prevention procedures and practices may present ethical challenges.

Disease prevention strategies are generally divided into primary (risk avoidance), secondary (risk reduction), and tertiary (early identification and complication reduction). Primary prevention includes some primordial prevention (prevention of risk factors) and health promotion as well as specific interventions such as immunization. Quaternary prevention has been defined by the World Organization of Family Doctors (WONCA) as protecting people from overmedicalization.[48] Originally put forth to address over-investigation of those who are ill but have no disease (upper right of Figure 3.1)[49] it has been expanded to consider the potential harms of screening.

Screening procedures are applied to unselected populations seeking to identify those who unknowingly have a disease or are at increased risk of a disease. Case finding applies screening in the context of a patient–doctor relationship. The assumption behind both procedures is that diseases exist in a continuum with a pre-symptomatic period during which there exists an intervention which changes the course of the disease. Such tests should have acceptable sensitivity and specificity, be shown to have clear benefits in changing the outcome and be acceptable to the public. The evidence-informed information about screening tests is constantly changing and organizations such as the U.S. Preventive Services Task Force (USPSTF),[50] the Canadian Task Force on Preventive Health Care (CTFPHC),[51] and the National Health Service (NHS)[52] in the UK are tasked with maintaining databases to inform practitioners and the public.

Recommendations may also come from specialty groups. Because these various recommendations may differ or even conflict they can be a source of confusion and uncertainty for both patients and practitioners. Any benefits of screening depend upon follow up, diagnosis and institution of appropriate therapy. There are also harms that may arise from screening, including false positive results, incidental findings that lead to a cascade of investigations and being over-diagnosed all of which affect quality of life.[53-56] In a national survey of elderly people in the United States, there was very high enthusiasm and uptake of cancer screening tests, despite 38% reporting at least one false positive screening test. Among the public there exists unrealistic perceptions of the benefits of screening tests.[57] This creates the conditions for what is described as a basic conflict between evidenced-based medicine and patient-centered care; between patients who seek the reassurance perceived to come with tests and their physicians who are encouraged to try to reduce unnecessary and potentially harmful procedures and tests.[58] This may be worsened by clinicians' own misunderstanding of the benefits and harms of screening[59] and hampers their ability to communicate risks to patients.[60] Screening tests may move asymptomatic patients from the upper left of Figure 3.1 to the area overlapping with perceived poorer health by labeling them as having the potential for disease. Concern has been raised about the development[61] of "surveillance medicine".

> It was no longer necessary for individuals to feel ill and seek medical attention to become patients. They could be identified through testing to have risk factors and be deemed medically abnormal. The individual's subjective experience became unnecessary to making a diagnosis.[62]

The emergence of so-called "partial patients", those who felt well until placed in a risk category is a consequence of this emphasis on screening and has added greatly to the work of practitioners. Initiatives such as Choosing Wisely[63] are designed to provide evidence to both practitioners and the public on appropriate use of screening and diagnostic tests. Generally, clinicians demand stronger evidence of benefit and safety for preventive strategies than for treatment protocols for existing disease conditions. As a rule, patients are more willing to accept the risk of side effects of treatment for a condition that is causing symptoms than the risks of a procedure that might only prevent harm in the future.

A particular challenge is the discussion about when it is time to stop screening; when patients reach an age or health category in which the benefits of screening are outweighed by the negative effects.[64]

Approaching this topic is best carried out in the context of a relationship of trust, helping the patient review their personal health priorities and how these change over time.

Immunization is a powerful method of primary prevention of disease and illness and perhaps the premier example of a low cost, high value tool in health care. Nonetheless, while the benefits of mass vaccinations to population health are clear, at the individual level there are many individuals who are skeptical of the personal benefits compared to perceived risks. While it is important for clinicians to acknowledge the risks of adverse vaccine reactions, their rare occurrence needs to be placed against the greater risk of vaccine preventable diseases. Vaccine hesitancy may be best understood as the middle ground of attitudes and beliefs ranging from active advocates at one end to absolute refusers at the other end. The continuum in the middle ground includes those who accept recommended vaccinations but are skeptical, those who accept some but not all vaccines, and those who delay getting vaccinated. The roots of vaccine hesitancy are highly variable and include cultural, ethnic, and religious beliefs; past experience; and, increasingly, social media.[65] Understanding where on the continuum a vaccine hesitant patient lies – the fears and misunderstandings – is needed to begin a discussion seeking common ground.

Every contact can include education on the benefits of a healthy diet and exercise if only in the form of posters and handouts. It can also include screening for health risks such as hypertension or sedentary lifestyle and early detection of disease such as breast cancer or diabetes. In addition, it includes tertiary prevention to reduce the impact of disease on the patient's function, longevity, and quality of life.

DEFINING THE GOALS

Once the patient and clinician have reached a mutual understanding and agreement about the problems, the next step is to explore the goals and priorities for therapy; if these are divergent it may be a challenge to find common ground. For example

- The patient requests genetic testing to alleviate her fears of having breast cancer, while the doctor knows there are no present risk factors or family history to warrant such tests.
- A patient, suffering from unremitting back pain, demands an MRI; yet the doctor feels that this is likely mechanical back pain that will resolve spontaneously.
- The doctor advises the patient to take a number of medications following his myocardial infarction to prevent a recurrence, yet the patient declines, believing that diet and exercise will suffice.

If clinicians ignore their patient's expectations and ideas about treatment and/or management, they risk not understanding their patients, and the patients in turn will be angry or hurt by this perceived lack of interest or concern. Some patients will become more demanding in a desperate attempt to be heard; others will become withdrawn and will feel abandoned. Patients may be reluctant to listen to their clinicians' treatment recommendations unless they feel that their ideas and opinions have been heard and respected.

"A Caregiver's Voice" in Box 6.1 illustrates the importance of the exploration of the patient's perspectives of the treatment.

BOX 6.1: A Caregiver's Voice

Bridget L Ryan

OVERHEARD ON CARDIOLOGY

I am in my mother's room in the cardiology floor of our hospital where she is receiving care. I have been surprised at how often I hear conversations about patients taking place just outside Mom's door. I hear a young voice saying, "Mr Walters still won't take his Warfarin. I told him that you said he had to if he wants to get better". I hear another voice – maybe a bit older, "I've spoken to him and his wife about this repeatedly. Tell him I am not going to discharge him unless he starts taking his medication".

My heart aches for Mr Walters and his wife. I know how scary it is being here. I long to go out into the hall and say, "Have you asked Mr Walters why he does not want to take his medication?"

It is impossible for a clinician to find common ground with a patient if they have not explored the patient's perspectives on the suggested treatment.

Timing is important. If the physician inquires about the patient's perspectives too early in the interview, the patient may think that the doctor doesn't know what is going on and is avoiding their responsibility to make a diagnosis. On the other hand, if the practitioner waits until the end of the interview, time may be wasted on issues unimportant to the patient. The clinician may even make suggestions that will have to be retracted. Practitioners need to actively engage their patients and explicitly inquire about their expectations. For example, a clinician might say, "Can you help me to understand what we might do together to get your diabetes under control?" Often, it is helpful to pick up on patients' cues that hint at their feelings, ideas, or expectations. For example, "I have had this back pain for 3 weeks now and none of the pain medication you recommended has helped. I just can't bear the pain!" The clinician should avoid becoming defensive in trying to justify previous advice. Instead, it is more helpful to address the patient's frustration and the implied message that something must be done: "You sound fed up with the length of time this pain has dragged on. Are you wondering if it is something serious or if there might be a better treatment?"

Often patients find it awkward or difficult to provide suggestions about the treatment of their diseases. Some patients may feel that their opinion lacks validity and value, while others may defer to the authority of the "expert" clinician in the decision-making process, not wanting to offend. Physicians need to encourage patients' participation with statements such as "I'm really interested in your point of view, especially since you are the one who has to live with our decision about these treatments". It is important for doctors to clearly explain the treatment options and to engage patients in a conversation about the pros and cons of different approaches. It is also important to acknowledge and address the patient's questions and concerns so that they feel heard and understood. In exploring the patient's thoughts about a specific plan, questions such as the following can be very useful: "Can you think of any difficulties in following through on this?" "Is there anything we can do to make this treatment plan easier for you?" "Do you need more time to think this over?" "Is there anybody you would like to talk to about this treatment?" Unfortunately this phase of the consultation, essential for establishing common ground, is often done badly because not enough time is spent on it. Physicians routinely spend only 1 minute out of a 20-minute consultation discussing treatment and planning but overestimate the time they spend by a factor of nine.[66]

It is important to create a climate for discussion that makes it easier for patients to express their ideas and include their disagreements with the physician's recommendations. Patients need to feel that their opinions matter.[67] Ultimately, the patient is in control of whether or not they follow through with the plan, and the clinician may only discover their disagreement in the follow-up visit. It is far better to discuss differing opinions openly in the initial visit, explore the patient's reasons for their ideas, and together look for a plan that both can accept. Because plans generated by patients are much more likely to be adhered to,[68, 69] they are often preferable to plans developed solely by the physician, even if the physician's plans are based on guidelines. A plan rejected by the patient (even silently) is no plan at all. Patients may only hint at their disagreement, perhaps nonverbally, and clinicians need to be observant for any signs that the patient is not fully committed to the plan and should address the patient's concerns in an open and nonjudgmental manner.

Ford et al. note that although most patients want to be well informed about their medical condition, not all patients wish to take an active role in treatment planning. However, once they are better informed about the treatment options and their consequences, they are more inclined to be involved in decisions about management. "Over half of patients who wanted to make or share decisions felt they had not been involved".[70] McKinstry[71] conducted a study of patients' preferences for a directed or shared style of consultation using pairs of video vignettes of five common scenarios. Preferences varied by age, socioeconomic status, and medical condition. Patients with an injured leg preferred a directed approach, and those with depression preferred a shared approach.

'A Patient's Voice' in Box 6.2 illustrates how crucial the patient's priorities are in the situation of a long-standing chronic condition.

According to a Cochrane review of decision aids,[72] they can be used by patients to improve their understanding of their options, the benefits and harms of each, and the values they place on benefits, harms, and medical uncertainties. This helps to prepare patients to participate more actively in discussions with health care providers. However, Nelson et al. urge caution in using decision aids:

> They may interfere with a patient's implicit decision-making strategies, send the wrong message to patients about the goals of decision making, or lead patients to believe that they can reduce or eliminate uncertainty when confronting decisions that are by their very nature uncertain.[73]

They suggest it might be preferable to teach people early in life how to tolerate uncertainty and ambiguity. Over the past 30 years, health coaching programs have developed in North America, Europe, and Australia.[74] Similar to decision aids, the health coach prepares patients before their visit to a physician by helping to clarify their priorities, developing their skills in raising questions and concerns, and developing their skills in presenting their opinions about investigation and management to their physician. Following the consultation with the physician, the health coach assists the patient to implement their management plans and to strengthen their self-confidence, often using motivational interviewing techniques. A number of reviews of the effectiveness of coaching showed positive effects on patients' knowledge, information recall and participation in decision-making.[75]

Establishing the goals of treatment must also take into account the expectations and feelings of clinicians. Sometimes clinicians are concerned that patients may ask for something they disagree with because they are not comfortable with confrontation or saying no. As a result, they may prefer to avoid the issue, but then finding common ground will not be achieved. Clinicians

---

BOX 6.2: A Patient's Voice

Lorraine Bayliss

I have lived with the worst of the chronic health conditions that are 24 hours a day, 7 days a week for the last 51 years (type 1 insulin-dependent diabetes). I will never forget meeting with other people living with diabetes in a group who were under 30 years old. I had never met the others, but the doctor gave us a spot to come together once a month. We were with others who walked in our shoes. This support was critical.

Over the years, the endocrinologist always started the visit saying: "What are the greatest challenges you are currently facing and how can I best help you?" Although lab results were relevant, my identified priorities were listened to and addressed.

My point is that lab results give data but also giving patients the tools for better self-management through listening to their articulated challenges and providing appropriate support is so critical.

can become frustrated and disheartened when patients do not adhere to treatment protocols and management plans. But what physicians call "noncompliance" may be patients' expressions of disagreement about treatment goals – it may be patients' only option if they feel unable to discuss their disagreement. As Quill and Brody observe: "Final choices belong to patients, but these choices gain meaning, richness, and accuracy if they are the result of a process of mutual influence and understanding between physician and patient".[76] The following two case examples illustrate some challenges in defining the goals for treatment and/or management.

CASE EXAMPLE

As a 32-year-old single mother, Tabitha led an active and busy life caring for her three children, aged 7, 9, and 13, as well as working part-time as a teacher's assistant. A simple slip on a small patch of ice resulted in a broken wrist requiring extensive surgery. Her entire right arm was immobilized in a cast with "Frankenstein like" pins protruding from her arm. Her life was turned upside down; unable to perform routine tasks, she could not care for her children or work. The healing process was slow and painful. Her confidence and hope that she would recover was becoming severely tested. Tabitha felt that she had been reduced to a disease, stating: "I felt I was given no part in my care except to bring my arm in for appointments". She felt diminished and excluded in decisions about her treatment and rehabilitation. Her ability to voice her concerns and expectations became weaker, in striking parallel with her damaged limb: "I could not express how motivated I was to be included as someone who could influence my own health and healing. Also, in my view the doctor did not seem to appreciate or understand my feelings".

The serious misunderstandings between Tabitha and her surgeon arose because there was a failure to find common ground. As Tabitha later reflected: "I needed the physician to have a greater understanding of what I was concerned about and the relevance of my questions . . . No one asked me anything about what I needed".

CASE EXAMPLE

Anjali, aged 64, smiled pleasantly as the doctor outlined the various options for dealing with her kidney failure. However, she had no intention of ever going on dialysis. The very thought of being hooked up to some machine three times a week was unbearable for Anjali. Just let me die peacefully and with dignity, Anjali thought.

Anjali was defending herself from the terror she experienced when realizing how serious her illness was – talking about dialysis was too frightening! Until the physician could connect with some of her mixed feelings, she would not be willing to discuss the management of her renal failure.

Realizing that Anjali seemed distracted, Dr O'Brien, her nephrologist, commented: "You seem to have other things on your mind. Can you tell me how you are reacting to this kidney trouble?" Anjali, caught off guard by Dr O'Brien's change in direction, paused a few moments, and replied, "Well, I don't like it one bit! But I've had a good life, and I will muddle through as best I can. I'm not ready to end my days attached to some infernal machine". Dr O'Brien responded, "So your independence is very important to you and whatever treatment I recommend must take that into account?" Anjali nodded affirmatively, "That's for sure, Dr O'Brien".

   Agreeing on those overall goals of management was the first step in treatment planning. Anjali may or may not accept dialysis, but it would need to be on her terms. If she sees it as a way to provide some increased quality of life, she will accept the inconvenience and distress of long-term dialysis. In the future, when dialysis becomes necessary, the doctor and Anjali will need to explore the pros and cons of independence, quality of life, and length of life.

Flach et al.,[77] in a study comparing provision of preventive services at Veteran's Administration ambulatory facilities, found that more preventive services were provided in facilities where patients had a better opportunity to discuss issues of importance to them and where there was greater continuity of care. It may take several contacts between patient and clinician to understand what really matters to the patient and their wishes for health promotion or preventive procedures. Just as in the learner-centered approach to medical education (see Chapter 11 in this book), the first step is a needs assessment. This will be based partly on the patient's medical conditions, health behaviors, and health risks based on age and sex. The following three questions are helpful in gleaning the patient's perspective of health behaviors:

1. All of us at one time or another do things that aren't good for us. It might be something like not wearing a seat belt or perhaps drinking more than we think we should. What behaviors are you doing that might put you at risk?
2. Most of us forget to take our medication or follow through with diet or exercise at some point or another. What difficulties have you had with managing or treating your _____?
3. What are you doing these days that you believe is contributing to your health?[78]

The answers to these questions provide clinicians with an understanding of patients' awareness of behaviors that might influence their health. However, awareness is not enough. In order to change behavior, patients must want to change, know how to change, and have the necessary environmental resources and social supports to change. Typically, people go through a number of stages in making a change – precontemplation (they are not even thinking about change or have decided not to change), contemplation (thinking about it but not changing because of strong ambivalence), preparation (having decided to change and getting ready), action (in the early phase of behaving in the new way but vulnerable to relapse), maintenance (becoming more comfortable with the change but still needing to work on it), and identification (seeing oneself as changed).[79, 80] Identifying the patient's stage of change is a helpful step in finding common ground. People think about and experience change differently in each stage and need different help from their healthcare practitioners. For example, in the precontemplative stage, the clinician should ask the patient if it is all right to mention some of the reasons for concern about their behavior in order to advise the patient about their risks. In the contemplative stage the clinician assists the patient to consider the advantages and disadvantages of changing their behavior. Only when the patient reaches the preparation stage, or beyond, is it worthwhile to spend time discussing strategies that might make it easier to change. Providing detailed instructions on a healthy diet to a patient in precontemplation would be a waste of time for everyone.

CASE EXAMPLE

The scene in the mass vaccination center was one of carefully controlled chaos with anxiety hanging like a mist. In a building the size of an airport hangar were 48 stations, each separated by a carefully measured six meters. At each station sat a vaccinator with a basket of syringes already loaded with vaccine, while a line of people stretched to the entrance of the building.

"I'm not sure I want to have this vaccine".

Dr Carel looked up from the tablet he was holding to see a dark haired, tired, middle-aged woman wearing a black parka, standing with her arms firmly crossed across her chest and appearing to be near tears. He carefully placed the syringe he was holding back in the basket and turned to face the woman.

"Tell me about your concerns", he said, gesturing to the empty chair she was standing next to: "We're not doing anything unless you're comfortable".

Vaccination fears have a history stretching back to the time they were first introduced in the 18th century, but the introduction of new mRNA vaccines for SARS-CoV-2, along with a host of misinformation spread on the Internet, had added a new layer of anxiety. With daily coverage of the rising number of hospitalized patients and deaths, people in quarantine and closure of schools and businesses, there was wide appreciation of the threat of the pandemic, but in some people's minds, doubts about the safety of the vaccines loomed. In addition, the more that distant health authorities recommended vaccine or required proof of vaccination, the more individual autonomy was challenged, reminding all that though we are individuals, we are also part of a collective, a community—the body politic. "The natural body meets the body politic in the act of vaccination, where a single needle penetrates both".[81]

Dr Carel was knowledgeable about how vaccines work, the outcomes of the clinical trials, and reported side effects. He was also aware that quality control measures are stringent in vaccine manufacture. He was confident that they were a necessary part of responding to the pandemic. Nevertheless, he was also aware that even some healthcare workers were against vaccination and that this added to the confusion of the public.[82]

Vaccine hesitancy is a complex phenomenon that is context specific and varies with time, place, and even different vaccines.[83] Key reasons for hesitancy are complacency, inconvenience in accessing vaccination, and lack of confidence in them.[84] In the midst of a worldwide pandemic and rising cases, complacency was not a problem, and while it wasn't convenient to line up at a mass vaccination clinic, great efforts were made to ensure that the process ran smoothly. The hesitancy orbited around the uncertainty of a new vaccine technology, one that had delivered effective vaccines in record time but left lingering unanswered questions about length of protection and side effects.

Dr Carel listened as Eunice expressed her fears of the vaccine, about which she only knew what she had seen on the news and on her social media. Her vaccine fear was almost as great as her fear of becoming infected with the SARS-CoV-2 virus. He inquired about her general state of health, including any contraindications to the vaccine. As she became more relaxed, she related that she was most afraid of severe side effects. After a short pause, Dr Carel told Eunice that he had received the vaccine 2 weeks ago, and while he did have a sore arm and mild headache, both side effects resolved quickly. She nodded and quickly added that she had responsibilities and couldn't afford to be sick. Picking up on the cue he asked:

> "Do you have family at home? Someone you care for?"
>
> "Yes, my elderly mother. I have to stay healthy for her".
>
> Eunice stared briefly at the floor, then her gaze lingered on the line of people waiting for their shot. She removed her parka and rolled up her sleeve.
>
> "OK. Let's do it".
>
> In this case, the clinician recognized that Eunice was not a vaccine refuser. She needed to place her fear of vaccine side effects against her need to stay healthy. For her, at this time, health meant being able to attend to the needs of her mother. By taking time to listen and reassure her, he helped her confirm a decision toward which she was already leaning.

Although, in typical medical consultations, time is short and serious medical conditions take priority, it is important to consider how to reduce the risk of new problems and to prevent patients' conditions from getting worse. Simple interventions, like making sure the patient's immunization is up-to-date, take little time. Assuring that the patient's nutritional needs are addressed before surgery can improve wound healing and recovery. Because many patients have medical conditions that cannot be cured, the primary goal of treatment is to minimize the impact of the disease on the patient's life. In particular, the goal is to reduce the symptoms and functional deficits that are interfering with the patient's ability to pursue their aspirations, goals, and purposes.

Disease symptoms or unhealthy behavior blocking the achievement of important life goals are an obvious target for health promotion and prevention.

The case example of Rex was presented in Chapter 3. He had coronary artery disease, a recent myocardial infarction, and a bypass surgery. Dr Wason identified symptoms of depression, which he clarified by exploring Rex's sadness about his losses and limitations and his fears about another myocardial infarction. Together they agreed it would be helpful to include Rex's wife in further discussion. In addition, Dr Wason had identified obesity and an elevated cholesterol. The doctor also gently explored Rex's health perceptions as basic groundwork for his health promotion and disease prevention plan. Dr Wason had explored Rex's sense that he was "no longer a healthy man," that family winter activities were very important to him, and that he was looking for guidance and reassurance about resuming lovemaking.

After the exploration of Rex's perceptions and risk factors, the work of finding common ground could continue. The doctor created a complete health promotion and disease prevention plan, which he will present to Rex in bite-sized portions over their future monthly visits. The plan includes the following points:

- *Lifestyle modification:* Dr Wason will continue to monitor and discuss with Rex his diet and exercise programs.
- *Secondary prevention:* Dr Wason will continue, and monitor as relevant, such medications as acetylsalicylic acid, statins, angiotensin-converting enzyme inhibitors, and beta-blockers.
- *Primary prevention:* Dr Wason will present and discuss four immunizations (annual flu shots, pneumonia vaccine, herpes zoster vaccine, COVID-19 vaccine), as well, he will recommend colon cancer screening.

Dr Wason fully recognizes the complexities of including health prevention in the ongoing contacts with Rex as he recovers from his bypass surgery.

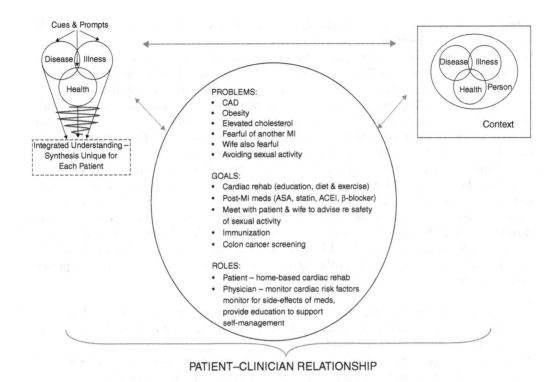

Figure 6.1 Finding Common Ground, Including Prevention and Health Promotion Activities

Figure 6.1 organizes the health promotion and disease prevention plan described in the previous paragraph into the conceptual framework of finding common ground, using Rex as the example. The figure demonstrates how prevention can be seamlessly incorporated into the care of patients with chronic conditions.

Although Dr Wason's plan was based on current guidelines, it remains tentative until discussed and confirmed with Rex and should also include consideration of alternative or additional interventions suggested by Rex. Applying the patient-centered approach allows practitioners like Dr Wason to find the methods of health promotion and preventive care that most appropriately match the patient's world – their health beliefs, values, preferences, priorities, aspirations, and resources. The practitioner's knowledge of this world helps in making a judgment about which health promotion or disease prevention strategy provides the most appropriate fit.

DEFINING THE ROLES OF PATIENT AND CLINICIAN

Inherent in articulating the roles to be assumed by the patient and clinician is a definition of mutual responsibility for the actions that will follow. These may be quite simple, such as "I want to see you again in one month to check that this new medication is lowering your blood pressure". Implicit in this statement is the patient's use of the medication as prescribed and the doctor's desire for future follow up. Certain situations, however, may be more complex and therefore require an explicit statement of the roles to be assumed by the patient and the doctor.

Sometimes there is profound disagreement about the nature of the problem or the goals and priorities for treatment. When such an impasse occurs, it is important to look at the relationship between the patient and the clinician and at their perception of each other's roles. (The nature and characteristics of the relationship will be dealt with in-depth in Chapter 7, while here we focus on problems in role definition.) Doctors, perhaps with a cancer patient, may see themselves wanting to bring about remission and may expect the patient to assume the role of a passive recipient of treatment. Patients, however, may be seeking a physician who expresses concern and interest in their values and preferences and who is prepared to treat them in the least invasive manner, viewing them as autonomous individuals with a right to have a voice in deciding among various forms of treatment. This is not such a dilemma for doctors when the various forms of treatment are equally effective, but physicians are understandably concerned when the patient chooses a treatment that the physician considers either less efficacious or even harmful.

Evolution of the patient–clinician relationship over time, as described in Chapters 4 and 7, allows the doctor to see the same patient with different problems in different settings over a number of years and also to see the patient through the eyes of other family members. The physician's commitment is to "be present" with the patient throughout their illness. Patients need to know that they can count on their doctors to be there when they need them. This ongoing relationship colors everything that happens between them. If there are difficulties in their relationship or differing expectations of their roles, they will have problems in working together effectively. The following points are examples of this:

- The patient is looking for an authority who will tell them what is wrong and what they should do; the physician, on the other hand, wants a more egalitarian relationship in which clinician and patient share decision-making.
- The patient longs for a deep and meaningful relationship with a parental figure who will make up for everything the patient's own parent never gave; the doctor wants to be a biomedical scientist who can apply the discoveries of modern medicine to patients' problems.
- The physician enjoys a holistic approach to medicine and wants to get to know patients as people; the patient seeks only technical assistance from the doctor.

Finding common ground about a patient's role in the decision-making process does not necessarily imply that the patient will assume an active role. Patients' levels of participation in decision-making may fluctuate depending on their emotional and physical capabilities. Thus, clinicians need to be flexible and responsive to potential changes in their patient's involvement. Some patients may be too sick or too overwhelmed by the burden of their illness to actively participate in their care. Others may find decisions about treatment options too complex and confusing, hence abdicating the decision-making to the clinician. When patients are receiving care from multiple healthcare professionals, they assume different roles and relationships with each. Roles within and across the healthcare team may also influence the patient's care, as we discuss in detail in Chapter 8.

THE PROCESS OF FINDING COMMON GROUND

In the process of finding common ground it is the clinician's responsibility to provide their medical expertise in defining the diagnosis. This may be as clear-cut as "You have a strep throat" or ultimately more complex and uncertain such as "There are several possibilities for what your symptoms suggest and a number of options for the next steps including more testing or waiting to see how your condition unfolds. Do you have a preference?" Sometimes the patient's story starts out simply and evolves into something unexpected. For example, consider a healthy-looking 35-year-old man presenting with a recent history of a single episode of palpitations lasting 15 minutes and associated with a feeling of anxiety. The history and physical examination revealed no abnormalities, but the patient was very worried and had discontinued his daily exercise program for fear it might damage his heart. He had surfed the Internet and decided he needed an electrocardiogram, stress test, Holter monitoring, and numerous blood tests. Because the tachycardia occurred right after receiving "bad news", the physician decided that the single episode of tachycardia was unlikely serious and, if the electrocardiogram was normal, nothing further was needed. After the physician explained his conclusions, the patient was somewhat relieved, but he still requested additional investigation. Recognizing that the patient needed additional reassurance, the physician agreed to order a stress test, but he explained the risk of a false positive result. He was reluctant to order more tests that he considered unnecessary, but he agreed to discuss this again after the stress test. The doctor explored further the story of the "bad news" and learned that the patient's best friend had recently died in a motor vehicle accident. They had often worked out together and had even run a marathon together a few months previously. Now it made sense why the patient needed all the additional investigation. Until he was convinced that his heart was okay he would live in fear that, like his friend, he was vulnerable. Although the additional testing may not be necessary from a strictly biomedical perspective, it was needed to assist the patient to get on with his life. In follow-up visits, the physician will invite the patient to talk more about his friend and his reaction to his loss. What started out as benign palpitations potentially needing only reassurance revealed a life-altering experience requiring that the physician support the patient to come to terms with a major loss.

In exploring patients' stories (the meaning of health to them; their life aspirations; their symptoms, feelings, and ideas; how illness interferes with their activities; and their hopes for treatment) physicians are able to discern a probable diagnosis and the impact of the illness experience. The therapeutic plan must address the whole story, not just the disease, and illness must be consistent with the patient's beliefs and aspirations. While explaining their understanding of the patient's predicament, it is important that physicians are open to patients' questions and alert to verbal and non-verbal cues that they are confused, upset, or anxious about what they are hearing. It is important to provide the patient with an opportunity to ask questions and offer suggestions. This must be more than simply clarifying the physician's plans but a genuine offer to reconsider and revise the approach to treatment if it is not congruent with the patient's values and preferences. Sometimes when the physician asks, "What do you think?" some patients may respond with "I don't know – you're the doctor!" Doctors need to answer with a comment such as "Yes and I will provide you with information and my opinion, but your ideas and wishes are important in making our plan together". This is the basis of a true sharing of ideas.

The patient and clinician can then participate in a mutual discussion of their shared understanding of the problem and how it can best be addressed. At the conclusion of their discussion of treatment options and goals, it is the clinician's responsibility to clarify explicitly the patient's understanding and agreement. It is during this summation that the practitioner and patient can make specific their respective roles in achieving the mutually agreed upon treatment goals. This may be as simple as agreeing on how follow-up plans will be arranged or as complex as a discussion of how a patient with cancer in the palliative phase needs the doctor to assume a caring role rather than a curative stance.

If disagreements arise, clinicians must avoid getting into power struggles. Instead, they must listen to the patient's concerns or opinions, as opposed to dismissing the patient as obstinate or difficult. When conflicts do arise, the grid shown in Box 6.3 may be a useful tool. How do both the patient and the clinician view the problem(s), the goals of treatment, and their respective roles? Why are these divergent and can their differences be resolved? This grid also helps the clinician to check if important information is missing, such as the patient's experience of illness or specific issues relevant to the patient's unique context.

BOX 6.3: Finding Common Ground

Issue	Patient	Doctor
Problems		
Goals		
Roles		

The next case example illustrates the key concepts of finding common ground: defining the problems, the goals, and the roles of the patient and doctor. It also emphasizes the fundamental importance of a trusting relationship between patient and clinician.

CASE EXAMPLE

When Dr Matise first met 28-year-old Lyle, the smell of alcohol and cigarettes permeated the examination room. Standing at just over 6 feet and weighing approximately 300 pounds, Lyle was an imposing presence. He was unshaven and dressed in a T-shirt and torn jeans. His language was peppered with expletives. Lyle's stated reason for the visit was to have his cholesterol checked.

Lyle revealed how he was unhappy with his weight and was beginning to worry about his health. Lyle stated, "I asked my last doctor why the hell do I sweat so much, and the doc said to me, 'Lyle, look at it like this, imagine a 150-pound man carrying another 150-pound man everywhere he goes . . . that's why you sweat so much'". Lyle snorted, "Shit, what kind of an answer is that!"

His obesity had worsened over the last year after Lyle had been laid off work. He had completed ninth grade and maintained that "education isn't worth a damn unless you end up with a job that pays good money!" Indeed, Lyle had made good money; he had worked his way up from manual laborer to foreman at the steel plant. That was until the plant closed down. "Hell, I'd worked at the plant since I was 16", lamented Lyle, "those guys were like family to me". Unable to manage his mortgage payments after being laid off, Lyle had moved into a rundown trailer owned by his mother. He was now spending most of his days smoking and drinking with "good buddies" who shared a similar life perspective.

Lyle's cholesterol had never been previously investigated, but he had heard "talk of cholesterol" on television. Now with his purported concerns about his own health, Lyle was curious about his own cholesterol. Lifestyle questions revealed the following. "I'm a meat-and-potatoes guy, doc!" explained Lyle. He also reported being a pack-a-day smoker since his teens, and he drank a "case of 24" a week. While alcohol abuse was a consistent pattern for his father and his two brothers, Lyle did not view his own alcohol consumption as a problem.

It was readily apparent to Dr Matise that Lyle was facing many serious issues. The plant closing had resulted in his feeling bitter and angry, although Lyle denied these emotions. However, from Dr Matise's perspective, Lyle's loss of work and his home were seemingly related to an increase in his eating, smoking, and drinking. Despite his gruff exterior, Lyle seemed scared. When Dr Matise asked Lyle directly how he wanted to proceed in addressing his concerns about his weight and cholesterol, Lyle appeared reluctant to make any alterations to his current lifestyle.

From Lyle's story, Dr Matise had gleaned how his patient's past interactions with other healthcare professionals had been tenuous. While there were multiple health issues requiring attention, these would only be tackled when Lyle was ready and once a more firm and trusting relationship was established. For now, finding common ground would consist of focusing directly on Lyle's cholesterol, including learning what he knew about cholesterol and what steps Lyle was prepared to take in addressing this issue.

Dr Matise hoped that during future rechecks of Lyle's cholesterol he could further develop the relationship with his patient. Formation of a strong patient–doctor relationship would increase the likelihood of finding common ground regarding the many issues still confronting Lyle.

STRATEGIES TO ASSIST FINDING COMMON GROUND

The development of specific interviewing approaches such as motivational interviewing and informed decision-making provide useful strategies to assist patients and clinicians in the process of finding common ground. Motivational interviewing reflects the same spirit of collaboration we encourage with an emphasis on acceptance, compassion, and building a partnership.

It is not something done by an expert to a passive recipient, a teacher to a pupil, a master to a disciple. In fact, it is not done "to" or "on" someone at all. Motivational interviewing (MI) is done "for" and "with" a person. It is an active collaboration between experts. People are the undisputed experts on themselves. No one has been with them longer or knows them better than they do themselves. In MI, the helper is a companion who typically does less than half of the talking. The method of MI involves exploration more than exhortation, interest and support rather than persuasion or argument. The interviewer seeks to create a positive interpersonal atmosphere that is conducive to change but not coercive.[85]

Motivational interviewing began in the 1980s with a focus on addictive behaviors such as alcoholism and smoking, and it is now widely used in many settings to assist people wanting to make many types of behavioral change.[86-88] For example, a person may desire to be a non-smoker but be unwilling or unable to tolerate the struggle to quit. They are often paralyzed by their ambivalence about quitting – on the one hand they recognize the benefits of quitting but on the other hand they enjoy smoking and find the withdrawal symptoms intolerable. Motivational interviewing challenges the "righting reflex", a clinician's almost automatic attempt to help people fix what's wrong by telling them what to do. Some clinicians will endeavor to frighten patients into changing by quoting fearful statistics about the harmful effects of smoking; others may try to make them feel guilty for not quitting. Although well intentioned, these approaches usually fail. "MI is about arranging conversations so that people talk themselves into change, based on their own values and interests".[89]

Practitioners commonly intervene by providing information about smoking, tips on how to quit, and pharmacological aids such as nicotine patches, sticks, or bupropion. This is often helpful if it matches the patient's ideas about quitting, but the patient might have other ideas about what might work better. Effective clinicians begin by establishing rapport using interviewing methods such as open-ended inquiry, reflective listening, and empathy. They develop an alliance with patients that is collaborative and relational.[90] Next, they encourage the patient to discuss the behavior they wish to change, what they have already tried, and what they might have successfully used for other behaviors in the past. They will pick up on any change talk (tentative thoughts about the need or desire to change, reasons to change, or how they might change) and help patients explore and flesh out their ideas, identifying how they might tackle any barriers and how they might incorporate any helpful resources in their setting. The key to success is for the ideas to come from the patient, not the clinician.

Another helpful interviewing technique is to ask about the patient's confidence and degree of importance in making change.[88] For example, if a patient expresses a desire to get into better shape, ask about their conviction: "How important is it for you to get into better shape?" Scaling can be incorporated by asking: "On a scale from zero to ten, how would you rate its importance to you?" If the patient rates it five, the clinician could follow with: "What would it take for you to say seven or eight?" This helps to clarify the patient's values and motivation and may even generate change talk. Similarly, the clinician can ask about the patient's confidence in making the desired changes. This technique also helps clinicians decide where to concentrate their efforts. If the patient is strongly motivated but lacking in confidence, then the interview should concentrate on finding effective strategies for change; on the other hand, if the patient is confident they could change if they wanted to but feels ambivalent, then the focus should be on exploring what would enhance the patient's motivation.

Several authors advocate the use of shared decision-making techniques in patient care.[91-97] Elwyn and colleagues[91] propose a three-step approach to shared decision-making consisting of "team talk", "option talk", and "decision talk". In step one, "team talk", the clinician invites the patient to work together and supports them as the patient becomes aware of the choices. Essential to this step is eliciting the patient's goals in order to guide the decision-making process. "Option talk" is step two, and here the clinician and patient discuss various alternatives, through the use of risk communication principles. The third step is "decision talk" where the clinician uses their experience and expertise to guide the patient in making a decision(s) which mirrors their informed preferences. Throughout the decision-making process the clinician uses active listening and encourages collaboration.[91] Légaré and her research team have been leaders in the development of patient decision aids such as curated Internet sites, pamphlets, videotapes, working with a health coach,[98] and, most recently, the role of artificial intelligence.[99] These patient decision aids are not meant to serve as a substitute for the interaction between the patient and clinician in the shared decision-making process but rather to improve patient knowledge and risk perception resulting in improved patient decision-making.[100] Discussing how patients prefer to handle decisional conflict (what they do when they are confronted with opposing ideas and uncertainty) may help them to resolve such dilemmas. Légaré et al.[98] highlight how COVID-19 testing raised profound decisional conflict in the wake of unprecedented decisions about "vaccination, COVID-19 testing, social isolation and moving family members to or from residential care".[98] Misinformation on these issues and others related to the pandemic were perpetuated in the media. Furthermore public health mandates often trumped individual decisions and preferences.[101-103]

Recent research examining the process of shared decision-making with patients who are potentially vulnerable (e.g. patients with polypharmacy,[104] black patients receiving type 2 diabetes care,[105] patients undergoing lung cancer screening,[106] patients with complex care needs,[107] and patients with breast cancer[108]) suggests that clinicians are failing to fully elicit patients' preferences and priorities.

It is important to understand that, in this approach, the clinician is not simply a servant doing whatever the patient requests but, rather, a partner who brings medical expertise and evidence to the discussion about treatment. Being explicit about these issues enhances patients' opportunities for an effective partnership with clinicians, as they explore choices together and come to a mutual decision that best matches the patients' preferences and is congruent with the best available evidence and clinical wisdom.[91]

> In a truly shared decision, physicians and patients mutually influence each other, each potentially ending up in a place different from where they began, with different understandings than either would have reached alone. It is not a matter of who has power and who does not. It is a matter of mutual influence.[109]

The strategies described here can be very useful in finding common ground, but they must always be applied in the context of patient-centered practice. As stated previously, patients may not feel well enough or confident enough to be active participants in decisions about their care. They may choose to abdicate their responsibilities and hand them over to the clinician. This is patient-centered care, as it respects the needs and preferences of the patient in that specific circumstance. However, the situation may change and would necessitate that clinicians be responsive and flexible to an alteration in the patients' degree of involvement in the process of finding common ground.

CONCLUSION

Finding common ground requires that patients and physicians reach a mutual understanding and mutual agreement on the nature of the problems, the goals and priorities of treatment, and their respective roles. Sometimes patients and clinicians have divergent views in each of these areas. The process of finding a satisfactory resolution is not one of bargaining or negotiating but, rather, of moving toward a meeting of minds or finding common ground. Sometimes it means agreeing to differ, but always it means respecting one another.

As Boudreau et al. suggest, the single overarching goal of care is "the wellbeing of the patient and, more specifically, improvement in the patient's functions to allow the patient to pursue his purposes".[110] As such, it is essential to involve patients in planning their treatment and determining priorities for care, since only the patient is aware of how their diseases are blocking the achievement of what matters most to them. Placing these considerations in the center of patient care transforms the clinical method by urging physicians to recognize that they are called on to do more than stamp out and prevent disease; they are called on to join with patients in addressing the full impact of disease and its prevention in patients' lives.

Thus, the process of finding common ground between the patient and the clinician is an integral and interactive component of the patient-centered clinical method. Finding common ground is the lynchpin or place of convergence, where all of the components of the patient-centered clinical method come together. To find common ground, the clinician must take into consideration all aspects of the patient-centered clinical method: knowing the patient's health, disease, and illness experience; appreciating the person and their life context; and constantly building on the patient–clinician relationship. As McLeod cogently notes:

> When we listen to, accept, and validate the illness story, when we interpret the illness in terms of its symptomatic pathophysiology, when we explain treatment plans and prognosis, and, most importantly, when we define the patient's own role in the healing process, then trust, compassion, and a human connection between the patient and doctor becomes possible.[111]

AGREEING TO DISAGREE

Eng Sing Lee

First Impression and Subsequent Encounters

It was the height of the H5N1 epidemic in 2009; I was on duty in the acute cluster seeing only patients complaining of upper respiratory tract infection with or without fever. The physical separation of the clinic into a different area of practice was to ensure that other patients who came to the clinic were not infected with the H5N1 virus. Recollections of SARS (severe acute respiratory syndrome) still sent chills down my spine.

I came to know Mr Lam when he visited the clinic insisting to see his doctor who was off duty on that day. I was covering for his regular doctor and unfortunately, I was working in the acute cluster. I was gowned up in full personal protection equipment – goggles, full gown, gloves, N95 mask, surgical cap, and shoe overlay.

Mr Lam spoke to me on the phone but indicated he was actually outside the clinic. He said that it was a trivial matter. All he had wanted was a letter for his employer explaining that he had sprained his ankle and would not be able to walk in the examination hall but could still invigilate. He did not want to jeopardize his health by seeing me in the H5N1 cluster, which I concurred. I agreed to have a quick look at his ankle just outside the clinic.

I de-gowned, threw away all the contaminated attire into a special bin, did the necessary hand-rub, and met him outside the clinic. Mr Lam was a slightly overweight gentleman and looked more like a businessman than an educator. It was a mild sprain on his right ankle, and I agreed that resting and elevation of the affected limb was the best course of action.

I did my hand-rub and re-gowned with a new set of attire before going back to the long queue of patients suspected to have the H5N1 virus. Shortly thereafter, the telephone rang and Mr Lam said that he wanted some words changed in the letter stating that the way I written the letter had put him in a bad light. This happened twice before he was satisfied with the letter, with me de-gowning and re-gowning each time!

I was surprised to see Mr Lam on my patient list a month later. He had decided to change his chronic disease follow up to my clinic session as it was more convenient for him. Mr Lam had recently attained his PhD in education and made it very clear to all the clinic staff that he would like to be greeted as "Dr Lam" in the future.

Over the next few years, his medical consultations with me were usually tough battles for "finding common ground". Dr Lam's lipid profile and blood pressure were well-controlled but his diabetes was not. His diabetic condition swung between poorly controlled to very poorly controlled. Dr Lam was, however, still cheerful as he rejected all my suggestions regarding new medications or important referrals. We agreed to disagree on his management, but I would not fail to dish out my concerns and advice at every encounter. He became more appreciative of my suggestions and would sometimes surprise me by accepting some of them.

A Misunderstanding?

During a regular follow-up visit in 2012, he looked radiant, slimmer, and so much happier. Miraculously, with no change in his medication, Dr Lam's diabetes had improved to a level never seen in the past decade. He was very happy about his achievement. I was pleasantly surprised with all the improvements and looked forward to our next appointment a few months later.

Just as I was going to bid him goodbye and slot him in for another appointment, I checked his routine electrocardiogram. It showed a very different and significant change from his previous year's electrocardiogram. I queried Dr Lam about chest complaints and feelings of breathlessness, and he said he never felt better. I was perplexed and persuaded him to repeat the electrocardiogram again, just in case it was a fluke printout. The second printout showed exactly the same tracing as the first.

Despite my persuasion, he refused to see the cardiologist. He would come back to me if he felt unwell. As he departed the office, he cheerfully explained that according to Dr Oz high doses of cinnamon would help protect the heart. I replied that I was not convinced with non-evidenced-based claims, but he retorted that I worry too much.

Dr Lam sent an email about his new blog, then left a phone message a week later because I had not replied. He never came back to the clinic and never sent me another email. He must have been upset with me and cancelled his appointment, I thought.

The Revelation

I next saw Dr Lam with his wife 6 months later. He was in a wheelchair with a large ulcer on his right Achilles tendon area. He looked very frail and was slumped in the wheelchair. I noted a large sternotomy scar right in front of his chest. I was quite taken aback!

"What happened?" I asked, totally puzzled.

Mrs Lam did most of the talking this time.

A few days before our planned consultation, Dr Lam suffered debilitating central chest pain in the middle of the night. Mrs Lam called the ambulance immediately, and Dr Lam was taken to the nearest hospital. Dr Lam underwent emergency cardiac bypass surgery and slipped into a coma after the operation for 2 weeks. The doctors were giving up hope, but Mrs Lam refused to have him extubated or life support switched off.

"It was really scary to hear the doctors persuading my wife to agree to switch off the machine . . . it was the first time in my life that I felt really frightened", Dr Lam said.

I noticed that Dr Lam was different. He almost cried when he shared how much his wife had been through during his hospitalization. He had been told that he would never be able to walk again.

My assumption that Dr Lam was upset with me had been wrong. Dr Lam had specially made this long trip from his home to let me know his condition as soon as he felt well enough to travel. I patted Dr Lam on his shoulder and felt a lump in my throat, unable to speak properly for several seconds. He saw my eyes tearing and smiled sadly.

At the back of my mind, I was asking myself, should I have pushed him harder to see a cardiologist. Doubts came but they did not stay long. I did continue to worry that Dr Lam could become depressed due to being isolated and having lost much of what brought meaning to his life.

Postscript

Dr Lam walked into the clinic today with a walking stick. "You know, Dr Lee, when have you ever been able to convince me to do the things I have decided not to do? I know you have a good heart and really care about me. I am in control, as always". He grinned jokingly.

"He is back to normal!" I exclaimed silently in my heart. My worry that he would get depressed was unfounded. "Well, sugar check at the next visit then. No more excuses". I beamed.

THE CYCLE OF LIFE

Caroline Villa Martignoni Rebicki

Piotr, a 66-year-old man, came to the clinic for an appointment for the first time in a couple of years. He seldom came to the clinic, preferring the easy access and the 'round-the-clock' availability of pharmacies for health advice. This was the first time we had met. Piotr presented himself with the characteristic formality and politeness of his generation, removing his hat from his head as he entered the office in a sign of respect. His pale blue eyes revealed concern, but his words were calm and controlled. Piotr had noticed large tender lumps in his neck and came to see what I thought it could be. He was a smoker and had a history of heavy alcohol consumption, which he cut down in fear of losing his driving permit. He disclosed little of his past history of depression that had required the use of antidepressant medication. Similar to many of the eastern-European descendants who settled in southern Brazil (Polish in this case), Piotr was the stoic type. We agreed to further investigations with laboratory imaging. He seemed pleased with the straightforward approach and further testing. To my surprise he came back the next afternoon with the ultrasound results (this meant that he had paid for an emergency exam, confirming that he was indeed concerned despite his apparent lack of emotional expression).

Piotr had worked in his family's vegetable field every day since he was able to carry a shovel, hoe, or a rake. Piotr was also a husband and a father but never spoke of his family. Maybe Piotr felt that such personal information was of no use in our meetings. I can only imagine the impact of the scan result in his mind, and yet again, the expression in his eyes did not match his voice. The idea of entering the world of the sick must have been so terrifying for this strong man that his first reaction was to question the results. "Maybe they just got it wrong, Doctor!" he argued. I felt that the seriousness of his condition did not allow for too much time to ponder, and I arranged for a specialist to see him within a couple of days.

Two days was not enough time for Piotr to prepare for what the specialist would recommend. The day after the specialist appointment he dropped by the clinic (informality, a sign of disturbance of his usual self, I thought) and asked to see me. I was aware of the content of his encounter with the specialist monitoring it through the electronic medical record. The hematologist requested that he be admitted to the hospital immediately in order to undergo a biopsy. Piotr was not oblivious to the hypothesis of cancer, and it frightened him.

Eric Cassell wrote: "The universal concept of cancer in the metaphor (in allusion to ideas of Alexander Solzhenitsyn in his book *The Cancer Ward*) makes clear the striking effect of illness without hope in removing man from control of his own life. Cast into the hospital world of doctors and nurses, the individual is impotent in the face of the medical array because he needs it to maintain the hope of survival. Dignity is a luxury of the healthy, and self-respect requires a constant struggle. Control in this other world is in the hands of others".[112]

Piotr had not come to discuss treatment options, nor could he admit that he needed a safe place to emotionally crash. Not Piotr, he still wanted to hold on to whatever control of his life remained. He entered my office, took off his hat and closed the door behind him. He thanked me for caring about him. He wanted me to know that he had made up his mind and that he was not going to be hospitalized. Piotr felt the diagnosis was his fate, and he accepted it. He told me that if he was not able to work, he would rather die. It would devastate him to become a burden to his wife and children. Control and independence were not negotiable to Piotr.

I felt frustrated. How could I convince this strong man that his life was seriously threatened if he did not consent to the biopsy, and how could I *impose* it without shattering his autonomy? It occurred to me that if he were my father, I would invest in crossing that line. Countertransference is an interesting phenomenon: with it one becomes, perhaps, dangerously involved; without it one might become too cold, distant, and impersonal – ultimately, impotent to heal. I reassured him that we (the clinic staff and I) would be there no matter what his decision was and that he was entitled to change his mind at any point along the way. We agreed to visit again in a week, and I told him we would call to check on him.

As we talked in the weeks that followed, something changed. We had become partners in this journey. I believe that's when we both reached the sacred turf of common ground. I had accepted his choice, and he had learned that he could trust me. Only then Piotr agreed to have the biopsy. He talked more about his family, his beautiful grandchildren, and his daughter's upcoming wedding. It was around this time that his health started to deteriorate at a rapid pace. He still refused hospitalization but accepted supportive care only. I began to understand what my role was in this relationship. Finding common ground with Piotr meant that I needed to step aside and let him be free to show me how to care for him. Commitment to his autonomy was essentially what he expected of me.

Almost 4 months after our first visit, I received a call from the family that Piotr had passed away that night. The results from the biopsy were still not available at that date. They wanted me to know that he was grateful for the time I spent with him and that he felt respected and heard.

This week Piotr's son brought his newborn baby girl to the clinic for a well baby visit and shared with me what seemed like the missing puzzle to Piotr's story. He told me that 2 days prior to his death, Piotr walked his youngest daughter down the aisle at her wedding, stood for pictures with the family, and watched the family dance and celebrate. The next morning he asked to be hospitalized. The medical record noted that he was admitted with signs of acute renal failure and died the following night.

Piotr's pièce de résistance was his need for control over his life. He believed it was his duty to stay strong until he felt that the cycle of life was complete. He walked beside his youngest daughter to the altar, standing tall. His job was done. Only then could he let go. As the meaning of his name implied Piotr had been the "rock" of his family.

Piotr reminded me that to be a family doctor is a privilege and an honor. He invited me to become a part of his story in his final days along with the important others in his life. In turn, he became a beautiful and indelible part of my story as a healer apprentice, and for this precious lesson I will always be grateful.

REFERENCES

1. Loxterkamp D: A change will do you good. *Ann Fam Med.* 2009 May–Jun;7(3):261–263. Doi: 10.1370/afm.976.
2. Tuckett D, Boulton M, Olson C, Williams A: *Meetings Between Experts: An Approach to Sharing Ideas in Medical Consultations.* London: Tavistock Publications, 1985.
3. Mold JW: *Goal-Oriented Medical Care: Helping Patients Achieve Their Personal Health Goals.* Chapel Hill, NC: Full Court Press, 2020: xxi.
4. Chin JJ: Doctor-patient relationship: From medical paternalism to enhanced autonomy. *Singapore Med J.* 2002;43(3):152–155.
5. Tauber AI: *Patient Autonomy and the Ethics of Responsibility.* Cambridge, MA: MIT Press, 2005.
6. van den Brink-Muinen A, van Dulmen SM, de Haes HCJM, et al: Has patients' involvement in the decision-making process changed over time? *Health Expect.* 2006;9:333–342.
7. Levinson W, Kao A, Kuby A, Thisted RA: Not all patients want to participate in decision making – a national study of public preferences. *J Gen Intern Med.* 2005;20:531–535.
8. Coulter A: What's happening around the world? In: Edwards A, Elwyn G (eds). *Shared Decision-Making in Health Care. Achieving Evidence-Based Patient Choice.* Oxford: Oxford University Press, 2009: 159.
9. Korsch B, Negrete V: Doctor-patient communication. *Sci Am.* 1972;227:66–74.
10. Stewart MA, Buck CW: Physicians' knowledge of and response to patients' problems. *Med Care.* 1977 Jul;15(7):578–585. Doi: 10.1097/00005650-197707000-00005. PMID: 875502.
11. Starfield B, Wray C, Hess K, Gross R, Birk PS, D'Lugoff BC: The influence of patient-practitioner agreement on outcome of care. *Am J Public Health.* 1981 Feb;71(2):127–131. Doi: 10.2105/ajph.71.2.127.
12. Coulter A: *The Autonomous Patient – Ending Paternalism in Medical Care.* London: Nuffield Trust, 2002.
13. Fong J, Longbecker N: Doctor-patient communication: A review. *Ochsner J.* 2010;10:38–43.
14. Braddock III CH, Edwards KA, Hasenberg NM, Laidley TL, Levinson W: Informed decision making in outpatient practice: Time to get back to basics. *JAMA.* 1999 Dec 22–29;282(24):2313–2320. Doi: 10.1001/jama.282.24.2313.
15. Long KL, Ingraham AM, Wendt EM, Saucke MC, Balentine C, Orne J, Pitt SC: Informed consent and informed decision-making in high-risk surgery: A quantitative analysis. *J Am Coll Surg.* 2021 Sep;233(3):337–345. Doi: 10.1016/j.jamcollsurg.2021.05.029.
16. Stevenson FA, Barry CA, Britten N, Barber N, Bradley CP: Doctor–patient communication about drugs: The evidence for shared decision making. *Soc Sci & Med.* 2000 Mar 1;50(6):829–840.
17. Britten N, Stevenson FA, Barry CA, Barber N, Bradley CP: Misunderstandings in prescribing decisions in general practice: Qualitative study. *BMJ.* 2000 Feb 19;320(7233):484–488. Doi: 10.1136/bmj.320.7233.484.
18. Dowell J, Jones A, Snadden D: Exploring medication use to seek concordance with 'non-adherent' patients: A qualitative study. *Br J Gen Pract.* 2002;52(474):24–32.
19. Dowell J, Williams B, Snadden D: *Patient-Centered Prescribing – Seeking Concordance in Practice.* Oxford: Radcliffe Publishing, 2007.
20. Stewart M, Brown JB, Donner A, McWhinney IR, Oates J, Weston WW, Jordan J: The impact of patient-centered care on outcomes. *J Fam Pract.* 2000 Sep;49(9):796–804.

21. Antonovsky A: *Health, Stress, and Coping: New Perspectives on Mental and Physical Well-Being*. San Francisco, CA: Jossey-Bass, 1979: 12–37.
22. McWhinney IR, Freeman TR: *McWhinney's Textbook of Family Medicine*. Oxford, New York: Oxford University Press, 2016: 274.
23. Champion VL, Skinner CS: The health belief model. In: Glanz K, Rimer BK, Viswanath K (eds). *Health Behavior and Health Education: Theory, Research, and Practice*. 4th edition. San Francisco, CA: Jossey-Bass, 2008.
24. Street RL, Haidet P: How well do doctors know their patients? Factors affecting patient understanding of patients' health beliefs. *J Gen Intern Med*. 2011;26(1):21–27.
25. Street RL, Haidet P: How well do doctors know their patients? Factors affecting patient understanding of patients' health beliefs. *J Gen Intern Med*. 2011;26(1):21–27.
26. Kleinman, A: The illness narratives. In: *Suffering, Healing and the Human Condition*. New York, NY: Basic Books; 1988.
27. Wood ML: Naming the illness: The power of words. *Fam Med*. 1991;23(7):534–538.
28. Cassell EJ: *The Nature of Suffering and the Goals of Medicine*. 2nd edition. Oxford: Oxford University Press, 2004.
29. McWhinney IR, Freeman TR: *McWhinney's Textbook of Family Medicine*. 4th edition. Revisions by T. Freeman. New York, NY: Oxford University Press, 2016 Jan 1: 232.
30. Hodges BD: Clinical commentary. In: Atkins CGK (ed). *My Imaginary Illness*. Ithaca, NY: Cornell University Press; 2010: 160–161.
31. Gill VT, Maynard DW: Explaining illness: Patients' proposals and physicians' responses. In: Heritage J, Maynard DW (eds). *Communication in Medical Care – Interactions between Primary Care Physicians and Patients*. Cambridge: Cambridge University Press, 2006: 117.
32. Brody H: 'My story is broken; can you help me fix it?' Medical ethics and the joint construction of narrative. *Lit Med*. 1994;13:79–92.
33. Launer J: *Narrative-Based Primary Care – A Practical Guide*. Abingdon, Oxon: Radcliffe Medical Press, 2002.
34. Roter DL, Hall JA: Physicians' interviewing styles and medical information obtained from patients. *J Gen Intern Med*. 1987;2:325–329.
35. Edwards A, Elwyn G: *Shared Decision-Making in Health Care – Achieving Evidence-Based Patient Choice*. Oxford: Oxford University Press, 2009: 20.
36. Kroenke K: A practical and evidence-based approach to common symptoms: A narrative review. *Ann Intern Med*. 2014 Oct 21;161(8):579–586. Doi: 10.7326/M14-0461.
37. Gask L, Dowrick C, Salmon P, Peters S, Morriss R: Reattribution reconsidered: Narrative review and reflections on an educational intervention for medically unexplained symptoms in primary care settings. *J Psychosom Res*. 2011 Nov;71(5):325–334. Doi: 10.1016/j.jpsychores.2011.05.008.
38. McAndrew LM, Friedlander ML, Alison Phillips L, Santos SL, Helmer DA: Concordance of illness representations: The key to improving care of medically unexplained symptoms. *Educ & Couns Psychol Fac Scholarsh*. 2018;17. https://scholarsarchive.library.albany.edu/edpsych_fac_scholar/17.
39. Steinmetz D, Tabenkin H: The 'difficult patient' as perceived by family physicians. *Fam Pract*. 2001 Oct;18(5):495–500. Doi: 10.1093/fampra/18.5.495.
40. Hartz AJ, Noyes R, Bentler SE, Damiano PC, Willard JC, Momany ET: Unexplained symptoms in primary care: Perspectives of doctors and patients. *Gen Hosp Psychiatry*. 2000 May–Jun;22(3):144–152. Doi: 10.1016/s0163-8343(00)00060-8.
41. Stone L: Managing medically unexplained illness in general practice. *Aust Fam Physician*. 2015 Sep;44(9):624–629.

42. Anastasides N, Chiusano C, Gonzalez C, Graff F, Litke DR, McDonald E, Presnall-Shvorin J, Sullivan N, Quigley KS, Pigeon WR, Helmer DA, Santos SL, McAndrew LM: Helpful ways providers can communicate about persistent medically unexplained physical symptoms. *BMC Fam Pract.* 2019 Jan 16;20(1):13. Doi: 10.1186/s12875-018-0881-8.

43. Lorig K and Associates: *Patient Education – A Practical Approach*. 3rd edition. Thousand Oaks, CA: Sage Publications, 2001.

44. Lorig K: Self-management education: More than a nice extra. *Med Care.* 2003;41(6):699–701.

45. Lorig KR, Holman HR: Self-management education: History, definition, outcomes, and mechanisms. *Ann Behav Med.* 2003;26(1):1–7.

46. Holman H, Lorig K: Patient self-management: A key to effectiveness and efficiency in care of chronic disease. *Public Health Rep.* 2004;119:239–243.

47. The US Burden of Disease Collaborators: The state of US health, 1990–2016: Burden of diseases, injuries, and risk factors among US states. *JAMA.* 2018;319(14):1444–1472. Doi: 10.1001/jama.2018.0158.

48. Jamoulle M: Information et informatisation en médecine générale. In: *Inf.-G-Iciens.* Namur, Belgium: Presses Universitaires de Namur, 1986: 193–209.

49. Martins C, Godycki-Cwirko M, Heleno B, Brodersen J: Quaternary prevention: Reviewing the concept: Quaternary prevention aims to protect patients from medical harm. *Eur J Gen Pract.* 2018 Jan 1;24(1):106–111.

50. US Preventive Services Task Force: https://uspreventiveservicestaskforce.org/uspstf/home.

51. Canadian Task Force on Preventive Health Care: https://canadiantaskforce.ca/.

52. National Health Service (NHS) in the United Kingdom: www.nhs.uk/conditions/nhs-screening/.

53. Welch HG, Schwartz L, Woloshin S: *Overdiagnosed: Making People Sick in the Pursuit of Health*. Boston, MA: Beacon Press, 2012.

54. Heleno B, Thomsen MF, Rodrigues DS, Jørgensen KJ, Brodersen J: Quantification of harms in cancer screening trials: Literature review. *BMJ.* 2013 Sep 16;347.

55. Harris RP, Sheridan SL, Lewis CL, Barclay C, Vu MB, Kistler CE, Golin CE, DeFrank JT, Brewer NT: The harms of screening: A proposed taxonomy and application to lung cancer screening. *JAMA Intern Med.* 2014 Feb 1;174(2):281–286.

56. Gérvas J: Quaternary prevention in the elderly. *Revista Espanola de Geriatria y Gerontologia.* 2012 Oct 11;47(6):266–269.

57. Hoffmann TC, Del Mar C: Patients' expectations of the benefits and harms of treatments, screening, and tests: A systematic review. *JAMA Intern Med.* 2015 Feb 1;175(2):274–286.

58. Korenstein D: Patient perception of benefits and harms: The Achilles heel of high-value care. *JAMA Intern Med.* 2015 Feb 1;175(2):287–288.

59. Hoffmann TC, Del Mar C: Clinicians' expectations of the benefits and harms of treatments, screening, and tests: A systematic review. *JAMA Intern Med.* 2017 Mar 1;177(3):407–419.

60. Wegwarth O, Schwartz LM, Woloshin S, Gaissmaier W, Gigerenzer G: Do physicians understand cancer screening statistics? A national survey of primary care physicians in the United States. *Annals Intern Med.* 2012 Mar 6;156(5):340–349.

61. Liang H, Zhu J, Kong X, Beydoun MA, Wenzel JA, Shi L: The patient-centered care and receipt of preventive services among older adults with chronic diseases: A nationwide cross-sectional study. INQUIRY: *J Health Care Organ, Provis Financ.* 2017 Aug 4;54:0046958017724003.

62. Armstrong D: The rise of surveillance medicine. *Sociol Health Illn*. 1995;17:393–404.

63. Choosing Wisely®: *A Watershed Moment in Health Care*. www.choosingwisely.org/our-mission.

64. Schoenborn NL, Boyd CM, Lee SJ, Cayea D, Pollack CE: Communicating about stopping cancer screening: Comparing clinicians' and older adults' perspectives. *The Gerontologist*. 2019 May 17;59(Supplement_1):S67–S76.

65. Dubé E, Laberge C, Guay M, Bramadat P, Roy R, Bettinger JA: Vaccine hesitancy: An overview. *Hum Vaccines Immunother*. 2013 Aug 8;9(8):1763–1773.

66. Waitzkin H: Doctor-patient communication: Clinical implications of social scientific research. *JAMA*. 1984;252:2441–2446.

67. Street RL: Aiding medical decision-making: A communication perspective. *Med Decis Making*. 2007:10:550–553.

68. Rollnick S, Miller WR, Butler CC: *Motivational Interviewing in Health Care – Helping Patients Change Behavior*. New York: Guilford Press, 2008.

69. Miller WR, Rollnick S: *Motivational Interviewing: Helping People Change*. 3rd edition. New York: Guilford Press, 2013.

70. Ford S, Schofield T, Hope T: Are patients' decision-making preferences being met? *Health Expect*. 2003;6:72–80.

71. McKinstry B: Do patients wish to be involved in decision making in the consultation? A cross sectional survey with video vignettes. *BMJ*. 2000;321:867–871.

72. Stacey D, Bennett CL, Barry MJ, et al: Decision aids for people facing health treatment or screening decisions (Review). *Cochrane Database Syst Rev*. 2011;(10):CD001431. Doi: 10.1002/14651858.CD1431.pub3.

73. Nelson WL, Han PKJ, Fagerlin A, Stefanek M, Ubel PA: Rethinking the objectives of decision aids: A call for conceptual clarity. *Med Decis Making*. 2007;27:609–618.

74. O'Connor AM, Stacey D, Légaré F: Coaching to support patients in making decisions. *BMJ*. 2008 Jan 31;336(7638):228–229.

75. Coulter A, Ellins J: Effectiveness of strategies for informing, educating and involving patients. *BMJ*. 2007;335:24–27.

76. Quill TE, Brody H: Physician recommendations and patient autonomy: Finding a balance between physician power and patient choice. *Ann Intern Med*. 1996 Nov 1;125(9):763–769. Doi: 10.7326/0003-4819-125-9-199611010-00010.

77. Flach SD, McCoy KD, Vaughn TE, et al: Does patient-centered care improve provision of preventive services? *J Gen Intern Med*. 2004;19:1019–1026.

78. Institute for Healthcare Communication: *Choices and Changes: Clinician Influence and Patient Action. Workshop Syllabus*. New Haven, CT: Institute for Healthcare Communication, 2010: 36–37.

79. Prochaska JO, DiClemente CC: *The Transtheoretical Approach: Crossing Traditional Boundaries of Therapy*. Homewood, IL: Dow/Jones Irwin, 1984.

80. Prochaska JO: Decision making in the transtheoretical model of behavior change. *Med Decis Making*. 2008;28:845–849.

81. Biss E: *On Immunity: An Inoculation*. Melbourne: Text Publishing, 2015 Jan 28.

82. Dzieciolowska S, Hamel D, Gadio S, Dionne M, Gagnon D, Robitaille L, Cook E, Caron I, Talib A, Parkes L, Dubé È, Longtin Y: Covid-19 vaccine acceptance, hesitancy, and refusal among Canadian healthcare workers: A multicenter survey. *Am J Infect Control*. 2021 Sep;49(9):1152–1157. Doi: 10.1016/j.ajic.2021.04.079.

83. MacDonald NE; SAGE Working Group on Vaccine Hesitancy: Vaccine hesitancy: Definition, scope and determinants. *Vaccine*. 2015 Aug 14;33(34):4161–4164. Doi: 10.1016/j.vaccine.2015.04.036.

84. Dean: COVID-19 vaccine hesitancy: What to say to allay patients' concerns. *Nurs Stand*. 2021;36(1):22–24. Doi: 10.7748/ns.36.1.22.s12.

85. Miller WR, Rollnick S: *Motivational Interviewing: Helping People Change*. 3rd edition. New York: Guilford Press, 2013: 15.

86. Bischof G, Bischof A, Rumpf HJ: Motivational interviewing: An evidence-based approach for use in medical practice. *Dtsch Arztebl Int*. 2021 Feb 19;118(7):109–115. Doi: 10.3238/arztebl.m2021.0014.

87. Spencer JC, Wheeler SB: A systematic review of motivational interviewing interventions in cancer patients and survivors. *Patient Educ Couns*. 2016 Jul 1;99(7):1099–1105.

88. Zolezzi M, Paravattil B, El-Gaili T: Using motivational interviewing techniques to inform decision-making for COVID-19 vaccination. *Int J Clin Pharm*. 2021 Dec;43(6):1728–1734. Doi: 10.1007/s11096-021-01334-y.

89. Miller WR, Rollnick S: *Motivational Interviewing: Helping People Change*. 3rd edition. New York: Guilford Press, 2013: 4.

90. Hardcastle SJ, Fortier M, Blake N, Hagger MS: Identifying content-based and relational techniques to change behaviour in motivational interviewing. *Health Psychol Rev*. 2017 Mar;11(1):1–16. Doi: 10.1080/17437199.2016.1190659.

91. Elwyn G, Durand MA, Song J, Aarts J, Barr PJ, Berger Z, Cochran N, Frosch D, Galasiński D, Gulbrandsen P, Han PKJ, Härter M, Kinnersley P, Lloyd A, Mishra M, Perestelo-Perez L, Scholl I, Tomori K, Trevena L, Witteman HO, Van der Weijden T: A three-talk model for shared decision making: Multistage consultation process. *BMJ*. 2017 Nov 6;359:j4891. Doi: 10.1136/bmj.j4891.

92. Towle A, Godolphin W: Framework for teaching and learning informed shared decision making. *BMJ*. 1999 Sep 18;319(7212):766–771. Doi: 10.1136/bmj.319.7212.766.

93. Charles C, Gafni A, Whelan T: Decision-making in the physician-patient encounter: Revisiting the shared treatment decision-making model. *Soc Sci Med*. 1999;49:651–661.

94. Elwyn G, Edwards A, Kinnersley P, Grol R: Shared decision making and the concept of equipoise: The competences of involving patients in healthcare choices. *Br J Gen Pract*. 2000 Nov;50(460):892–899.

95. Elwyn G, Charles C: Shared decision-making: The principles and the competencies. In: Edwards AG, Elwyn G (eds). *Evidence-Based Patient Choice: Inevitable or Impossible?* Oxford: Oxford University Press, 2001: 118–143.

96. Edwards A, Elwyn G: *Shared Decision-Making in Health Care – Achieving Evidence-Based Patient Choice*. Oxford: Oxford University Press, 2009.

97. Légaré F, Ratté S, Stacey D, Kryworuchko J, Gravel K, Graham ID, Turcotte S: Interventions for improving the adoption of shared decision making by health-care professionals. *Cochrane Database Syst Rev*. 2010 May 12;(5):CD006732. Doi: 10.1002/14651858.CD006732.pub2. Update in: *Cochrane Database Syst Rev*. 2014;9:CD006732.

98. Légaré F, Stacey D, Forest PG, Archambault P, Boland L, Coutu MF, Giguère AMC, LeBlanc A, Lewis KB, Witteman HO: Shared decision-making in Canada: Update on integration of evidence in health decisions and patient-centered care government mandates. *Z Evid Fortbild Qual Gesundhwes*. 2022 Jun;171:22–29. Doi: 10.1016/j.zefq.2022.04.006.

99. Abbasgholizadeh Rahimi S, Cwintal M, Huang Y, Ghadiri P, Grad R, Poenaru D, Gore G, Zomahoun HTV, Légaré F, Pluye P: Application of artificial intelligence in shared decision making: Scoping review. *JMIR Med Inform*. 2022 Aug 9;10(8):e36199. Doi: 10.2196/36199.

100. Elwyn G, Cochran N, Pignone M: Shared decision making – the importance of diagnosing preferences. *JAMA Intern Med.* 2017 Sep 1;177(9):1239–1240. Doi: 10.1001/jamainternmed.2017.1923.

101. Menear M, Garvelink MM, Adekpedjou R, Perez MMB, Robitaille H, Turcotte S, Légaré F: Factors associated with shared decision making among primary care physicians: Findings from a multicentre cross-sectional study. *Health Expect.* 2018 Feb;21(1): 212–221. Doi: 10.1111/hex.12603.

102. Becerra-Perez MM, Menear M, Turcotte S, Labrecque M, Légaré F: More primary care patients regret health decisions if they experienced decisional conflict in the consulta-tion: A secondary analysis of a multicenter descriptive study. *BMC Fam Pract.* 2016 Nov 10;17(1):156. Doi: 10.1186/s12875-016-0558-0.

103. Thompson-Leduc P, Turcotte S, Labrecque M, Légaré F: Prevalence of clinically signifi-cant decisional conflict: An analysis of five studies on decision-making in primary care. *BMJ Open.* 2016 Jun 28;6(6):e011490. Doi: 10.1136/bmjopen-2016-011490.

104. Mangin D, Risdon C, Lamarche L, Langevin J, Ali A, Parascandalo J, Stephen G, Trimble J: 'I think this medicine actually killed my wife': Patient and family perspectives on shared decision-making to optimize medications and safety. *Ther Adv Drug Saf.* 2019 Apr 5;10:2042098619838796. Doi: 10.1177/2042098619838796.

105. Zisman-Ilani Y, Khaikin S, Savoy ML, Paranjape A, Rubin DJ, Jacob R, Wieringa TH, Suarez J, Liu J, Gardiner H, Bass SB, Montori VM, Siminoff LA: Disparities in shared decision-making research and practice: The case for black American patients. *Ann Fam Med.* 2023 Mar–Apr;21(2):112–118. Doi: 10.1370/afm.2943.

106. Melzer AC, Golden SE, Ono SS, Datta S, Crothers K, Slatore CG: What exactly is shared decision-making? A qualitative study of shared decision-making in lung cancer screen-ing. *J Gen Intern Med.* 2020 Feb;35(2):546–553. Doi: 10.1007/s11606-019-05516-3.

107. Poitras ME, Hudon C, Godbout I, Bujold M, Pluye P, Vaillancourt VT, Débarges B, Poirier A, Prévost K, Spence C, Légaré F: Decisional needs assessment of patients with complex care needs in primary care. *J Eval Clin Pract.* 2020 Apr;26(2):489–502. Doi: 10.1111/jep.13325.

108. Savelberg W, Smidt M, Boersma LJ, van der Weijden T: Elicitation of preferences in the second half of the shared decision making process needs attention; a qualitative study. *BMC Health Serv Res.* 2020 Jul 9;20(1):635. Doi: 10.1186/s12913-020-05476-z.

109. Hanson JL: Shared decision making. Have we missed the obvious? *Arch Intern Med.* 2008;168(13):1368–1370.

110. Boudreau JD, Cassell EJ, Fuks A: A healing curriculum. *Med Educ.* 2007;41:1193–1201.

111. McLeod ME: Doctor-patient relationships: Perspectives, needs, and communication. *Am J Gastroenterology.* 1998;93(5):676–680.

112. Cassell EJ: *The Healer's Art.* Third printing. Cambridge, MA: MIT Press, 1995: 44.

7

The Fourth Component: Enhancing the Patient–Clinician Relationship

MOIRA STEWART, JUDITH BELLE BROWN, AND THOMAS R FREEMAN

INTRODUCTION*

In 2005 and 2014, our books asked, why is the value of the patient–clinician relationship not more widely embraced?[1, 2] Even in those relatively calm times, societal values did not, on the whole, support or nurture relationships, but rather society valued individual accomplishment above community, valued science over art, valued analysis over synthesis, and valued technological solutions over wisdom. But now in post-pandemic, contrarian mid-2020s, there has been an upsurge of technology and confrontation followed swiftly by a clarion call that health care may become "endangered", its survival threatened, unless it cleaves to its core as "caring professions" emulating its central purposes of "compassion and human connectedness".[3] We remind ourselves of:

> lessons of lasting value: the importance of listening to patients before we lecture them. The indispensability of courage as we speak up for those who cannot. Humility as the best means to master our mistakes. The enormous return on investment that follows every generous, selfless and faithful act. The healing that occurs when patients are restored to their self-identified community. It is from a sense of belonging that humans derive their sense of purpose and meaning, identity, and self-worth, and the strength to overcome adversity. For [the health professional] . . . connection is our currency.[4]

In *A Fortunate Woman*, the clinician's work on her relationships with patients, has been described as a moral and ethical enterprise so that she:

---

* Some of the material in this chapter is adapted from Stewart's article "Reflections on the Doctor–Patient Relationship: From Evidence and Experience" (2005).

DOI: 10.1201/9781003394679-9

relates the process to her capacity for hope. 'What is the right thing to do? How can we, how can I, do better?' This engagement with the morality of her work, as well as the practical and clinical, underpins every aspect of the doctor's approach to general practice and to her patients . . . the key word here is 'practice'. Her life's work is not simply about the application of a body of knowledge to an assortment of human objects. Nor is it the static state of being a qualified doctor who holds that body of knowledge. It is iterative, a virtuous activity in the true Aristotelian sense: a pursuit meaningful in and of itself, both ethically and interpersonally. It is becoming rather than knowing, and its lifeblood is trust. Looked at this way, each . . . consultation becomes a waypoint on a journey, rather than a clinical destination.[5]

The day-to-day tasks of medicine are accomplished through the interaction of patient and clinician during a visit, the "essential unit of medical practice".[6] Or, to put it another way, "coursing like a river underneath these discrete visits, is the ongoing relationship, manifesting dimensions more enduring than the qualities of any one visit, dimensions such as trust, caring, feeling, power, and purpose".[7] Loxterkamp, as well, has used the river as a metaphor for patient–clinician relationships:

It may be said that I buoyed him (the patient) at his low point, helped him through rocky times – saw around a bend in the river that he, for one dark moment, could not. Together we let the river carry us, knowing it was stronger and swifter than our solitary effort to swim ashore.[8]

In a long-term practice, like Morland describes, the relationship is anchored not only in time but also in the community:

At the centre of it all, is that two way relationship between doctor and patient. Each of these interactions is necessarily pragmatic, current, but they also have deep roots that over time intertwine the individual with the collective, the present with the past.[5]

Medical, nursing, and psychotherapeutic literature contains references to processes that have as a goal a strong patient–clinician relationship: a working alliance or a therapeutic alliance. The relationship requires "skills as varied as highly technical, psychologically insightful and personally empathetic".[9] "The primary agent of treatment is the clinician".[9] These relationships "provide the foundation for those pillars of good healthcare, trust, rapport and empathy".[5]

COMPASSION, CARING, EMPATHY, AND TRUST

The word compassion derives from the root word meaning "suffering with" and suggests the requirement of human presence.[10] It stresses the emotional connection through identifying, acknowledging, and acting on suffering.[11, 12] In contrast, empathy can be seen as a "necessary pre-requisite for compassion"[12] and, although empathy draws on a history of feeling, it has also been defined cognitively and behaviorally as understanding the patient's situation, communicating that understanding, and acting on it in a helpful way.[13, 14]

The doctor, arriving late and already anticipating her (the doctor's) next three moves, could deflect the ambiguity of his (the patient's) averted eyes and nervous hands by writing a prescription and moving to the next room, where a strep test has already turned positive. Or she could gamble her balancing act on five unscripted minutes that could open a can of worms.

At that moment of indecision, why would a patient risk self-disclosure or the doctor relinquish the safety of higher ground? Their choice often reflects a mutual leaning towards relationship: trust that here one's true self can safely emerge; reassurance that their galloping fears will be calmed through the clinician's touch, words, and familiar surroundings; companionship that ends the exile of illness and offers a promise of deliverance to some recognizable shore; some sign that there is shelter here, and restorative good will. And mindfulness of what matters most. Why do we live? What is our sacrifice for? When is there more to cherish than the time stretched between us?

The investment of these moments, whose consequence ripples in ever widening arcs, matters as much as any lifesaving heroics. These are the moments that make life worth saving. They unveil the worth of a living thing, an intrinsic value that can never be priced or marketed or proved beyond the affirmation of a handshake or nod of thanks.[15]

In contrast, however, not all doctors "lean towards relationship".

Brian McDonald, a young man in his early 20s already had two visits to the family doctor and had been diagnosed with mononucleosis. After 3 weeks he became too weak to get out of bed, and the doctor made a house call to the patient's home where he lived with his parents. Even before examining Brian, the doctor stated, "If I had a room like this, I'd want to stay here all the time too!"

Anna Ferriera, a young pregnant woman, was in her eighth month when she developed signs of toxemia of pregnancy. When entering her bedroom at her home, the doctor remarked, "So you've taken to your bed already, have you?"

A patient participant in a qualitative study[16] was of patients with medically unexplained symptoms (MUS), "uncomfortable" with the clinician as shown in Box 7.1.

BOX 7.1: A Patient's Voice

Juul Houwen

Patients felt uncomfortable when GPs did not show empathy. Some patients with MUS felt irritated when GPs "were busy with their computers". Patients wanted the opportunity to tell their story and expected GPs to question them in greater depth about their symptoms. In cases where the GP did not do a thorough exploration, patients were dismayed:

P: "I wasn't impressed with this, you know. Where he said at a certain point that everyone, you know . . . basically it comes across as saying that everyone deals with their complaints in their own way, right? . . . And if push came to shove – suppose there wasn't another solution – well, I would find that really awful. And then I thought, hang on, what are we talking about?"

I: "So what should the doctor . . . what should he have said?"

P: "Well, he shouldn't have said that, I reckon. No, I wasn't impressed. It came across to me as if, well, maybe you should grin and bear it a bit more. Which I thought was a shame. Because then I think, heavens, no one else can know how you feel. I know perfectly well that there are hypochondriacs, but I'm not one of them".

quoted from Houwen J.[71]

The lack of respect, compassion, empathy, or support reflected in these short narratives may have negative consequences for patients' self-respect and inner resources just when patients need them most. Our self-absorption as professionals, whether or not it is recognized, can interfere with care in so many ways. Current emphasis on technology and efficiency in medical practice provides fertile ground for this problem to grow: "Technologies have introduced distance between healthcare providers and patients. This distance has often been a threat to compassion. Health professionals need to be aware of this distance and find new ways to foster presence".[17] The distancing due to technologies is covered in Chapter 9 of this book. Speaking of the tendency of doctors to distance, McWhinney has said:

> The temptation is to avoid the patient with very good excuses, such as by giving all our attention to the physical examination or pretending to ourselves that we have no time to visit them. But the patient is usually not deceived by such ways and means, perceiving perfectly well that we are frightened to face them. We may even be tempted to abandon the patient without explanation. Yet it is essential that we continue being present to these suffering patients.
>
> If we speak of suffering, we will not be tempted to distance ourselves from the experience. Facing a patient's suffering in this way, not from behind a barrier or as an expert practicing a certain technique, but as one person to another, is perhaps our most difficult task. But there are rewards, as when we witness the joy of recovery or emergence from despair. Not being tied to a particular disease, organ system or technology makes it easier for family doctors to step out of our abstractions and open ourselves or our patients.[18]

However, doctors may be mistaken if they think that compassionate care is always more difficult and more taxing. On the contrary, sometimes our difficulty is that we fail to understand that what the patient wants is something very simple: a recognition of their suffering or perhaps only our presence at a time of need.

For generations, medical students have been taught, "don't get involved". In the conventional clinical method, the doctor is assumed to be a detached observer, prescriber of treatment, and user of technologies. Remaining uninvolved may protect doctors from some very disturbing things, especially as they encounter the depth of a patient's suffering. However, it also has a personal price. Hodges has said, "my personal suspicion is that the current epidemic of burnout among health professionals is largely driven by the diminution of human contact in our work environments".[17] To remain uninvolved, physicians have to build up protective shells to suppress their feelings. This lack of openness creates difficulties in relationships, not only with patients but also with colleagues. To suggest that one can remain uninvolved is also a fallacy. One cannot help being affected in some way by the encounter with suffering, even if the result is avoidance and denial.

This book advocates for more emotional involvement of the clinician with the patient than is the case in conventional medicine. However, it recognizes the multiple roles of practice and the need for the clinician to integrate and synthesize. The clinician must possess:

> that willingness to invest in the moment, that instinctive ability to occupy, reflect and respond to the here and now, both emotionally and intellectually sits at the heart of the doctor–patient relationship. . . . Building good relationships calls for both spontaneity and judgement. Summoning [with each patient visit] empathy, precision, collaborative decision-making and shrewd risk management . . . [it] is about looking and listening with the/utmost care, wringing every verbal and non-verbal vestige of meaning . . . to knit it all together over time. It is a job that requires both heart and head . . . in delicate balance.[5]

To empower and support clinicians to discuss and address suffering in their patients, Phillips et al. suggest clinicians "systematically investigate, organize, and understand the patient's experience . . . Understanding the patient's view of self and the impact of their illness are the foundations of patient-centred care and create a starting point to facilitate healing".[19]

Patient–clinician interactions while providing a "glimpse of the stability, continuity and connection" do not sacrifice the medical "skill, intellect and aspiration".[5] The multifaceted nature of patient–clinician relationships has been observed for decades. Enid Balint and colleagues[20] pointed out that for doctors it is important to move back and forth from objective observation to empathetic identification, in the same sort of weaving back and forth that we recommended in Chapter 3 and which we replicate here in Figure 7.1.[21] However, what is too often forgotten with this sort of dichotomous thinking is the injunction to integrate the elements. Cassell (2013) reminds us of the seminal quote from Feinstein that the work of a doctor requires the "oscillating" recommended by Balint but also, after that, "not just a conjunction but a true synthesis of art and science, fusing the parts into a whole".[9, 22]

Selwyn eloquently reflects on a career of almost sacred presence:

Each time I sit with a patient, it is as if everything in both of our lives has brought us to this exact moment, which can be an opportunity for the mundane or, at times, the almost sacred. Sometimes we connect only briefly, or perhaps miss each other's meaning, and continue superficially through our daily routine. But sometimes, when a certain question, phrase, or gesture opens a door, we may have a glimpse into a whole new room that is suddenly open to light and understanding. Like a glance in a crowd between strangers, sometimes everything aligns, the extraneous is stripped away, and we can look deeply into someone's soul. Random yet precise, a series of interactions, of fleeting moments that occasionally verge on timelessness. These moments can't be forced or created; the best we can do is to learn to witness, patiently, with humility, and not let

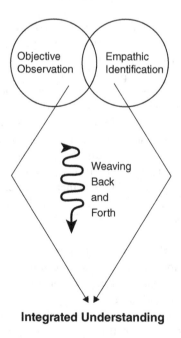

Figure 7.1 Connecting with Patients

ourselves or our judgments get in the way of the process – to learn to be present, attentive, and open to the story that is waiting to be told.[23]

Perhaps the kernel of the caring relationship from the patient's point of view is trust. Breast cancer patients have difficulty understanding the vast amounts of information they need to assimilate before treatment decisions can be made, especially in their understandable state of anxiety and fear. Women with breast cancer say that they cannot make sense of all the facts and figures regarding options, unless they work with a trusted physician.[24]

In response to a lack of conversation about infertility as a side effect of her leukemia treatment, the patient says:

> As much as I appreciated their support, the absence of communication on something so important felt like a breach of trust early in our patient–doctor relationship.[25]

Trust takes time to develop in a working relationship based on respect. Trusting relationships, therefore, require personal continuity.[26] The sources of trust in medical practice include a just society, moral integrity, continuity of care, sharing power, compassion, authenticity, and competence:

> Trust is an individual's belief that the sincerity, benevolence, and truthfulness of others can be relied on. Trust often implies a transference of power, to a person or to a system, to act on one's behalf, in one's best interest.[27]

POWER IN THE PATIENT–CLINICIAN RELATIONSHIP

Health care's role in reducing disparities and in providing a glue that helps hold society together has long been recognized.[28-30] There are a variety of mechanisms helping this role: an ethical stance of sharing power, i.e. a belief that the patients have a right to share in decisions about their life course,[31, 32] and a thoughtful and humble stance by the clinician seeking to marry medical expertise with personal humility in moving the relationship from patient dependence to mutual interdependence.[32, 33] A key hindrance to sharing power is the individual patient's reduced capacity during the illness, as amply demonstrated by Dr W Wayne Weston's "A Patient's Voice" in Box 7.2, in which he simply was not ready to contribute to making decisions about medication options quickly, even though he was a medical doctor himself.

BOX 7.2: A Patient's Voice

W Wayne Weston

HEART ATTACK – A DOCTOR'S EXPERIENCE

1:00 am and all is not well! I awaken with burning pain across the front of my chest. My initial reaction is fear: "I wonder if this is my heart." But I can't stand the fear and immediately decide it must be heartburn and go downstairs for some antacid. It doesn't help and I become fearful again. Then I vomit and convince myself it must be a stomach problem. But the pain gets worse. Finally, I can't stand the pain any longer and ask my wife to call for an ambulance. I decide it is probably a heart attack and take an aspirin. The ambulance arrives in five minutes. The attendants start an IV, give me nitroglycerine and take me directly to the hospital where I work. It feels odd to be on the stretcher receiving care rather than providing care. The fear is gone – partly because the pain is so bad that all I can think about is getting relief and partly because I feel I am in good hands. I see a familiar face, the chief of the ER, looking on and feel safe. One of the team members does an ECG and the resident holds it up in front of me where I can easily see the telltale ST elevation indicating an acute MI. They start a nitro drip and administer tPA.

I don't remember anyone discussing my diagnosis or treatment in the ER. It could well have happened, but the experience was such a blur I blotted out much of it. If I gave consent, it was not very informed. But I am not sure I would want to hear about the risk of stroke or death at that time. Finally, the tPA does its job and "busts the clot", my chest pain dissolves, and I go to sleep.

Next day I meet my cardiologist and hear about my heart attack and learn that I also have diabetes. I am so glad to be pain free and alive that I am at peace with this news. I am initially treated with insulin four times a day as well as beta-blockers, ramipril and aspirin to protect my heart, Pravachol to lower my cholesterol, and injections of low molecular weight heparin to prevent a new clot from forming. Again, there is very little discussion of the pros and cons of any of this treatment although I know from professional experience that this is standard therapy.

Later, they decide it is time to switch to oral drugs for my diabetes and tell me they will start glyburide. When I suggest I would prefer metformin they are hesitant but agree. Next day my gout flares up and I ask for NSAIDs. The medication immediately arrives. I am impressed with the rapid response and surprised that there is no discussion.

On the day before discharge my cardiologist discusses the pros and cons of warfarin for a few months and asks if I have any questions or alternative suggestions for therapy. This is the first time anyone has opened up the options, and I am not ready. Although he is sitting down and appears unrushed, I know how busy he is and am hesitant to start a long discussion of the pros and cons of all the different drugs I am on. Despite my professional education and my knowledge of evidence-based medicine, I am intimidated by my vulnerability and don't want to impose on my physician. I want to be a "good" patient.

In reflecting on this experience, I am struck by how vulnerable I felt. Although I spoke up about the treatment of my diabetes and gout (they didn't seem to know how to treat these conditions in the coronary unit), I felt very reluctant to question the treatment of my heart. As an advocate for patient-centered care, I realized how hard it is for patients to have a voice in decisions even when physicians are friendly and invite dialogue. Perhaps doctors need to take the time over several visits to open up the options and to explicitly address a patient's reluctance to question authority. As I return to practice I realize, more fully, the tremendous power differential between patients and doctors and use my experience to try to bridge that gap and encourage my patients to give voice to their ideas and concerns.

Similarly, Janet Sutherland's case emphasizes a patient's diminution in the face of illness and slow recovery.

CASE EXAMPLE

Janet Sutherland, a health care worker in her late 30s, recently broke her arm in a car accident. Her world was shattered, as were the bones in her arm. For 10 weeks she was unable to care for her two preschool children, drive the car, or work. By this time, her confidence in herself was deteriorating because she felt responsible, not only for the accident but also for the fact that her bones were not healing as quickly as expected. Moreover, the confidence and trust in the family doctor were also waning because the decisions they made together (regarding the type of surgeon she would be referred to, the type of anesthetic she would receive, and the type of follow-up care) were never realized. The information about the surgery too was conflicting. Janet expressed these fears, "Why was nothing as it should be? Why was I not recovering? Was something being hidden? Why can't I get better – I need to get better!"

The central issues of lack of control over the recovery and over the health care created a sense of powerlessness. As angry as Janet became at herself, she was doubly angry at the doctors, including the family doctor. The ebbing trust and the increasing powerlessness united in a crisis of care. It took weeks of work on the part of this patient to gain insight into her own issues. It took a new willingness on the part of all the physicians to listen and to solve problems mutually with the patient, before both the healing of the person and the healing of the bones became evident.

Recent reviews of the literature have found that *the* most common element in frameworks describing patient-centered care is "sharing power and responsibility".[32, 34] This aligns with the rise in interest in shared decision-making, which is similar but not identical to Component 3, Finding Common Ground, described in Chapter 6. The quality of a relationship within which finding common ground is possible includes a readiness of clinician and patient to become partners in care. Their encounters are truly meetings between experts.[35] However, each partnership is unique and may include permutations and combinations employing varying degrees of control along many dimensions and changing over time. One example would be the adolescent who needs information (from the expert doctor) but who also maintains control of management (envisioning herself as expert on her life) because she yearns to be treated as an adult, but at the same time she needs guidance. An ability on the part of the clinician to remain open and alert to these shifting needs for control is an essential aspect of an ongoing partnership.

Scott and colleagues found that physicians were able to eloquently describe these shifts. One physician noted "an intuitive understanding about when and how to push patients based on assessments of patients' needs and strength of relationships". Another said, "sometimes you're a coach and sometimes you're the boss and sometimes you're the sibling and sometimes you're the doctor".[36]

The resulting therapeutic alliance is related in complex ways to the healing of patients, suffering the loss of their central purpose – that is, sense of control over themselves and their world or loss of control of their life. We will see later in this chapter a connection between healing and key dimensions of wellness, health, and wholeness aligning this discussion with the health promotion role of clinicians. This connection between the dimensions of trust in the therapeutic alliance, the taking and giving of control, and regaining a central purpose in life is best illustrated in the following qualitative longitudinal study. Bartz[37] characterized the evolution of relationships of nine Indigenous patients with diabetes with one physician over time, using terms such as disease focus, misunderstandings, mistrust, detachment, and hopelessness.

To control the environment, the doctor adopted various strategies that constrained the interactions, including use of a diabetic protocol form and a medicalized way of knowing patients. Paradoxically, these strategies produced varying degrees of mistrust, clinical nihilism, interpersonal distance, and loss of control in relationships with these patients.[38]

One sees the negative implications of continued attempts to exert medical control. Another alternative in situations of misunderstanding and mistrust may be consciously to share power, to be humble, to move away from medical conversation, and to be curious about the patients' beliefs and the meaning of the situation to the patient.[33, 39, 40]

By facilitating the telling of their life stories over time, doctors share with their patients the process whereby they reconstruct themselves through the experience of their suffering. In sharing this, "doctors are also open to change, experiencing their own vulnerability and powerlessness . . . (an acknowledgement of which) may be one of the most powerful things doctors do to facilitate healing in patients . . . the strength borne from the awareness of shared weakness".[41]

CASE EXAMPLE

Mrs Patrick was an elderly woman who had arthritis, irritable bowel syndrome, and a cancer of the breast 6 years ago. The doctor, in his late 30s, had been Mrs Patrick's family physician for the past year. This insightful patient and doctor found a way to accommodate her seemingly contradictory needs. On the one hand, her advanced age and physical problems left her insecure enough to require explicit reassurance. The doctor provided the reassurance after appropriate questioning and physical examination and by exploring the nature of her symptoms. On the other hand, she needed to maintain control over some aspects of her life and health; this manifested itself in her controlling the choice and the order of topics during the encounter with her family doctor. She always brought a written list of her complaints. Although this family physician thoughtfully interpreted her behavior, other doctors might have been offended by her somewhat bossy manner and might have failed to see it as an important coping mechanism.

CONTINUITY AND CONSTANCY

There extends behind every encounter the doctor has, on every day of her working life, not just a medical history but also a personal history, a winding corridor of experience and emotion, the patient's whole life. In any given consultation, she is afforded but a fragment, a scintilla of that history. It is one of the joys of being a long-serving family doctor in a community like this, that she has both the time and the opportunity to piece the fragments together, over years and across families and generations. . . . Reduce any of your patients to their affliction, the tumorous breast, incompetent heart valve or lazy pancreas, and it's akin to regarding a book as nothing more than paper and ink.[5]

Personal continuity is necessary for a healing relationship.[42] Herbert[43] has described the power of continuing relationships as a way to reveal the patient's untold story. Continuity of relationships has been shown to accrue many benefits.[44] The benefits to clinicians include joy in their work, as revealed in qualitative studies[45] and in this quotation:

> It is equilibrium that makes the work sustainable. . . . brings the richest rewards of the job. For being there, available most days for your patients, is one of the key elements in building relationships, and strong, rooted relationships don't just help patients. They also help the doctor.[5]

There is powerful evidence of the benefits of personal continuity for patients as well as clinicians; it affects the bottom line. Pereira Gray says, "Continuity of care is associated with lower mortality rates".[46] This benefit transcends cultures and occurs regardless of the physicians' speciality. In addition, continuity influences patient trust, autonomy, and shared decision-making as well as clinician empathy and understanding of the patients' values.[45]

Despite the benefits of continuity, in all medical disciplines and in most Western countries, policy decisions have resulted in marked disruptions in continuity of care, particularly during the COVID-19 pandemic. Patients have described the harms of discontinuity in terms of anxiety, loss of trust, experiencing conflicting advice, and fear of safety; their health care suffers from over-investigation and missed opportunities for prevention.[45]

Not only does the system put barriers in the way of continuity of care but also physicians themselves consciously or unconsciously close doors or at worst abandon patients. Nonetheless, it remains doctor's responsibility to be constant in their commitment to the well-being of the patient. The required commitment is not easily achieved because the doctor may experience feelings of failure and have to encounter a patient's anger or other expressions of mistrust. Cassell describes constancy in the following way:

> Constancy to the patient is necessary. Constant attention and maintained presence are not difficult when things are going well. It requires self-discipline to maintain constancy when the case is going sour, when errors or failures have occurred, when the wrong diagnosis has been made, when the patient's personality or behaviour is difficult or even repulsive, when impending death brings the danger of sorrow and loss because emotional closeness has been established. When constancy is absent or falters, too frequently, patients lose that newfound part of themselves – the doctor – that promised stability in the uncertain world of sickness arising from their relationship.[47]

Lucassen's case, entitled "A Man and A Woman", found at the end of this chapter, illustrates constancy in the face of physical suffering, deprivation, and squalor; the clinicians' commitment is to not distance themselves, not to abandon, but to remain present.

HEALING AND HOPE

The most important aspect of healing the suffering patient is "understanding suffering".[9] Healers must bridge between the world of the sufferer and the well world. To begin to do this, the clinician must understand that "all suffering is unique and individual" (attend to the particulars of each patient); "suffering involves self conflict" (understand that the patient simultaneously fears rejection from their family while craving acceptance); "suffering is marked by loss of central purpose" (attend to the person that was before the illness so that all hope is not lost in "the redirection of purpose" solely to the medical needs such as pain relief); and "all suffering is lonely" (understand that the ill experience "social deprivation and isolation even in the midst of others"). A clinician might ask, "What is there in all this that you find particularly distressing?" "Ask your questions and then be quiet and wait for the answers – and be patient"[9] (quotes are from Cassell, 2013: 225–6).

Stein[48] too writes about the distance across the chasm that opens between the ill and the healthy. "What patients trust about me – or any doctor – is the ability to understand that the moment they become ill they are apart, different, separate from the healthy, that relationships have changed and will change again, that life is cruel".

He enjoins doctors to welcome the revelation:

> The revelation of terror is an admission that disruption and incoherence now rule, and it is a disclosure made to a relative stranger, your doctor, who you can only hope will welcome such honesty. But such a revelation assumes your doctor can and will understand your admission in all its shadings, its context and weight.[48]

He stresses the revelation's importance:

> Doctors hold the world in place for patients . . . establish the legitimacy of their claims. We offer human contact and concern. The best we can do as doctors is to turn ourselves into a reflection of our patients' pain. The doctor's job is to make pain shareable. The impossibility of sharing . . . the pain is . . . a contributing factor in its essential horror.[48]

One patient's perspective is to encourage a courageous stance by the clinician. He, the patient, wishes clinicians would welcome uncomfortable disclosures: "I have never heard an ill person praised for how well she expressed fear or grief or was openly sad" (Arthur Frank, quoted in Stein[48]). Perhaps, our society in general needs to be more accepting of expressions of sadness. Has anyone ever said to you: "I love you for your tears?"

Stein describes another courageous moment for both the patient and the clinician:

> "What if I survive and my brain does not?" I responded with chances and odds so small they were impossible to summon or calculate. We went over it again and again. I could see his mind buckle and flex, assert and cringe. But by asking questions, patients feel less powerless, and by answering them, doctors try to alleviate terror. I know there is no drastic remedy for terror, but what patients want and need badly is, as Reynolds Price wrote, "the frank exchange of decent concern." I try never to turn away from conversation. I give looks of mild encouragement. I offer words, nothing altogether convincing, but at least amulets of hope.[48]

If offered in an emotionally connected way, such attention and conversation is experienced by the patient as consolation and comfort; it makes the suffering more bearable, and it marks a transition to a more hopeful place.[36, 49] "If therapeutic relationships possess a certain unquantifiable magic, it is the magic of hope. . . . Hope hinges on the presence of another and the reassurance that yes, we are knowable".[50]

In an ongoing patient–clinician relationship the process of healing has been described as following certain paths. For a group of patients who suffered alcoholism and/or suicide attempts but survived, the steps in their healing relationships were listening, trust, willingness to change, acquisition of life skills, and control.[51] For a group of chronically ill older persons, the process, akin to health promotion, included trust, connecting, caring, mutual knowledge, and mutual caring.[52] One sees a synergistic benefit to both patient and clinician in these accounts of healing.

SELF-AWARENESS AND PRACTICAL WISDOM

It would not be surprising to find that clinicians working in our instrumental society (and in healthcare systems much more prone to rules and accountabilities than a decade ago), feel a little embattled, perhaps running against the predominant current. Cassell,[9] as well as Kinsella and Pitman,[53] express their alarm and quickly suggest solutions highly relevant to this book.

A relevant dilemma and reflection was presented by Miksanek,[54] whose paper described a series of "difficult" patients – they were difficult in that they did not permit him to practice in a manner approved by the rule-oriented healthcare system. Frank,[55] in reviewing and applauding the clinician (Miksanek), noted that, although discouraged, the clinician was courageous in showing constancy and ongoing commitment to these patients. Furthermore, the clinician also took time to reflect on the dissonance arising from the fact that his practice was out of step with the current system's expectations.

In the face of such anomalies how can a professional react? We offer two themes in response to this question: mindfulness and practical wisdom.

Scott et al.'s study of healing revealed that:

Mindfulness, a constant awareness of the encounter at multiple levels . . . Is this a story of shame and they need you to listen? Is this a story of fear and they need you to be there with them? Is this a story of blame . . . or self-blame and they need to hear that it wasn't their fault? I mean, what is the story? So what role do they need you to be in?[56]

To hear the story, the clinician is advised to remain silent while at the same time giving attention, maintaining a stable focus and having clarity (unbiased perception).[57] It is recommended that this "receptive stance holds back . . . analytic thinking, in favour of a more contemplative process, in which the mind acts more like a receptor, receiving ideas images and feelings and being moved by them".[58]

Whatever the source, self-awareness and self-knowledge are as imperative to current practice as they were decades ago. As Howard Stein[59] observed, "one can truly recognize a patient only if one is willing to recognize oneself in the patient". McWhinney had a similar message: "We cannot begin to know others until we know ourselves. We cannot grow and change as physicians until we have removed our defences and faced up to our shortcomings".[60]

CONCEPTS OF SELF FOR THE PATIENT AND THE CLINICIAN

Dowrick considers "that recovering a sense of self, both for patients and doctors, is an essential prerequisite" for health care today.[61]

A pragmatic definition of the self is proposed by Heath: "the recipient and the holder of all subjective experience built up in stories and memories over a life time, an agent with at least some ability to shape and influence that experience".[62]

Definition of Self of the Clinician

When swimming against the stream of the steadily more instrumental healthcare environments, clinicians must rise above the understandable tendency to blame the patient or rage against the system. The question becomes: "To what extent can the capacity to disengage from . . . an overactive mind, contribute to how practitioners might reframe the problems of practice and discern wise action in practice",[63] or as Cassell puts it: one needs "the skill of a quiet mind" to pay "attention to your own words, mannerisms and presentation to the patient".[9] It helped the clinician, in the book *A Fortunate Woman*, to learn that "less experienced doctors had a higher proportion of heart sink patients . . . and that externalizing this as the patients' problem was fundamentally flawed".[5] "This discovery radically changed the doctor's approach to certain troubling . . . patients, who no longer rattled her cage . . . and over time it made her happier in the job".[5]

Patienthood, the Self of the Patient

The role of the patient is becoming more recognized, with the recent swing from office to community, from being cared for to self care and self management. Patients "are increasingly accountable . . . have agency . . . mobilise capacity . . . absorb adversity". Dowrick calls this "the proactive work of patient hood".[64]

The Dyad: Specifics of Relationship Building

The interactions of patients with clinicians bring the two distinct persons together in a joint enterprise of deep connection.

> Understanding and recognising the other, the patient, as a self with intrinsic worth, offers liberation from restricted . . . attachments . . . and reduces the risk of doctor-centred encounters. . . . It encourages us to engage with the selves of our patients, with skill, curiosity and wonder.[64]

Iona Heath suggests two important aspects of relationship building: attention and dialogue, as channels using the self of the clinician to help patients.

> Attention is essential and is profoundly rewarding to both patients and clinician . . . failures of attention to the subjective reality of the patient can have serious repercussions. . . . If crucial dimensions of the subjective experience are ignored, a key aetiological factor may be missed so that the diagnosis becomes partial or inadequate, or even wrong.[62]

Attention to the subjective experience of a patient starts with a willingness to share but "the actual work of recovering the self, depends on dialogue".[62]

Heath goes on to say that clinicians have a responsibility:

> to attempt to relieve distress and suffering and, to this end, to enable the sick to benefit from advances in biomedical science while protecting people from its

harms. Clinicians need to be able to see and hear each successive patient in the fullness of their humanity, to minimise fear, to locate hope (however limited), to explain symptoms and diagnosis in language that make sense to each different patient, to witness courage and endurance and to accompany suffering. There is no biomedical evidence that I know of that helps with any of this.[62]

TRANSFERENCE AND COUNTERTRANSFERENCE

All human relationships – and in particular, therapeutic relationships – are influenced by the phenomena of transference and countertransference. Many of the dimensions (i.e. compassion, power, constancy, healing, and self-awareness) of the patient–doctor relationship are influenced by transference and countertransference.

Transference is a ubiquitous phenomenon that is pervasive in our daily lives and happens outside of our conscious awareness.[65–67] Transference is a process whereby the patient unconsciously projects, onto individuals in their current life, thoughts, behaviors, and emotional reactions that originate with other significant relationships from childhood onward.[65, 66] In other words, past experiences that individuals have held in their unconscious are projected "onto a new experience, acting like a kind of colored filter which changes the appearance of the experience".[66] This can include feelings of love, hate, ambivalence, and dependency. The greater the current attachment, such as a significant patient–clinician relationship, the more likely that transference will occur. Transference, while often perceived as a negative phenomenon, actually helps build the connection between patient and practitioner.[68] Frequently, clinicians are intimidated by the concept of transference, which has its roots in psychoanalytic theory, viewing it as something mysterious and to be avoided. However, knowledge of the patient's transference reaction, either positive or negative, assists the clinician in understanding how patients experience their world and how past relationships influence current behavior.

Transference can occur during any stage of the patient–clinician relationship and be activated by any number of events. For example, when the capabilities of seriously ill patients are impaired or when patients are overwhelmed by the ramifications implied by a specific diagnosis, they may respond to their clinician in an uncharacteristic manner. They may return to a position of dependency and neediness, which is more a reflection of unresolved past relationships than of their current relationship with the clinician. During this time of crisis, patients may seek the care and comfort that was absent in the past. Conversely, they may respond by becoming distant and aloof, indicating the return to a stoical stance adopted in their early years when they were forced to assume a position of pseudo-independence and self-sufficiency. Take, for example, the story presented in Chapter 4 of Isabel, whose early years were plagued by disappointment and abandonment. Would her transference reaction be one of hostility and distancing behavior toward the clinician to avoid rejection again? Conversely, would Isabel exhibit a positive transference in response to the trust, empathy, and caring she experiences in the relationship with her clinician? Indeed, her transference reactions may fluctuate depending on her degree of vulnerability and sense of safety in the therapeutic relationship.

Like transference, countertransference is an unconscious process that occurs when the clinician responds to patients in a manner similar to significant past relationships.[65, 66, 69] Practitioners need to be alert to what triggers certain reactions – that is, unresolved personal issues, stress, or value conflicts. It is here that self-awareness, coupled with the ability for self-observation during the consultation, is paramount.

Internal manifestations of countertransference are reflected in the practitioner's emotional responses, such as anger, sadness, boredom, anxiety, fear, arousal, envy, and gladness;[65, 66, 68, 69] whereas, behavioral or external manifestations of countertransference include, for example, not listening attentively, misjudging the patient's level of feeling, excessive advice giving, becoming overly identified with the patient's problem, gaining vicarious pleasure in the patient's story, engaging in power struggles with the patient, running late, or running overtime.[65, 66, 68]

The origins and significance of practitioners' countertransference are as varied and complex as their patients. For example, the clinician who finds himself repeatedly giving advice to depressed female patients may be attempting to rescue the patient from her sorrow in a way similar to how he responded to his own mother's chronic angst. The demanding and obstinate behaviors of a patient may in turn activate behaviors on the part of the physician, such as avoidance or engaging in power struggles, responses that may have been characteristic of the doctor's relationship with her domineering father.

While historically countertransference was perceived as a negative phenomenon that needed to be "managed" and at best eradicated, more recent conceptualizations of countertransference indicate how clinicians' successful understanding of their countertransference reactions can assist them in both understanding their patients and the therapeutic relationship.[65, 69] Schaeffer writes: "Countertransference opens the door to 'a slice of life': the client's life, the therapist's own life, and the life that client and therapist share in the therapeutic process".[65]

The primary tool for effectively using transference and countertransference to aid and deepen the patient–clinician relationship is self-awareness. Such self-knowledge is a requirement for the clinician's accurate recognition of both transference and countertransference. Self-evaluation and working with others may help practitioners gain valuable insights which will ultimately strengthen relationships with patients and also increase their own comfort and satisfaction in their provision of care.[70]

CASE EXAMPLE

"Why is this woman so frustrating?" Dr Fournier blurted out loud. Alone in her car she felt embarrassed, but at the same time relieved by her outburst. After leaving her home visit with Mrs Cirneski, she felt exasperated and unsure about how to best move forward in the care of her 85-year-old patient.

Mrs Cirneski had multiple chronic conditions, including congestive heart failure, chronic obstructive pulmonary disease, diabetes, and arthritis. In the past few months, there had been several admissions to hospital and it had taken some time to untangle Mrs Cirneski's complex medical problems. For the most part Dr Fournier had felt as if she had been lurching from one health crisis to the next. Just when Dr Fournier thought her patient's health had stabilized and the appropriate treatment regimens were in place, the bottom fell out. Mrs Cirneski was diagnosed with a recurrence of her breast cancer – she was riddled with metastases.

As Mrs Cirneski rapidly declined, home visits became necessary, which were often chaotic and difficult to navigate. Her little bungalow was often crowded with neighbors and friends who had come to sit with Mrs Cirneski and bring her plate after plate of her native food. Frequently, one or more of her 11 grandchildren would be at her bedside, looking at old photo albums that bore witness to Mrs Cirneski's life and family. On one hand Dr Fournier deeply appreciated the outpouring of support being showered on her patient; on the other hand, trying to "doctor" in this utter confusion unsettled her.

Dr Fournier was baffled by her emotional response to this warm and well-loved woman. No other patient in her practice elicited similar distress. As Dr Fournier arrived at the clinic, she resolved to discuss her unease with a colleague. Later that day, following a busy afternoon treating coughs and colds, fevers and rashes, and muscle sprains, Dr Fournier shared her struggles with one of her partners.

As Dr Fournier began to recount her story of caring for Mrs Cirneski, her eyes welled up with tears. Initially taken aback by this uncharacteristic emotional response, it dawned on Dr Fournier how Mrs Cirneski's life had many parallels to her own Grandmamma.

Like her patient, Dr Fournier's grandmother had emigrated from her homeland, married, raised a large boisterous family, and been a pillar in her community. Her grandmother had also suffered from many health issues, similar to Mrs Cirneski. However, the startling revelation, as Dr Fournier's story tumbled out, was how she had been abroad at the time of her Grandmamma's final illness and eventual death. Dr Fournier had not returned home for her funeral – a decision she had always regretted.

Slowly Dr Fournier began to understand the emotional challenges she faced in caring for this woman who very much resembled her beloved Grandmamma. This insight offered Dr Fournier a deeper appreciation of how she could truly care for her patient and be with her until the end – amidst all the joyful chaos.

CONCLUSION

The interactive components of the patient-centered clinical method occur within the ongoing relationship. The relationship serves the integrating function and is accomplished through a sustained partnership with a patient that includes compassion, sharing power, continuity, constancy, healing, hope, awareness of the self, and transference/countertransference.

Three cases conclude this chapter. All three represent continuity and healing relationships.

The first of the three cases, "About Christine", illustrates constancy with a patient when the clinician knows the solution to the problems is beyond control.

ABOUT CHRISTINE

Jennifer K Johnson

I first met Christine when she was 14 years old. She was a foster child placed in the care of a single female patient in my practice and new to the community I worked in. I didn't see Christine often at first, other than to prescribe her birth control in her later teens. Looking back, it might have helped to try to know her better in those vulnerable years. Perhaps I could have affected the course her life took in some small way. Maybe it was already too late, given the abuse she experienced as a child.

Christine's home of origin was destructive right from the beginning. Over the years she told me her story, but always in a disconnected, factual way without emotion. Her father was addicted to drugs, and although he did not abuse Christine, he was verbally and physically abusive to her older brother who, when older, sexually abused Christine as a child. As well, Christine's father had repeatedly told her how her mother had been jealous of the attention he showered on Christine. As a result, she neglected Christine, letting her cry in her crib for hours without responding for the first few years of her life.

When her father and mother separated, Christine's mother arranged for Christine to work as a prostitute as a young teen to generate income to support the fragmented family. In desperation Christine ran away and became involved in a violent street gang in the nearby city. The police intervened, and Christine was put in foster care.

I recall Christine being friendly and direct whenever she came into the office – a style uncommon for a teen, but it made her very likable and easy to talk to. I learned much later that Christine's behavior was manipulated by her foster mother during the time they lived together. She did this by rewarding desired behavior with Percocet tablets. Christine told me this was when her battle with opiate addiction started.

After Christine left this foster home, she started using street drugs. Long after an ankle fracture healed, Christine insisted she still needed to take opiates to manage her pain during her shifts as a personal support worker. When I stopped prescribing these medications, Christine confessed she had started buying opiates on the street. It wasn't long after this confession that she found a drug rehab program and enrolled herself.

Over the years that followed, Christine also struggled intensely with her mood. She did not come into the clinic regularly but rather in bursts of effort to get better. Instead of reporting sadness or anxiety, she consistently described her mind as "not being right". Although she did not endorse psychotic symptoms, she was not well mentally. It was a challenge for her caregivers because it was difficult to separate her mood problems from the effect of the illicit drugs she was regularly using again. Despite the efforts of psychiatrists and counsellors to help her over the years, Christine did not get better. Diagnoses ranged from bipolar and ADHD to depression and anxiety. Her compliance with prescribed medications was suboptimal. Visits continued to be crisis driven, brief, and intense.

The chaos of Christine's life revealed itself most acutely when she moved in with an abusive man and started a family. In the office she was seen to be loving and attentive to her children on some visits, while on other visits she was agitated, distracted, and clearly overwhelmed. I witnessed adequate parenting when she was "clean", her children clearly attached, but inevitably Children's Aid became involved when her very young children were seen by neighbors as unattended.

Inspired to be the parent she wanted to be for her children, Christine went back to rehab again! This cycle repeated itself many times. Unfortunately, the bad times became worse, and for a while she resorted to prostitution to get money for street drugs. Her abusive husband punished her for the drug use and banned her from any methadone program. Her stints in rehab became longer, sometimes for months, with only short periods of abstinence in between. It was a dark time for Christine, and she rarely came in to see me. She moved rental homes often and was admitted for a while to a psychiatric facility for suicidal ideation in a city far from her home.

It was during a healthy period when she returned home that Christine decided to leave her husband and moved with her children to a shelter. She knew the hold her ex-husband had on her was making her sicker. Although she managed for a while after, living in her own place with her children, the drugs inevitably caught up with her. When Christine's children failed to show up at the elementary school, Children's Aid stepped in to investigate and once again found them neglected. It was sad the day her children were taken away from her and placed in protective custody. Christine reached out to me to help, but I couldn't stop them from having to go.

We have had frequent visits since that day more than a year ago. Christine is part of a methadone program now. She no longer spends entire days fixated on how she will get drugs. She is hopeful and comes in to report on her progress and to give me urine samples for drug testing that go directly to Children's Aid. She has reembraced the religion of her childhood and connected to family in a community an hour away. She says she is determined this time. She has picked herself up once again.

Numerous times I have witnessed Christine rising after falling and doing well without illicit drugs for a while. Christine's life has taught me how truly chronic addiction is. I no longer have expectations regarding her ever getting better, although I never give up hope. We have a good relationship and exchange big hugs whenever she comes into the clinic. She has a great sense of humor, wildly changing hair color, and a big laugh.

Through all these years together, I have learned that what Christine needs from me is to be nonjudgmental and a stable force in her life. I think as her family doctor, I am a familiar face, a trusted person, someone standing still, as her life spins. We don't pretend that we have the kind of relationship where she comes in seeking advice, and I respond by giving it. Our relationship is different than many of my other patient–doctor relationships. I try to make a safe place in my office where she can say out loud what has happened to her, tell me where she is going next, how tomorrow will be different . . . that she will manage someday to assemble her life into something strong enough and big enough to safely hold her kids. These stories of becoming well are incredibly important. She is not telling me the lies people with addictions sometimes tell. I believe instead that this repeated practice of describing her life as she would like it to be generates possibilities where she is in control of her life and able to stand strong and resilient. By listening and being there for these rituals, I am a witness to her hopes.

I know Christine hasn't had a lot of healthy relationships in her life, so I believe our patient–doctor relationship is the biggest thing I can offer her. She trusts my door is always open, even though she knows the limits of my power to help her.

Although I am saddened that Christine will quite possibly return to her self-destructive ways in time, I regularly remind her of the strong and healthy part of herself that thrives despite her horrible past. I think patient–physician relationships, like this one, stand out from other patient–physician relationships because they are emotionally intense, but also because we bring to them some of best of what we have to offer as family physicians – our acceptance, long-term commitment, and love.

This next case by Reis shows that clinicians often face intractable situations where their singular power is the ongoing health relationship.

YOU COULDN'T HAVE PREVENTED THIS

Olivia Reis

Erin pulls me aside at the end of the day. As the full-time nurse extraordinaire of our unit, she has her finger on the pulse of the entire practice. "I just wanted to check in", she says, eyes full of sadness. "I saw the Kooples leaving exam room eleven . . . Kate looked awful".

Kate did look awful. It was my first thought as I entered the exam room earlier that afternoon. Her skin was dull, face thin. Yet she was buzzing with energy, poised on the edge of her seat, her tired eyes focused. My second thought went to the stacks of papers, neatly tucked inside her arm.

Dan wouldn't make eye contact. His eyes pointed down, focused on the large hands folded in his lap. As he hunched in his too-small office chair, I could feel his discomfort. He is a very kind man by nature, not one for conflict. But I know this year has been painful for him, too. Kate has told me he never sits still, just jumps from one project to another. A busy mind doesn't have time to process.

I know Jamie the least. As the Kooples' youngest son, he was a part of the practice I inherited. But young adults don't often require frequent care. The first time we met was on that day, last year. I have since communicated to his parents multiple times that my door is open. But Jamie and I don't have a history, and I appreciate it's hard for him. I mean, doctors are supposed to help, aren't they? I don't imagine he felt I helped much when he found Cam's body in their garage. He sits stiffly, his back toward the door, facing his mother.

I take a deep breath. Try to convey with my eyes that I am here to listen.

Kate starts. In a nervous, pleading voice. "I need to ask this. I need to understand. I've been reading and re-reading the journal Cam left . . . and it just doesn't make sense". She glances at Dan. He doesn't look up. "Dan doesn't agree", she whispers. Dan still doesn't look up. Jamie nods. Kate continues, "Do you think it was the meds? I mean the Ativan he got in the ER. I've combed through his journal. And it seems to me the symptoms could have been the meds. Look . . ." she fans out the papers then. Dozens of pages. Photocopies of Cam's journal, marked up with her writing. Print offs of Google searches and blogs recounting personal experiences of benzodiazepine withdrawal. "I mean; how do you know? If the symptoms are caused by mental illness, or by the medication itself? How many people kill themselves from anxiety? I have anxiety myself! I know what it's like, and I would never do this, and he never said anything! I just don't understand".

I take a deep breath and think of how to respond. But it's Jamie who speaks next.

His grief is dripping off him. The room is suffocating. He seems to be more comfortable with anger, and when he speaks his voice has a quiet edge. "It's not hard to find, you know. Just type it into Google. You can withdraw even after one dose. There are so many stories of suicides. Of families reporting the same thing. I just wish doctors knew this. Didn't you learn about medication safety? You should tell people about the side effects when you give a prescription".

We sit in a moment of silence. Then "If Cam knew . . . maybe, he wouldn't have felt so alone. Maybe this wouldn't have happened".

I take another deep breath. There is a lot to unpack here.

Cam was given Ativan. Initially in the ER and then by myself with the guidance of a psychiatrist. He had severe anxiety, and I believe comorbid depression. I had tried for months to get him on a long acting antidepressant. I had communicated with him clearly that a benzodiazepine was not appropriate mono-therapy. I always discuss side effects of medication. Further, I do not think that Cam committed suicide due to benzodiazepine withdrawal. He was given a small prescription to use as needed with panic attacks; this was not a chronic scheduled medication.

Cam was very ill. It has been hard for his family to come to terms with this, given the measures Cam took to protect his loved ones from the depth of his suffering. The symptoms that Kate has pulled from his journal are the initial symptoms he presented to me with: feelings of doom, racing thoughts, obsessive concerns for his health, sensations of chest pain, and shortness of breath. The diagnosis was clear. We have had this discussion before, but I am not sure this is the information they need today. Today, the Kooples are grieving. The 1-year anniversary is approaching, and they are no closer to understanding than they were last year. I doubt they will respond kindly to a conversation describing the difference between evidence-based medicine and blog posts.

So I don't say any of this. Instead, I take another breath. Listen.

"I am not trying to place blame", Kate tears up, "it just doesn't make sense, and I need to know". This time, her voice cracks.

My heart bleeds for them. For Kate, in a time trap, reading and re-reading her son's journal, searching fruitlessly for answers. For Dan, still staring at his hands, tear marks tracking down his ruddy cheeks, desperately searching for distractions. For Jamie, who I think of often. What a trauma, to find the body of your big brother, hanging in the cold.

What the Kooples don't know is that I have done this too. I've combed through Cam's entire chart. Replayed every visit in my head, what if's eating me alive. If only he met the criteria for certification and admission. If only I could ensure he took his SSRI. If only I could have found a way to spark some hope in him. If only he told me, even just once, that he was considering suicide. His picture hangs in my office. A handsome 30-year-old man, next to the photos of newborns I delivered this year. A stark contract of life and death. I grieve him. And I also wonder.

"Would it help?" I ask. "If Cam did commit suicide for a reason like drug withdrawal, would that help?" Kate nods. "I'm not looking for blame. I am just looking for a reason; I just need to understand".

I feel helpless today. I cannot offer a solution. We were all blindsided by Cam's death. It was calculated and meticulously planned. He orchestrated the kindest suicide possible. Consideration was put into every detail: a note advising Jamie to avoid the garage and call 911, letters to each family member reminding them of his love and dismissing them of any blame, parting gifts for his siblings. This was a long, planned, and secret process. It's unlikely we could have stopped it, yet we are likely to spend forever asking "what if".

I offer compassion the best way I know how. "I am sorry for your suffering. I am so deeply sorry". We talk about suicide. Similar to our previous conversations, I explain, "The evidence shows that people who truly intend to commit suicide often don't report it. I know you spoke with him daily, but there is no way you could have known". I look at Jamie. "Even though you lived together, you couldn't have known. You couldn't have prevented this".

I take a breath and say it one more time. "You couldn't have prevented this".

I worry that part of the drive to find a reason, be it medication or something else, is so that the Kooples can finally believe it is not their fault. Maybe they want to find a cause, a focus for their anger, to prevent being angry at themselves, or worse, at Cam. I can relate more than they know. I also want a reason.

I anticipate there will be more meetings like this. At the end of the visit, I remind Kate "You can always ask. You don't need to be afraid to come here, to talk to me. I want to do anything I can to help". Kate asks me to take her papers. "Please just read them. Look into this, it may be the cause. I may help someone else". I take them.

Later that day, in Erin's office, she offers me a kind smile as I take a deep, grounding breath. "Honestly Olivia, you couldn't have prevented this".

There is still a long road of healing ahead, for all of us.

Lucassen writes the final case in this chapter. It reveals the clinician's ongoing commitment to a suffering and impoverished couple.

A MAN AND A WOMAN

Peter Lucassen

The man and the woman lived together on the first floor of a small house in our village. They were in their early 70s. Several years ago, when the older brother of the man was living there also, there had been quarrels and even fights between the brothers. There were rumors about these issues in the village. But after the death of the older man, the house was quiet again.

The man called the practice. He had pain in his chest and had tried to call the out-of-hours service in the night, but the conversation, with all its questions, had been far too complicated for him. He couldn't explain what was wrong and thus waited for the practice to open and called on Monday at 8 o'clock. I make a house call and ring the doorbell. The woman opens the door. Behind her I climb the stairs. She wears a transparent nightgown and a diaper. The man sat at the table in his underwear that was once white. The woman lit a cigarette. The table was full of lighters, cigarettes, ashtrays, pills and capsules, an empty coffee cup, pencils, keys, playing cards, nail clippers, and a fishbowl with one goldfish. The man told me his story, it was unclear as ever, but the same as the previous time, although he almost never contacted the practice. For me, this was simple. I had to call the ambulance and send him to the hospital. A few days later, the man is home again with a less well functioning heart muscle.

In our village, I see them walk together on Sundays when they play keno. The woman first and after a few meters the man, short of breath. It's always the same.

A few months later. He called again and asked if I would visit him because his foot hurt. He hadn't slept for several nights because of the pain. He had been in the hospital for this problem but when he returned home, the foot was still hurting a lot. This is a very difficult problem for patients (and their doctors) with diabetes and narrow arteries in their legs. The air in the room had turned blue from smoke. The woman told me that they recently decided to open the window when smoking because this is healthier. They can't quit smoking. While I'm paying attention to his foot, the woman calmly continues preparing her bread and a cup of tea for her evening meal. After having finished dressing the wound and writing a prescription for painkillers, I politely refuse the woman's invitation for me to join their evening meal.

Half a year later. The man is at home. He is alone. She has left the door open. I go upstairs and greet him warmly. He says hello but less enthusiastically than before. He also does not give me the usual clap on my shoulder. His face was red. His mouth, never an example of cleanliness, is filthy. The upper part of his removable dentures hung halfway down his opened mouth; this only happens when the man is speaking. He fidgets with the hands. It seems as if he experiences this situation as strange. He takes a seat and says nothing, which is strange. I ask him all the medical questions. He responds shaking his head no. I ask him where his wife is and ask him to call her. He cannot push the right numbers. I try it myself. The woman rushes up the stairs invoking the Lord in pejorative terms. Stuttering raw and loudly in our dialect. I ask her how long a time her husband had been like this. Indignantly, she said not long. I am concerned and examine him as much as possible. I suspect a stroke. I send him to the hospital again. Two days later, I visit the man in the hospital. He does not say much, he is tired. When I say good-bye, he reaches out and squeezes my hand firmly. Several days later he dies.

Two weeks later. I planned to visit the woman to give her support after the death of the man. After ringing the doorbell, she comes down the stairs, opens the door and greats me enthusiastically. She gestures to me to come and see the house. She is very proud. Everything is white and clean, the dining room, the sleeping room, the kitchen, and the bathroom. Her daughter is sitting at the table, smoking a cigarette. She is very lean and wears a white shirt and white pants. We join her at the table. Her daughter has done all the work cleaning up the house. In the meantime, the woman was watching her daughter's children, did her laundry, did the shopping and the cooking. The woman fervently speaks about everything they did, about how she had enjoyed working and being together. And then, unexpectedly, she starts to cry.

The next time she comes to the practice, she calls me by my first name: "Peter, it's been 4 months now, and I miss him every day". She tells me about her physical complaints. I examine her and tell her what's wrong. Then I ask how she is doing. With both her hands she takes mine and there we sit, hands clasped across my desk. She held my hands firmly, warm, and long. We did not speak. With a smile on her face, she left the consultation room.

REFERENCES

1. Stewart M, Brown JB, Weston WW, McWhinney IR, McWilliam CL, Freeman TR. *Patient-Centered Medicine: Transforming the Clinical Method*. 2nd edition. Radcliffe Medical Press, Oxford, UK, 2003.
2. Stewart M, Brown JB, Weston WW, McWhinney IR, McWilliam CL, Freeman TR. *Patient-Centered Medicine: Transforming the Clinical Method*. 3rd edition. Radcliffe Publishing Ltd, Oxford UK, 2014.
3. Hodges BD, Paech G, Bennett J. *"Without Compassion There Is No Healthcare" Leading with Care in a Technological Age*. McGill-Queen's University Press, Montreal, 2020: xiii, 8.
4. Loxterkamp D. Whither family medicine? Our past, future, and enduring scope of practice. *Family Medicine*. 2019 Jul;51(7):555–558. Doi: 10.22454/FamMed.2019.633317.
5. Morland P. *A Fortunate Woman: A Country Doctor's Story*. CPI Group (UK) Ltd, Croydon, 2022: 56, 80–81, 105, 120, 128, 141, 214.
6. Spence JC. *The Purpose and Practice of Medicine: Selections from the Writings of Sir James Spence*. Oxford University Press, London, UK, 1960.
7. Stewart M. Continuity, care, and commitment: The course of patient-clinician relationships. *Annals of Family Medicine* 2004 Sep/Oct;2(5):388–390.
8. Loxterkamp D. The headwaters of family medicine. *The BMJ*. 2008;337:3.
9. Cassell E. *The Nature of Healing: The Modern Practice of Medicine*. Oxford University Press, New York, 2013: 19, 81, 83, 111, 225–226.
10. Hodges BD, Paech G, Bennett J. *"Without Compassion There Is No Healthcare" Leading with Care in a Technological Age*. McGill-Queen's University Press, Montreal, 2020: 20.
11. Phillips WR, Uygur JM, Egnew TR. A comprehensive clinical model of suffering. *Journal of the American Board of Family Medicine*. 2023 March–April;36(2):344–355.

12. Blane D, Mercer SW. Compassionate health care: Is empathy the key? *Journal of Holistic Healthcare*. 2011;8;3:18–21.
13. Mercer SW, Reynolds WJ. Empathy and quality of care. *British Journal of General Practice*. 2002 October;S9–S12. Quality Supplement.
14. Rudebeck CE. Imagination and empathy in the consultation. *British Journal of General Practice*. 2002;52:450–453.
15. Loxterkamp D. The headwaters of family medicine. *BMJ*. 2008 Dec 9;3, 337.
16. Houwen J, Lucassen PL, Stappers HW, Assendelft WJ, van Dulmen S, Olde Hartman TC. Improving GP communication in consultations on medically unexplained symptoms: A qualitative interview study with patients in primary care. *British Journal of General Practice*. 2017 Oct;67(663):e716–e723. Doi: 10.3399/bjgp17X692537.
17. Hodges BD, Paech G, Bennett J. *"Without Compassion There Is No Healthcare" Leading with Care in a Technological Age*. McGill-Queen's University Press, Montreal, 2020: 18, 21.
18. McWhinney IR. *A Call to Heal – Reflections on a Life in Family Medicine*. Benchmark Press, Saskatoon, Canada, 2012, 88.
19. Phillips WR, Uygur JM, Egnew TR. A comprehensive clinical model of suffering. *Journal of the American Board of Family Medicine* 2023 March–April;36(2):347.
20. Balint E, Courtenay AE, Hull S, Julian P. *The Doctor, the Patient, and the Group*. Routledge, London, 1993.
21. Virshup BB, Oppenberg AA, Coleman MM. Strategic risk management: Reducing malpractice claims through more effective patient-doctor communication. *American Journal of Medical Quality*. 1999;14(4):153–159.
22. Feinstein AR. *Clinical Judgement*. Williams & Wilkins, Baltimore, 1967.
23. Selwyn PA. The island. *Annals of Family Medicine*. 2008;6(1):78–79.
24. McWilliam CL, Stewart M, Brown JB, McNair S, Desai K, Patterson ML, Del Maestro N, Pittman BJ. Creating empowering meaning: An interactive process of promoting health with chronically ill older Canadians. *Health Promotion International*. 1997;12(2):111–123.
25. Jaouad S. *Between Two Kingdoms*. Random House, New York, NY, 2021, 61.
26. Mercer S. Empathy is key. In: *Working Towards People Powered Health: Insights from Practitioners*. NESTA, London, UK. 2012: 25.
27. Fugelli P. Trust – In general practice. *British Journal of General Practice*. 2001;51:575–579.
28. Jani B, Bikker AP, Higgins M, et al. Patient centredness and the outcome of primary care consultations with patients with depression in areas of high and low socioeconomic deprivation. *British Journal of General Practice*. 2012;62(601):e576–e581.
29. Jayadevappa R, Chhatre S. Patient centered care-a conceptual model and review of the state of the art. *Open Health Services and Policy Journal*. 2011;4(1).
30. Stewart M. Reflections on the doctor-patient relationship: From evidence and experience. *British Journal of General Practice* October 2005;55:793–801.
31. Bernstein SF, Rehkopf D, Tuljapurkar S, Horvitz CC. Poverty dynamics, poverty thresholds and mortality: An age-stage Markovian model. *PloS One*. 2018 May 16;13(5):e0195734.
32. Langberg EM, Dyhr L, Davidsen AS. Development of the concept of patient-centeredness – A systematic review. *Patient Education and Counseling*. 2019 Jul 1;102(7):1228–1236.
33. Moore GF, Audrey S, Barker M, Bond L, Bonell C, Hardeman W, Moore L, O'Cathain A, Tinati T, Wight D, Baird J. Process evaluation of complex interventions: Medical Research Council guidance. *BMJ*. 2015 Mar 19;350:h1258. Doi: 10.1136/bmj.h1258.

34. Sturgiss EA, Peart A, Richard L, Ball L, Hunik L, Chai TL, Lau S, Vadasz D, Russell G, Stewart M. Who is at the centre of what? A scoping review of the conceptualisation of 'centredness' in healthcare. *BMJ Open.* 2022 May 2;12(5):e059400. Doi: 10.1136/bmjopen-2021-059400.

35. Tuckett D, Boulton M, Olson C, Williams A. *Meetings Between Experts: An Approach to Sharing Ideas in Medical Consultations.* Tavistock, New York, NY, 1985.

36. Scott GS, Cohen D, DiCicco-Bloom B, Miller WL, Stange KC, Crabtree BF. Understanding healing relationships in primary care. *Annals of Family Medicine* 2008;6:315–322.

37. Bartz R. Beyond the biopsychosocial model: New approaches to doctor-patient interactions. *Journal of Family Practice.* 1999;48(8):601–607.

38. Bartz R. *Interpretive Dialogue: A Multi-Method Qualitative Approach for Studying Doctor-Patient Interactions.* Paper presented at the Annual Meeting of the North American Primary Care Research Group, San Diego, CA, 1993.

39. Charon R. *Narrative Medicine: Honoring the Stories of Illness.* Oxford University Press, Inc., New York, NY. 2006.

40. Bright FA, Boland P, Rutherford SJ, Kayes NM, McPherson KM. Implementing a client-centered approach in rehabilitation: An autoethnography. *Disability and Rehabilitation.* 2012;34(12):997–1004. Doi: 10.3109/09638288.2011.629712.

41. Goodyear-Smith F, Buetow S. Power issues in the doctor-patient relationship. *Health Care Analysis.* 2001;9:449–462.

42. Blane D, Mercer SW. Compassionate health care: Is empathy the key? *Journal of Holistic Healthcare.* 2011;8;3:18–21.

43. Herbert C. Stories in family medicine commentary: The power of stories. *Canadian Family Physician.* 2013 Jan;59:62–65.

44. Freeman GK. Progress with relationship continuity 2012, a British perspective. *International Journal of Integrated Care.* 2012;12;29:1–6.

45. Nowak DA, Sheikhan NY, Naidu SC, Kuluski K, Upshur REG. Why does continuity of care with family doctors matter? Review and qualitative synthesis of patient and physician perspectives. *Canadian Family Physician.* 2021 Sep;67(9):679–688. Doi: 10.46747/cfp.6709679.

46. Pereira Gray DJ, Sidaway-Lee K, White E, Thorne A, Evans PH. Continuity of care with doctors-a matter of life and death? A systematic review of continuity of care and mortality. *BMJ Open.* 2018 Jun 28;8(6):e021161. Doi: 10.1136/bmjopen-2017-021161.

47. Cassell EJ. *The Nature of Suffering and the Goals of Medicine.* Oxford University Press, New York, 1991: 78.

48. Stein M. *The Lonely Patient: How We Experience Illness.* HarperCollins, New York, 2007: 53, 77, 93, 139, 163.

49. Frank AW. *The Renewal of Generosity: Illness, Medicine, and How to Live.* University of Chicago Press, Chicago, 2004.

50. Loxterkamp D. The Headwaters of family medicine. *BMJ.* 2008;337:2575.

51. Seifert Jr MH. *Qualitative Designs for Assessing Interventions in Primary Care: Examples from Medical Practice. Assessing Interventions: Traditional and Innovative Methods.* Sage, Thousand Oaks, CA, 1992 Aug 20: 89–95.

52. McWilliam CL, Stewart M, Brown JB, et al. Creating empowering meaning: An interactive process of promoting health with chronically Ill older Canadians. *Health Promotion International.* 1997;12(2):111–123.

53. Kinsella EA, Pitman A (eds). *Phronesis as Professional Knowledge: Practical Wisdom in the Professions.* Sense Publishers, Rotterdam, Boston, 2012.

54. Miksanek T. On caring for 'difficult' patients. *Health Affairs*. 2008;27(5):1422–1428.
55. Frank AW. Reflective healthcare practice: Claims, phonesis and dialogue, chapter 4. In: Kinsella EA, Pitman A (eds). *Phronesis as Professional Knowledge: Practical Wisdom in the Professions*. Sense Publishers, Rotterdam, Boston, 2012.
56. Scott GS, Cohen D, DiCicco-Bloom B, Miller WL, Stange KC, Crabtree BF. Understanding healing relationships in primary care. *Annals of Family Medicine* 2008;6:315–322.
57. Back AL, Bauer-Wu SM, Rushton CH, Halifax J. Compassionate silence in the patient-clinician encounter: A contemplative approach. *Journal of Palliative Medicine*. 2009 Dec;12(12):1113–1117. Doi: 10.1089/jpm.2009.0175.
58. Kinsella EA. Practitioner reflection and judgement as phonesis, chapter 3. In: Kinsella EA, Pitman A (eds). *Phronesis as Professional Knowledge: Practical Wisdom in the Professions*. Sense Publishers, Rotterdam, Boston. 2012: 41.
59. Stein HF. What is therapeutic in clinical relationships? *Family Medicine*. 1985 Sep–Oct;17(5):188–194.
60. McWhinney IR. The need for a transformed clinical method. In: Stewart M, Roter D (eds). *Communicating with Medical Patients*. Sage, Newbury Park, CA, 1989: 82.
61. Dowrick C (ed). *Person-Centered Primary Care: Searching for Self*. Routledge, Abingdon, Oxfordshire. 2018: x.
62. Heath I. Subjectivity of patients and doctors. In: Dowrick C (ed). *Person-Centered Primary Care: Searching for Self*. Routledge, Abingdon, Oxfordshire, 2018: 77, 83, 87–88.
63. Kinsella EA. Practitioner reflection and judgement as phonesis, chapter 3. In: Kinsella EA, Pitman A (eds). *Phronesis as Professional Knowledge: Practical Wisdom in the Professions*. Sense Publishers, Rotterdam, Boston, 2012: 43.
64. Dowrick C (ed). *Person-Centered Primary Care: Searching for Self*. Routledge, Abingdon, Oxfordshire, 2018: 135.
65. Schaeffer JA. *Transference and Countertransference in Non-analytic Therapy. Double-Edge Swords*. University Press of America, Lanham, MD, 2007: 28.
66. Murdin L. *Understanding Transference. The Power of Patterns in the Therapeutic Relationships*. Palgrave Macmillan, Hampshire, UK, 2010: 9.
67. Berman CW, Bezkor MF. Transference in patients and caregivers. *American Journal of Psychotherapy*. 2010;64(1):107–114. Doi: 10.1176/appi.psychotherapy.2010.64.1.107.
68. Centeno-Gándara LA. Improving the physician-patient relationship utilizing psychodynamic psychology: A primer for health professionals. *Health Psychology and Behavioral Medicine*. 2021 Jan 1;9(1):338–349.
69. Hayes JA, Gelso CJ, Hummel AM. Managing countertransference. *Psychotherapy (Chic)*. 2011 Mar;48(1):88–97. Doi: 10.1037/a0022182.
70. Goldberg PE. The physician-patient relationship: Three psychodynamic concepts that can be applied to primary care. *Archives of Family Medicine*. 2000;9(10):116–148.
71. Houwen J. Improving GP communication in consultations on medically unexplained symptoms: a qualitative interview study with patients in primary care, chapter 3. In: Houwen J. *Clinical assessment as therapy in managing medically unexplained symptoms*. (Doctoral dissertation), Nijmegen, The Netherlands: Radboud Repository, 2022: 39.

PART THREE

Applications of Patient-Centered Principles in a Variety of Health Care Contexts

INTRODUCTION

MOIRA STEWART

This part of the book addresses the question of relevance of the patient-centered clinical method in the current health care context. Team-based care is pervasive and may be enhanced by patient-centered care. In an effort to reinforce team-based care, we propose a method for creating and sustaining a team using four components that are parallel to the patient-centered clinical method, in Chapter 8. Technology is ubiquitous in our world today, in general and in health care. In Chapter 9, we introduce the idea that patient-centered care uses prescriptive technologies in the service of humanistic care. The chapter presents ideas and tips for clinicians to improve patient-centered care when they use patient portals, electronic medical records, and virtual care by telephone and video.

DOI: 10.1201/9781003394679-10

8

Team-Centered Approach: How to Build and Sustain a Team

MOIRA STEWART, JUDITH BELLE BROWN, BRIDGET L RYAN, THOMAS
R FREEMAN, CAROL L MCWILLIAM, JOAN MITCHELL, LYNN BROWN,
LYNN SHAW, AND VERA HENDERSON

Acknowledging that health care often takes place in the context of teams rather than single practitioners, we ask the following questions: Does patient-centered care enhance team care or not? And does team care embellish or impede patient-centered care? Is it possible for these to be mutually reinforcing and if so, how?

Our past experience in articulating the parallels between patient-centered care and learner-centered education led us to consider whether a similar parallel process might be helpful in thinking through positive attributes and processes to enhance team function. Knowing that modeling a behavior or relationship is one effective way to educate a group of trainees or improve care in a health care organization, we propose a process of team development that mirrors the patient-centered clinical method, potentially enhancing both.

We present a parallel process of a team-centered approach based on the four components of patient-centered care. The team-centered approach is presented as a diagram in Figure 8.1 and outlined more fully in Box 8.1. The first two components – Component 1, exploring both the disciplines and the members' personal experiences of their discipline, and Component 2, understanding the whole person of the team member – focus on the individual team members, asking them to reflect on and share their own discipline and some of their life history and personal context. Components 3 and 4 consider the team itself and the attributes that characterize the team.

The first component encourages each team member to be ready to share and to learn about others regarding each member discipline's formal scope of practice as described by their respective licensing body. The implication of this component is that team members become prepared to explain their legal and sanctioned role of practice in relation to other clinicians. It is somewhat surprising how common it is that these roles are implicit, unlearned, and out of date. This first step toward seamless team care firmly grounds the team in the realities of their current policy context.

Simply knowing the official scope of practice of the other disciplines may not be enough. Another important feature of this component is for healthcare team members to share and learn about all members' personal experiences of their discipline – for example, their unique

DOI: 10.1201/9781003394679-11

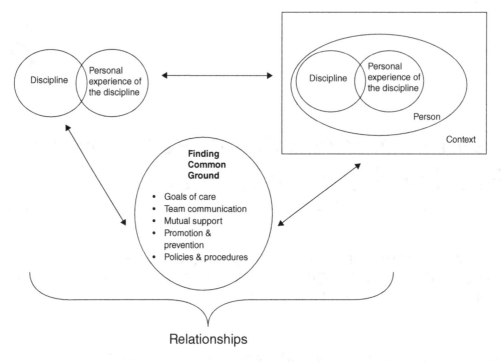

Relationships

Figure 8.1 Team-Centered Approach: The Four Components

BOX 8.1: Team-Centered Approach – How to Start and Sustain a Team

1 Exploring both the disciplines and the members' personal experiences of their discipline:
   - the discipline as described by the licensing body, scope of practice
   - the members' personal experiences of their discipline.

2 Understanding the whole person of each team member:
   - the "person" (life history and personal context, perceived ability to respond to change and manage conflict)
   - the context (opportunities and constraints of the team environment, time available for each individual).

3 Finding common ground – toward the shared language, culture, and philosophy of the team care:
   - underlying goals of care
   - formal and informal team communication (meetings, electronic medical record)
   - supporting one another's strengths, knowledge, and skills
   - promotion of team health and prevention of team dissonance, leadership issues
   - policies and procedures including regarding conflict resolution.

4 Enhancing ongoing team relationships:
   - sharing power
   - trust
   - empathy, respect, genuineness
   - individual clinicians' commitment to the team
   - self-awareness, awareness of others.

professional history and ways of thinking about health care. This sharing may open everyone's eyes to the myriad of ways formal roles can be enacted and utilized[1] and may bring the formal roles to life. Also, they may learn what they like about their role and what aspects they find challenging. Additionally, this exchange is especially important for teams who are at the beginning of their journey together. Knowledge of one another's formal discipline and experience within the discipline is an interprofessional competency outlined by the Canadian National Interprofessional Competency Framework.[2] Further, we contend that the mutual process of learning about each other's discipline promotes mutual respect and enables a more trusting interprofessional practice.[1, 3]

The second component stresses the need for understanding the whole person of each team member. The reflection, necessary for a team member in preparation for sharing their own story, may help prepare the clinician for the experience of being on a new team. Members will be encouraged to share relevant aspects of their life history, personal context, and their perceived ability to respond to change and manage conflict. As well, sharing one another's understanding of the team's current context, in terms of each member's perceptions of the opportunities and constraints of the team environment, may assist in getting the team started and, ultimately, sustain the team. The team's context can include such things as the location of team members (e.g., co-located or not)[3, 4] and the accessibility of team leaders.[1, 3] Such sharing fosters mutual understanding of team members as individuals, thereby enabling each to relate to the others in ways that promote effective team functioning. Also, studies show how social activities and opportunities for sharing life events are created and maintained by teams as they develop their unique routines and rituals. Social activities and sharing life events foster relationships and team cohesion.[1, 3, 5-7]

Also, social relationships in the workplace can contribute to both personal fulfilment and pride and to the maintenance of effective teams.[8]

The third component, finding common ground, represents the shift from the focus on the team members sharing their history and experiences to all team members co-creating the new team environment, moving toward a shared language, culture, and philosophy.[1, 3, 6, 9] Components 1 and 2 have provided some of the necessary building blocks of information and experiences from the past.

One element of the third component, finding common ground as a team, is to outline the underlying broad principles and goals of care. Some of this work may be explicitly shared early in the team's development; some of it may also become revealed as the team functions in its first weeks and months. A mechanism to encourage finding common ground as a team is to specify the formal and informal communication strategies of the team. For example, will team meetings occur and, if so, what is their agenda? Would team huddles suffice? Will the main communication strategy among the clinicians be the patient chart, usually an electronic medical record? If so, the approach to recording the clinical notes should be discussed and agreed upon. Regularly scheduled team meetings may be a vital mechanism for communication on the team. The need for meetings builds on findings reported in prior studies.[1, 3, 6, 7, 10-13] Craigie and Hobbs have described team meetings as a safe place to raise issues and to participate in a problem-solving process that is both respectful and collaborative.[11] These opportunities can both serve to build team cohesion and develop creative strategies for sustainment when teams are confronted by stress or conflict.[14] As meetings themselves can be a source of stress if inadequate time and remuneration become an issue,[15] and the location and timing of meetings can create tension on the team, particularly when certain agenda items are viewed by some members as mundane or not relevant to their role function.[16] Thus, clinical and administrative meetings may need to be held at separate times.[17] When this is not feasible it is important to create distinct agendas for each component of the meeting, including identification of the leadership or chair of designated agenda items. Teams must collectively agree upon required mandatory attendance by all members versus those meetings that are pertinent to specific disciplines only.[17] These issues need to be addressed in order for optimal communication to occur.

Informal communication is an important part of the daily interactions of the team members as they work together. Communication about patient care issues needs to be immediate. Ellingson has described this as "backstage communication," which occurs outside of formal team meetings and is essential in the provision of patient care.[18] Hallway consultations may remain the preferred means of communication for clinical as well as business matters that are time sensitive. As teams grow in size, the hallway consultation may not be an effective communication strategy for administrative or organizational matters, but it may remain critical for core team communication regarding patient care. Hence, the accessibility and physical proximity of team members is essential.[3, 19] When physical proximity is not possible, additional effort was be made to ensure opportunities for informal communication.[4] Approachability is also key.

Another element of finding common ground in a team is supporting each other's strengths, knowledge, and skills.[1] The extent to which this is done becomes one of the shared philosophies of the team. The team learns about these individual team members' attributes through successfully exploring the disciplines and members' personal experiences (Component 1) and understanding the other team members' personal and professional context (Component 2), but also by observing the contributions over time as part of finding common ground (Component 3).

Another element moving the team toward a shared language, culture, and philosophy may be the ways in which the team promotes team health and prevents team dissonance.[1, 3] Inherent in this element will be mutual agreement on policies and procedures through mutual discussion and efforts to test out approaches. For example, timely follow up of patients discharged from hospital to primary health care requires an organized approach, as various team members address different aspects of the community-based care.[20] Further, such policies need to attend explicitly to conflict resolution processes that can be followed early and equitably.

Role boundary issues, scope of practice, and accountability have been persistently identified as sources of team conflict in the literature.[21] Even though there is extensive documentation of these conflictual issues in the literature, accompanied by helpful suggestions on how to address them, they continue to disable team functioning in hospitals[22, 23] and in the community.[24] An important team strategy in addressing conflict may be the development and active use of conflict resolution protocols.[1, 3, 25] It is important to recognize that conflict is normal and inevitable in any group of individuals. Attempts to avoid it lead to misunderstandings and may contribute to errors in patient care. In effective teams, all members take responsibility for clarifying disagreements and misunderstandings and hold one another accountable for following through on commitments.[1] Teams may benefit from learning to use frameworks when discussions are particularly important.[1] These processes can help teams to find a common voice and can assist in broadening and strengthening the team's ability to succeed.

The fourth component of a team-centered approach is enhancing the ongoing team relationships. As clinical care transpires and team members gain experience with one another and with the cadre of shared patients, the ongoing relationships mature. One element of the team approach to relationships stems directly from the development of a common philosophy,[1, 3] one that encompasses sharing power. This is a requirement of a patient-centered approach, and it is equally germane to the team approach. Clinicians need to reframe their notion of particular aspects of care as belonging to their discipline – instead, recognizing that other disciplines have skills and interests in that domain too.[3] Team structures that place individuals in less powerful positions could be a barrier to team functioning. Prior work has focused primarily on the hierarchical relationship between doctors and nurses and the inherent conflict in this dyad.[21, 26] More widespread recognition of nursing as a professional discipline has contributed to an increase in the status of nurses within the healthcare system. While nurses may have achieved more equality in the team environment, other team members with less status remain vulnerable.[24] A literature review by Mickan and Rodger on characteristics of effective teamwork suggests that team functioning is impeded when the concerns and views of team members are devalued or dismissed.[27]

Another element, crucial in responsible clinical practice, is trust. Members must trust their team's processes if they are to provide superb communication and high-level clinical care. When trust is broken, the processes outlined in finding common ground such as conflict resolution must be implemented to restore trust among team members.

Aligned with trust are the three bedrocks of ongoing counseling relationships: empathy, respect, and genuineness. Studies suggest the importance of openness, willingness to find solutions, and respect.[1, 11, 16, 27, 28] Research has also suggested that humility is the foundation on which respect is enacted.[24]

Another element of ongoing team relationships is the commitment of each individual clinician to a shared approach. The degree to which the commitment is wholehearted and steady, in contrast to partial and inconsistent, will affect the team's potential; the potential will vary depending on how narrow or broad is the vision of interprofessional practice and the commitment of participating members to this approach.[1, 3]

All of these elements of enhancing ongoing team relationships depend to some extent on the ability of each team member to nurture self-awareness and gently encourage it in others. The self-knowledge that one feels threatened by some aspects of sharing clinical roles or that one responds (positively or negatively) to some types of individuals goes a long way to smoothing out rough patches in the early and continuing evolution of teams.

As in all patient-centered care, the patient is the focus. Therefore, the patient is considered a member of a healthcare team. We propose using the grid shown in Box 8.2 as one way of helping a team that is stumbling in its effort to provide patient-centered clinical care. This may be one of the tools to decrease conflict because it explicitly offers players, including the patient, the opportunity to clarify their health issues, goals of care, and roles they would propose to take on.

The following case is used to illustrate the grid as shown in Box 8.3.

BOX 8.2: Team Members' Perspectives of Health Issues, Goals, and Roles

	Health Issues	Goals	Roles
Patient and patient's family			
Dietician			
Nurse practitioner			
Family practice nurse			
Family physician			
Social worker			
Other health practitioner, such as pharmacist; psychologist; physiotherapist; occupational therapist			

BOX 8.3: Team Members' Perspectives Regarding Martina Morgan

	Health Issues	Goals	Roles
Patient	Difficulty accepting the diagnosis Experience of mother's diabetes Fears Overwhelmed "diabetes was final blow"	Reluctant to follow plan, frozen Felt need to regain control	Not willing or able to assume a role in her care yet
Nurse	Serious diabetes Potential for sequelae	Education about foot care	Health education Advocate for patient Go at patient's pace Try to find achievable plan
Family physician	Serious diabetes	Begin insulin injections Refer to specialist	Coordinator To achieve blood sugar control Try to find achievable plan
Social worker	Mother's diabetes Father's abandonment Diabetes as final blow	Explore strengths in the family Explore husband's fears	Communicate fears and family issues Advocate for patient Try to find achievable plan
Dietician	Serious diabetes Poor diet	Tight control of diet	Diet education Try to find an achievable plan

CASE EXAMPLE

Forty-two-year-old Martina Morgan had denied the symptoms she had been experiencing over the last several months including weight loss, frequent urination, and occasional blurred vision. When she finally went to her family doctor she declared, "I have diabetes." Mrs Morgan was in fact very familiar with diabetes, as her mother had been diagnosed with diabetes over 30 years previously and had suffered from numerous related complications. However, Mrs Morgan refused to accept the doctor's recommendation that she begin insulin injections to control her very high blood sugars. Furthermore, Mrs Morgan adamantly declined a referral to an endocrinologist because, from her perspective, interventions from such specialists had hastened her mother's deterioration. In response, the family doctor, serving in the role of coordinator, invited several other clinicians including the dietician, a family practice nurse, the social worker, and the nurse practitioner to assist in addressing Mrs Morgan's serious health problems. The doctor led the first meeting of the team of the five clinicians; the patient was not asked to attend. Because the team's focus was primarily on getting Mrs Morgan's diabetes under control, efforts to coordinate care leaned toward the medical model, such as modifying her lifestyle by attending to tight diet control, providing education about proper foot care, and exploring options for financial aid to assist with her financial difficulties. In spite of each individual team member's best intentions, over the next 4 months, Mrs Morgan remained reluctant to follow their recommendations and attempts at coordinating services faltered.

The more she didn't adhere, the more the primary healthcare team intensified their efforts to educate Mrs Morgan. Also, team members were focused solely on achieving their own professional goals, specific to their discipline. While they were not engaging in turf wars there was neither a shared language nor a shared vision for Mrs Morgan's overall care plan. What the team, collectively, had failed to ascertain was Mrs Morgan's meaning of health, life aspirations, experience of illness, and her current context.

A second meeting of the five clinicians was convened at the request of the nurse practitioner. A plan was made for all the clinicians openly to ask Mrs Morgan about her past experiences with diabetes, her beliefs, and her goals for care. The social worker planned a visit to the home to include other family members. It was only after some members of the team began to question and then listen to Mrs Morgan's other issues, not only her medical problems, that change began to occur.

Mrs Morgan had been raised in a very dysfunctional family. Her father had often been out of work, and he would frequently "disappear for months" leaving the family destitute. When Mrs Morgan was 16 years old her mother had a below-knee amputation due to complications of diabetes. Her progressively deteriorating eyesight meant she could no longer administer her insulin injections, and this responsibility fell on Mrs Morgan. Even though administering the injections into her mother's stumped limb repulsed her, Mrs Morgan dutifully assumed this task. The entire experience had been very difficult for her.

Thus the diagnosis of diabetes was overwhelming for Mrs Morgan. She was afraid and uncertain about her future. She had witnessed the effects of diabetes on her mother and was terrified that she would suffer the same long-term consequences of the disease. The only way she could handle her fear was to avoid even thinking about her diabetes. For Mrs Morgan, this was the "final blow" from her family of origin.

In meeting with Mrs Morgan's husband, the social worker learned that although Mr Morgan was supportive and understanding, he was struggling to cope. Further exploration by the social worker revealed that Mr Morgan was worried that his wife was going to have a hypoglycemic reaction in her sleep and die in bed next to him. Consequently, he was often awake in the night. He found it difficult to talk to his wife about his fears and was reluctant to reveal his terror that she might die.

In her work with Mrs Morgan on diabetic self-care issues, the nurse practitioner learned that Mrs Morgan desperately needed to regain some control over her life. The nurse practitioner began to appreciate the strong link between Mrs Morgan's struggles with her own diabetes and her past family relationships. She was immobilized by what she perceived the future would bring. Her past experiences had propelled her to future possibilities and her ability to exercise current options was frozen. The nurse practitioner's task, along with other members of the team, was to help weave the past, present, and future together into an acceptable and achievable care plan for Mrs Morgan. They had to connect with her by acknowledging her story, empathizing with her terror, and, together with the patient, discovering some small steps she could tolerate as a beginning in reducing the harm caused by her diabetes.

Eventually, the social worker, visiting nurse, Mrs Morgan, and her husband began to move toward a more collaborative and interdisciplinary team approach regarding Mrs Morgan's care. They now understood the multiple reasons for Mrs Morgan's nonadherence, but it was still a hard sell to the rest of the team. A third meeting, including the five clinicians and Mrs and Mr Morgan, moved the whole team from coordinated care to a more powerful position of sharing the patient's complex story, of adjusting goals to those the patient can accept and deal with, and working at the patient's pace. The team members could begin to find ways to interact with Mrs Morgan that were empathetic to her context, compatible with her capacity, and which opened new doors to caring.

One recognizes that using a grid such as those shown in Boxes 8.2 and 8.3, may be useful for teams early on but may not be necessary for teams after they have gelled, and the role blurring makes the boxes less relevant. We suggest that treating other team members with the same principles as one treats patients, in a patient-centered or team-centered manner, could enhance both team functioning and patient-centered care, each reinforcing the other.

In the next case, the story of Francine, every team member held her story. The story and its updates were developed at team meetings and carried from the team meetings to the visits with the individual clinicians and back again. The synergy between narrative in health care and patient-centered care has been presented already in this book in Chapter 1. Narrative was the way the clinicians on this team encapsulated the information about Francine. Narrative was how Francine understood her life. The narrative was created at two levels: (1) between the patient and each clinician where the story was built together and verified repeatedly and (2) among the clinicians on the team where the story was twice removed and co-created with team members. When the team functioned well and worked at sufficient depth, the story was rich and true. However, teams can harden around a story and, to guard against such inflexibility, each team member may want to reflect or verify with the patient and report nuances back to the team. During weekly training seminars, a mixed group of doctors, nurses, social workers, and others wrote about their attachment to patients, their emotional responses to patients and families, and their attempts to imagine clinical situations from the perspectives of patients and family members; participants then read aloud their narratives to one another during a facilitated discussion.[29 (p. 307)]

In focus groups, participants reported the value of the training for team building and getting to know one another as people and their perspectives on care. They also reported that the experience "spilled over" into the team's function as a unit. In Francine's care, the team consciously held a healing narrative in mind, one of hope, in explicit contrast to the struggles she faced. As you will read, the team helped Francine identify unique health outcomes as sparkling events, opening up the possibility of a positive future.

THE TEAM WAS THE CONTAINER FOR HER STORY: CASE ILLUSTRATING A TEAM-CENTERED APPROACH

Lynn Brown

Francine was a petite woman of 41 who had experienced trauma throughout her life including witnessing the homicide of a parent, abuse in her family, and exploitation in adolescent and adult relationships. Born in a different language tradition and with little support to attend school, she found reading difficult and direction-finding overwhelming. She usually required someone to assist her in order to attend appointments.

The family lived in dense, subsidized social housing that was not safe. She described events in which she was exploited and directly threatened. These events triggered past trauma and despair. She was unable to earn her way out of this situation because of symptoms of post-traumatic stress disorder, pain, and educational limits. Physical injury to her back during a domestic assault had resulted in chronic pain, for which she had become reliant on opiates. This was an ongoing concern to her family physician. She was receiving the most basic and insecure social assistance income, frequently having to prove her inability to work and unable to manage the letters of instruction. This also triggered intense fear and despair.

Social supports were limited to one main friend who drove her to appointments. Her three adolescent children were her chief source of pride and hope for the future. She was committed to their having a better life and would rally repeatedly to perform the routines she knew they needed. Religious faith at times offered a perspective beyond her surroundings and through her art and painting she could express both suffering and hope.

Francine's family physician was her anchor. She trusted him as he had been a reliable professional in a life where trustworthiness was rare. He created a team for Francine consisting of himself, the social worker, and the nurses. Contacts with all team members were both planned and episodic, with numerous crises.

Francine was not ready to accept referrals for treatment programs. She believed she required medication for her pain. Her ideas about her health focused on the medication, with some moments when she could consider building into a different future. Her functioning when in despair was severely limited; at those times phone calls and even housework were not possible. When feeling better, her expectations of the team were that they would be interested in her children's accomplishments and that some suggestions or hope would be proffered. The team was her major source of support.

The nurses on the team would often assist by repeating information concerning appointments and at times rescheduling appointments that had been missed because of direction and transportation problems. They dealt with medication requests, at times desperate in nature, and provided an enthusiastic audience for the stories of her children. The family physician and the nurses offered some hope when she had lost hers.

The social worker spent many hours with her, sometimes at her home but mainly at the clinic, listening to her horrific story. It was clear that Francine could not participate in trauma therapy, as her life was so unsafe in the present. They began working together to find a more secure foundation for her and her family. It required hours to help her complete an application for a disability pension, which would be more secure and would provide somewhat more income. With each question on the application form, she would offer more of the details of her trauma, although this was not being directly asked. Intense, keening grief would follow. Some sessions were focused on her present despair based on her pain, both emotional and physical intertwined. Months after this, she gained the more established income of a disability pension. During the wait she would call to report the dangers in the housing environment, and the social worker began to work toward finding safer housing with crisis calls and concerns about her children intermingled. Finally a move to a safer neighborhood was accomplished after appeals, letters, and efforts to sustain her hope.

The team's presence was crucial to the social worker as she struggled to grasp what was trauma and what was medication related. The team members supported one another in understanding the story of this unique woman, and the challenges of her care were strengthening to all. It appeared that Francine's alliance with her family physician became a form of institutional transference in which all team members were seen as meriting trust. The team shared in monitoring her safety. During dark times she would call and seemed to expect there would be some helpful and knowing response from one of the team. Because she let the team know her, they became her enthusiastic audience in the times of victory. The team members were more able to respond because they knew the meaning of a positive development in a story of frequent sacrifice and turmoil. Although some services offered to her and her family were discipline-specific, all members of the team contributed to providing a container in which her story, the victories, and sadness could be held.

REFERENCES

1. Brown JB, Mulder C, Clark RE, Belsito L, Thorpe C. It starts with a strong foundation: Constructing collaborative interprofessional teams in primary health care. *Journal of Interprofessional Care* 2021 Jul–Aug;35(4):514–520. Doi: 10.1080/13561820.2020.1787360.
2. Bainbridge L, Nasmith L, Orchard C, Wood V. Competencies for interprofessional collaboration. *Journal of Physiotherapy Education.* 2010;24(1):6–11.
3. Brown JB, Ryan BL. Processes that influence the evolution of family health teams. *Canadian Family Physician.* 2018 Jun;64(6):e283–e289.
4. Ryan BL, Brown JB, Thorpe C. Moving from space to place: Reimagining the challenges of physical space in primary health care teams in Ontario. *Canadian Family Physician.* 2019 Sep;65(9):e405–e410.
5. Brown JB, Lewis L, Ellis K, Beckhoff C, Stewart M, Freeman T, Kasperski MJ. Research report: Sustaining primary health care teams: What is needed? *Journal of Interprofessional Care.* 2010;1–3. Early Online.
6. Brown JB, Ryan BL, Thorpe C, Markle EK, Hutchison B, Glazier RH. Measuring teamwork in primary care: Triangulation of qualitative and quantitative data. *Families, Systems and Health,* 2015 Sep 1;33(3):193–202. Doi: 10.1037/fsh0000109.

7. Szafran O, Torti JML, Kennett SL, Bell NR. Family physicians' perspectives on Interprofessional teamwork: Findings from a qualitative study. *Journal of Interprofessional Care* 2018 Mar;32(2):169–177. Doi: 10.1080/13561820.2017.1395828.

8. Hodson, R. Work life and social fulfillment: Does social affiliation at work reflect a carrot or a stick. *Social Science Quarterly.* 2004;85(2):221–239.

9. Marra M, Angouri J. Investigating the negotiation of identity: A view from the field of workplace discourse. In: Angouri J, Marra M (eds). *Constructing Identities at Work.* London: Palgrave Macmillan, 2011. Doi: 10.1057/9780230360051_1.

10. Apker J, Propp KM, Zabava Ford WS, Hofmeister N. Collaboration, credibility, compassion, and coordination: Professional nurse communication skill sets in health care team interactions. *Journal of Professional Nursing* 2006;22(3):180–189.

11. Craigie FC Jr, Hobbs RF III. Exploring the organizational culture of exemplary community health centre practices. *Family Medicine.* 2004;36(10):733–738.

12. Brown JB, Lewis L, Ellis K, Stewart M, Freeman T, Kasperski MJ. Mechanisms for communicating on primary health care teams. *Canadian Family Physician.* 2009 Dec;55(12):1216–1222.

13. Bodenheimer T, Ghorob A, Willard-Grace R, Grumbach K. The ten building blocks of high-performing primary care. *Annals of Family Medicine.* 2014 Mar;12(2):166–171. Doi: 10.1370/afm.1616.

14. Ruddy G, Rhee K. Transdisciplinary teams in primary care for the underserved: A literature review. *Journal of Health Care for the Poor and Underserved.* 2005;16(2):248–256.

15. Petrini C, Thomas R. Meetings, stressful meetings. *Training & Development.* 1995;49(10):11.

16. Freeth D. Sustaining interprofessional collaboration. *Journal of Interprofessional Care.* 2001;15(1):37.

17. Payne M. *Teamwork in Multiprofessional Care.* Chicago, IL: Lyceum Books, Inc., 2000.

18. Ellingson LL. Interdisciplinary health care teamwork in the clinic backstage. *Journal of Applied Communication Research.* 2003;31(2):93.

19. Harris MF, Advocat J, Crabtree BF, Levesque JF, Miller WL, Gunn JM, Hogg W, Scott CM, Chase SM, Halma L, Russell GM. Interprofessional teamwork innovations for primary health care practices and practitioners: Evidence from a comparison of reform in three countries. *Journal of Multidisciplinary Healthcare.* 2016 Jan 29;9:35–46. Doi: 10.2147/JMDH.S97371.

20. Brown JB, Ryan BL, Thorpe C. Processes of patient-centered care in family health teams: A qualitative study. *CMAJ Open,* 2016 Apr 1;4(2):E271–E276. Doi: 10.9778/cmaj.20150128.

21. Bailey P, Jones L, Way D. Family physician/nurse practitioner: Stories of collaboration. *Journal of Advanced Nursing.* 2006;53(4):381–391.

22. Grunfeld E, Whelan TJ, Zitzelsberger L, Willan AR, Montesanto B, Evans WK. Cancer care workers in Ontario: Prevalence of burnout, job stress and job satisfaction. *Canadian Medical Association Journal.* 2000;163(7):166–169.

23. Laschinger HKS, Shamian J, Thomson D. Impact of magnet hospital characteristics on nurses' perceptions of trust, burnout, quality of care, and work satisfaction. *Nursing Economics.* 2001;19(Part 5):209–220.

24. Brown JB, Lewis L, Ellis K, Stewart M, Freeman TR, Kasperski MJ. Conflict on interprofessional primary health care teams – Can it be resolved? *Journal of Interprofessional Care.* 2011;25:4–10.

25. Porter-O'Grady T. Embracing conflict: Building a healthy community. *Health Care Management Review.* 2004;29:181–187.

26. Zwarenstein M, Reeves S. Working together but apart: Barriers and routes to nurse-physician collaboration. *Joint Commission Journal on Qualitative Improvement.* 2002;28(5):242–247.

27. Mickan S, Rodger S. Characteristics of effective teams: A literature review. *Australian Health Review.* 2000;23(3):201–208.

28. Lemieux-Charles L, McGuire WL. What do we know about health care team effectiveness? A review of the literature. *Medical Care Research and Review.* 2006;63(3):263–300.

29. Sands SA, Stanley P, Charon R. Pediatric narrative oncology: Interprofessional training to promote empathy, build teams, and prevent burnout. *Journal of Supportive Oncology.* 2008;6(7):307–312.

9

Patient-Centered Approaches in the Face of New Technologies

MOIRA STEWART, BRIDGET L RYAN, AND THOMAS R FREEMAN

INTRODUCTION – TECHNOLOGY AND THE PATIENT-CENTERED CLINICAL METHOD

Technology is so pervasive that it has been suggested that we are a technological civilization. Just as the metaphor states that fish have no concept of life without water, our relationship with the world is lived through technology.[1] Technology is understood to be the way something is done; a method to accomplish a task and a practice that entails organization, procedures, a vocabulary and a mindset.[2] In this sense, wood carving or knitting are technologies. So too is the clinical method a technology, a way of assessing illness or risk of disease and instituting or recommending a remedy. It is a response to suffering. Franklin distinguishes between those technologies that are *prescriptive* and those that are *holistic*.[2] Prescriptive technologies are characterized by breaking down the process into parts with each part assigned to a different worker; control resides with management; decisions are made beforehand, and outcomes predefined. Clinical guidelines and care pathways are examples. Holistic technologies are recognized by having one worker in control throughout the process; decisions are made while the work progresses and are attuned to the entire environment. The patient-centered clinical method, for the most part, is a holistic technology, but this does not mean that it eschews guidelines and evidence-based medicine. A patient-centered clinician uses prescriptive technologies, shaping them in the service of holistic or humanistic care.

As newer technologies such as virtual visits, patient portals, artificial intelligence (AI) and machine learning become incorporated into clinical practice, the challenge is to ensure that they are assigned a place in the workflow that requires linear intelligence (e.g., tools and calculators to assist clinical decision making, access to current literature and guidelines and alerts), leaving to the human clinician those aspects – empathy, compassion, hermeneutic reasoning – that humans are most suited for. Healthcare technology must enhance trust in the patient–clinician relationship and support continuity of care.

A preoccupation with technology may hinder patient-centered care by delaying clinician responses to patient cues and slowing empathetic statements.[3] Keenan et al. suggest that, in the context of using technology, "additional actions or behaviours are required by health professionals to win . . . patient trust".[4]

DOI: 10.1201/9781003394679-12

If we fail to counteract the distracting influences of technology, worrying consequences might ensue, including the diminishment of the patient–clinician relationship. We know this relationship is essential because studies have found that patient–clinician relationships positively influence patient health outcomes for chronic disease, recovery from common symptoms and subsequent use of services and costs.[5, 6] As well, one can infer from the concerns of clinicians that they may become demoralized in the face of less fulfilling relationships.

One of the ways to mitigate these unacceptable consequences could be to shore up clinical practice and the teaching of residents.

ENHANCING THE PATIENT-CENTERED APPROACH WHEN USING PATIENT PORTALS AND ELECTRONIC MEDICAL RECORDS

Two aspects of pervasive information technology may have varied effects on patient-centered care. One is the sharing of information with patients through patients viewing a screen in the consultation room or through patient portals for communication between patient and clinician outside the office. For the most part, these technologies are considered positive advances by patients and there is evidence of effects on patients' sense of control,[7] adherence to medications, degree of engagement, self-management,[8, 9] improving recall and understanding of their plans of care,[7] and better preparing them for visits.[7] However, the clinician dictates the degree of success by actively including the patient.[10] The way a patient portal should be used is best established within the patient–clinician relationship and is seen by patients and clinicians as a supplement – not a replacement – for this relationship.[11] "A Patient's Voice" and "A Clinician's Voice" illustrate some of the personal views on this topic in Boxes 9.1 and 9.2.

The second aspect of information technology is the use of electronic medical records (EMRs), which have been shown to have positive influences on healthcare quality indicators such as higher guideline adherence, lower number of medication errors and lower adverse drug effects.[12] EMRs' success in reducing the number of lawsuits against hospitals has been demonstrated, but notably, this success is higher when the hospital demonstrates higher communication scores.[13] However, cautionary data on the negative effects of EMRs also have been accruing; while EMRs

---

BOX 9.1: A Patient's Voice

Patients voiced a cautious approach to portals: "We don't want to replace our wonderful health care professionals with just machines". – Patient 7. Patients imagined that these technologies would be part of their health care, not a substitute for in-person care: "the face to face . . . should still be available". – Patient 1.

One patient expressed that each patient–clinician dyad should have a conversation about how they would together use the portal: [The technology] "is going to be custom tailored to each person . . . it doesn't need to be a long process. [Doctor would say] 'Here's the things that we can do. These are things I think would work for you, are there any other things that you'd like to have access to?' [My provider] and I could [in] five minutes between us, figure out what would work". – Patient 4 (pg 538).

From: Ryan BL, Brown JB, Terry AL, Cejic S, Stewart M, Thind A.[11]

BOX 9.2: A Clinician's Voice

Clinicians have expressed their views on portals: "You have to make sure the relationship is going to be established first. I wouldn't 'portal' with [just] anybody". – Provider 2. And: "the trusting relationship can grow electronically . . . but I think it takes a lot of sensitivity on the provider's part". – Provider 3 (pg 537).

From: Ryan BL, Brown JB, Terry AL, Cejic S, Stewart M, Thind A. Houwen J. *Clinical Assessment as Therapy in Managing Medically Unexplained Symptoms*, chapter3. Radboudumc SBOH, Nijmegen, The Netherlands, 2022: 39.[11]

---

encouraged clinicians on biomedical questioning, they discouraged patient questioning, rapport and emotional support.[9, 14] Negative impacts on clinicians include inability of physicians to see patients' status over time, increased workload and loss of clinical reasoning support.[15] In fact, decision support systems embedded in EMRs have had negative effects on outcomes,[16] indicating a mismatch between clinicians' own decision-making and technology-supported decision support systems. Along the same line, the higher the number of EMR features, the higher the physicians' stress and the lower their satisfaction.[17] But the EMR, as a means solely of documentation, has positive impacts[16] on patient–clinician communication and other outcomes. Nonetheless, the more the keyboard activity and gazing at the computer by the clinician, the less patient-centered the visit and the less patient activation occurred.[18, 19] The main message here is that clinicians' facilitation of patient involvement mitigates the intrusiveness of the EMRs, leading to two conclusions: training on patient-centered skills in the context of EMRs is essential and better design of EMRs is needed to facilitate smooth patient–clinician conversations.[18] The reader can turn to a useful patient-centered approach in the context of EMRs as outlined by Duke, Frankel and Reis.[20]

ENHANCING THE PATIENT-CENTERED APPROACH IN TELEPHONE AND VIDEO CONSULTATIONS

Virtual care exploded due to the pandemic. Within this context, much literature has emerged discussing the relative merits of virtual care compared to in-person care. It is essential to understand how to safeguard patient-centered communication within these other modes of clinical interactions post-pandemic. Therefore, this section, based on a literature review conducted by Stewart and Ryan as part of the ViCCTR training program, Department of Family and Community Medicine, University of Toronto,[21] provides an evidence-based patient-centered approach for the provision of virtual care. The goal of this focused literature review is to assist clinicians and provide advice/recommendations from research or experts on how to enhance the patient–clinician relationship during telephone and video care.

Some of the broad goals of health care advocated by the patient-centered clinical method seem to be lacking in telephone and video consultations, such as surfacing complex issues, dealing with many problems simultaneously, taking time to listen for patient cues and following them up. Nonetheless, while face-to-face visits seem superior, telephone and video visits offer more rapport building.[22] Downes et al.'s systematic review[23] was cautiously optimistic about telephone consultations, saying that they are an appropriate alternative. Comparing telephone and video care shows no differences in terms of patient satisfaction and mortality, but video care was superior in terms of length, healthcare utilization, medical errors and diagnostic accuracy.[24] Although virtual care is considered more successful if the patient and clinician have a prior relationship, clinicians are confident that they are establishing positive relationships with new patients too.[25] Authors agree there can be positive patient–clinician relationships across a variety of modes of care such as face-to-face, telephone, video and email.[26, 27]

Patients notice the benefits of telephone and video consultations regarding saved travel time and convenience.[22] The most striking difference of telephone and video compared to face-to-face consultations is their length – 5, 6, and 9 minutes, respectively.[22] Also, the clinician provides much more information when face-to-face especially explaining the diagnosis and asking for patients' own health understanding. Therefore, these two aspects of telephone and video care need improvement in ways outlined further. Nonetheless, rapport-building statements have been found less commonly in face-to-face consultations and, surprisingly, most commonly in telephone consultations.[22] Therefore, rapport can be accomplished and guidance to encourage rapport is the raison d'etre of the next sections of this chapter.

General Patient-Centered Behaviors

To facilitate patient-centeredness with patients in the context of telephone and video consultations, the literature recommends reminding oneself of approaches used in face-to-face consultations, such as being comfortable making social talk,[28] being patient,[29] actively listening[29, 30] and being open to sensitive topics (patients do not resist sensitive topics on the video).[31] A specific skill that is similar for video and face-to-face consultations is adapting questions to the particular patient's history.[29, 32] Other specific skills require some adaptation, such as knowing how to deal with silence. There are fewer pauses for silence in telephone and video consultations, so this may need some intentional work to be more similar to face-to-face consultations, such as allowing the silence to extend as well as using "Mmm" on the telephone[30, 33] and moving occasionally and nodding on the video so the patient knows that the clinician is listening and the screen is not frozen.[28, 29, 34] Clinicians can create other cues to indicate that they are listening.[35] An important point is that the clinician looking sideways can be considered by patients to be a non-verbal cut-off.[28] Writers consider that video care facilitates understanding through non-verbal communication[22] such as eye contact with the computer's camera and through use of hands within camera range[29] and promotes reassurance through facial expressions, even virtually holding the patient's hand during an emotional moment.[29] Specific skills that have been found to be used more often in telephone and video consultations are open-ended questions and frequent statements explaining what is happening now or what is coming up next (called transition talk[22, 30]). Finally, the clinician will want to look for and address discrepancies between what is seen on the video and what the patient is reporting.[31]

Exploring Health, Disease, and the Illness Experience

As with face-to-face consultations, clinicians start with listening attentively to patients' strengths, lifestyle issues, problems and concerns expressed directly or as cues.[29, 30] They then ask follow-up questions about symptoms and functions that would typically be observed as the patient entered the room.[32] Specific to a video encounter, the clinician should ask patients to report any measurements they may have carried out at home, such as temperature, pulse, blood pressure, peak flow and/or hemoglobin A1$_c$.[30, 32] As well, it is important to observe carefully the patient's general appearance such as blushing, weight loss or gain and a mental state visible in the face. Studies show lower levels of clinicians seeking patients' understanding of their health and illness and confirming that their own understanding is correct[22, 30] in both telephone and video versus office visits, although telephone visits were better at this than video visits. Nonetheless, there is a need to improve how clinicians clarify the patients' ideas about their illnesses. Shaw et al.[30] showed that patients are more active in expressing both medical information and emotion during video visits than office visits, leading to an optimism regarding video care.

Understanding the Whole Person

Car et al. say, "Video consultations offer a window into a patient's home".[36] The clinician can watch for where medications are stored and watch for scatter rugs and other fall-inducing trouble. The clinician may notice something unexpected that the patient is unaware can be seen and will want to address these visuals sensitively.[29] The social context is also visible, maybe with family members in the room or, alternatively, signs of isolation.[31] The clinician should be ready to facilitate family members' participation, depending on patients' comfort levels.[31] In addition, video can be a window to patients' personalities as revealed in their faces.[31] Comparison studies of telephone and video care versus face-to-face care have noted an interesting contrast. Telephone and video care reveal more rapport building personal and social talk especially in the early stages of the visit; however, psychosocial issues are discussed less.[22, 30] Perhaps cues to psychosocial distress are not as noticeable or they are more often ignored, but whatever the reason, perhaps focused attention on eliciting psychosocial issues is needed in telephone and video consultations.

Finding Common Ground

Evidence in this review helps the clinician improve video care focusing on finding common ground, i.e., regarding the agreement on the nature of the problem, the discussion of roles of the clinician and patient and the discussion of treatment options. Because patients make fewer statements on information in telephone and video care than face-to-face care, the clinician should explicitly encourage patients to speak openly about defining their problems.[22] The clinician asking for the patient to confirm the clinician's understanding of the problems is actually more common in video care than in-person care, illustrated by such questions "okay?" "Have I got that right?"[30]

Evidence is contradictory on the amount of information the clinician offers in instructions and advice; clinician information giving was higher in video care than office visits in Shaw et al.'s study[30] but was lower in Hammersley et al.'s comparison study[22] of telephone, video and face-to-face visits. The information in the clinician's advice and instructions must be clear and explicit. Video care has been found to provide the space for patients to define their roles and begin to co-design care.[3, 31] On attaining agreement with the patient on goals of care, video visits are at least as good[37] if not better[38] than in-person visits. Such agreement is known to be a facet of patient-centered care that most affects patient outcomes.[39]

Enhancing the Patient–Clinician Relationship

Growing the relationship is considered by our clinical colleagues to be quite difficult in video care. Indeed, several authors have suggested that video care works better if the patient and physician have met before in person.[30, 40] However, it needs to be stressed that others have found that the relationship is capable of growing over time[38] and that repeated visits lead to a joint medical and personal history which nurture trust in the patient.[31]

Regarding the connectedness capable of being attained in video care, it does encompass a loss of the personal aspect of care compared to in-person care,[40] but, interestingly, this was not considered to be unacceptable to patients.[41]

Video care is better for rapport building than telephone care[40] and in-person care.[22, 40] The physician must genuinely pay attention and may use humor to build rapport.[31] To enhance rapport and trust, a clinician should regularly check whether the patient hears and understands, offer short intermittent summaries and check the patient's understanding.[34]

It may be more difficult in video care to show empathy. Ways to demonstrate empathy are (a) take the patients' statements seriously[40], (b) respond to the patients' emotion verbally and non-verbally,[40] and (c) take enough time.[31]

The bond, partnership and alliance between the patient and clinician are aligned with the patients' trust and confidence.[3, 26, 31, 37] Video care has shown better patient perceptions of the alliance than in-person care,[26, 37] and furthermore, patients felt their relationship was more equal with video care and felt empowered over time to co-design care.[31] They felt they could be honest in a discussion of distress.[3]

Regarding emotional topics and bad news, patients found that the distant and unobtrusive video care allowed them to "pour their heart out" and then feel better after.[31] Patients did not mind talking about sensitive topics on video.[31] Patients indicated that, for results of a test which might mean bad news, they preferred an earlier call or video visit rather than a later in-person visit.[41]

CONCLUSION

On the horizon, it may not be an either/or proposition regarding virtual versus in-person care. Likely, the future will see a mix of care modes utilized by clinicians and their patients. It will be important for patients and their clinicians to seek an appropriate mix of care modes that protects patient-centered principles and the patient–clinician relationship.

REFERENCES

1. Grant G. *Technology and Justice*. Anansi Press, Toronto. 1986: 11.
2. Franklin U. *The Real World of Technology*, Revised Edition. Anansi Press, Toronto. 1990: 2–3, 10–12.
3. Pealing L, Tempest HV, Howick J, Dambha-Miller H. Technology: A help or hindrance to empathic healthcare? *Journal of the Royal Society of Medicine*. 2018 Nov;111(11):390–393.
4. Keenan AJ, Tsourtos G, Tieman J. The value of applying ethical principles in telehealth practices: Systematic review. *Journal of Medical Internet Research*. 2021 Mar 30;23(3):e25698, 52.
5. Stewart M, Brown JB, Donner A, McWhinney IR, Oates J, Weston WW, Jordan J. The impact of patient-centered care on outcomes. *Journal of Family Practice*. 2000;49(9):796–804.
6. Stewart M, Ryan BL, Bodea C. Is patient-centered care associated with lower diagnostic costs? *Health Policy*. 2011 May;6(4):27–31.
7. Walker J, Leveille S, Bell S, Chimowitz H, Dong Z, Elmore JG, Fernandez L, Fossa A, Gerard M, Fitzgerald P, Harcourt K, Jackson S, Payne TH, Peez J, Schucard H, Stametz R, DesRoches C, Delbanco T. OpenNotes after 7 years: Patient experiences with on-going access to their clinicians' outpatient visit notes. *Journal of Medical Internet Research* 2019 May;21(5):e13876. doi: 10.2196/13876.

8. Delbanco T, Walker J, Bell SK, Darer JD, Elmore JG, Farag N, Feldman HJ, Mejilla R, Ngo L, Ralston JD, Ross SE, Trivedi N, Vodicka E, Leveille SG. Inviting patients to read their doctors' notes: A quasi-experimental study and a look ahead. *Annals of Internal Medicine.* 2012;157:461–470.

9. Rathert C, Mittler JN, Banerjee S, McDaniel J. Patient-centered communication in the era of electronic health records: What does the evidence say? *Patient Education and Counseling.* 2017 Jan 1;100(1):50–64.

10. Asan O, Young HN, Chewning B, Montague E. How physician electronic health record screen sharing affects patient and physician non-verbal communication in primary care. *Patient Education & Counseling.* 2015;98(3):310–316.

11. Ryan BL, Brown JB, Terry AL, Cejic S, Stewart M, Thind A. Implementing and using a patient portal: A qualitative exploration of patient and provider perspectives on engaging patients. *Journal of Innovation in Health Informatics* 2016 July;23(2):534–540.

12. Campanella P, Lovato E, Marone C, Fallacara L, Mancuso A, Ricciardi, W, Specchia, ML. The impact of electronic health records on healthcare quality: A systematic review and meta-analysis. *European Journal of Public Health.* 2016;26(1):60–64.

13. Sharma L, Queenan C, Ozturk O. The impact of information technology and communication on medical malpractice lawsuits. *Production and Operations Management.* 2019 Oct;28(10):2552–2572.

14. Kazmi Z. Effects of exam room EHR use on doctor-patient communication: A systematic literature review. *Informatics in Primary Care.* 2013;21(1):30–39.

15. Varpio L, Day K, Elliot-Miller P, King JW, Kuziemsky C, Parush A, Roffey T, Rashotte J. The impact of adopting EHRs: How losing connectivity affects clinical reasoning. *Medical Education.* 2015;49:476–486.

16. Buckman JR, Woutersen T, Hashim MJ. Avoidable mortality: The mediating role of communication in health IT. *Decision Support Systems.* 2022 Jun 1;157:113764.

17. Babbott S, Manwell LB, Brown R, Montague E, Williams E, Schwartz M, Hess E, Linzer M. Electronic medical records and physician stress in primary care: Results from the MEMO study. *Journal of the American Medical Informatics Association.* 2013;0:1–7.

18. Street RL Jr, Liu L, Farber NJ, Chen Y, Calvitti A, Zuest D, Gabuzda MT, Bell K, Gray B, Rick S, Ashfaq S, Agha Z. Provider interaction with the electronic health record: The effects on patient-centered communication in medical encounters. *Patient Education and Counseling.* 2014 Sep;96(3):315–319. doi: 10.1016/j.pec.2014.05.004.

19. Street RL Jr, Liu L, Farber NJ, Chen Y, Calvitti A, Weibel N, Gabuzda MT, Bell K, Gray B, Rick S, Ashfaq S, Agha Z. Keystrokes, mouse clicks, and gazing at the computer: How physician interaction with the EHR affects patient participation. *Journal of General Internal Medicine.* 2018 Apr;33(4):423–428. doi: 10.1007/s11606-017-4228-2.

20. Duke P, Frankel RM, Reis S. How to integrate the electronic health record and patient-centered communication into the medical visit: A skills-based approach. *Teaching and Learning in Medicine.* 2013;25(4):358–365.

21. Grundland B, Forsey J, Herzog LS, et al. Patient-centered care turns 30: Being informed by person and patient experience in virtual care, chapter 3. In Hilty D, Mishkind MC, Malik TS, et al (eds). *Virtual Mental Health Care for Rural and Underserved Settings.* Springer, Cham, 2022. doi: 10.1007/978-3-031-11984-2.

22. Hammersley V, Donaghy E, Parker R, McNeilly H, Atherton H, Bikker A, Campbell J, McKinstry B. Comparing the content and quality of video, telephone, and face-to-face consultations: A non-randomised, quasi-experimental, exploratory study in UK primary care. *British Journal of General Practice.* 2019 Aug 29;69(686):e595–e604. doi: 10.3399/bjgp19X704573.

23. Downes MJ, Mervin MC, Byrnes JM, Scuffham PA. Telephone consultations for general practice: A systematic review. *Systematic Reviews.* 2017 Dec;6(1):1–6.
24. Rush KL, Howlett L, Munro A, Burton L. Videoconference compared to telephone in healthcare delivery: A systematic review. *International Journal of Medical Informatics.* 2018 Oct;118:44–53. doi: 10.1016/j.ijmedinf.2018.07.007.
25. Ryan BL, Stewart M, Brown JB, Freeman T, Meredith L, Booth R, Cejic S, Choi Y-H, He J, Mathews M, Reichert SM, Richard L, Shariff S, Terry AL, Thompson K, Wilson H. *Family Physician Patient-Centered Virtual Care during COVID-19.* Family Medicine Forum [Virtual live presentation]. November 10, 2021.
26. Wehmann E, Köhnen M, Härter M, Liebherz S. Therapeutic alliance in technology-based interventions for the treatment of depression: Systematic review. *Journal of Medical Internet Research.* 2020 Jun 11;22(6):e17195. doi: 10.2196/17195.
27. McGrail KM, Ahuja MA, Leaver CA. Virtual visits and patient-centered care: Results of a patient survey and observational study. *Journal of Medical Internet Research.* 2017 May 26;19(5):e177. doi: 10.2196/jmir.7374.
28. Little P, White P, Kelly J, Everitt H, Mercer S. Randomised controlled trial of a brief intervention targeting predominantly non-verbal communication in general practice consultations. *British Journal of General Practice.* 2015 Jun;65(635):e351–e356. doi: 10.3399/bjgp15X685237.
29. Statton S, Jones R, Thomas M, North T, Endacott R, Frost A, Tighe D, Wilson G. Professional learning needs in using video calls identified through workshops. *BMC Medical Education.* 2016 Dec;16(1):1–7.
30. Shaw S, Wherton J, Vijayaraghavan S, Morris J, Bhattacharya S, Hanson P, Campbell-Richards D, Ramoutar S, Collard A, Hodkinson I, Greenhalgh T. *Advantages and Limitations of Virtual Online Consultations in a NHS Acute Trust: The VOCAL Mixed-Methods Study.* NIHR Journals Library, Southampton, UK, 2018 Jun.
31. van Gurp J, van Selm M, Vissers K, van Leeuwen E, Hasselaar J. How outpatient palliative care teleconsultation facilitates empathic patient-professional relationships: A qualitative study. *PLoS One.* 2015 Apr 22;10(4):e0124387. doi: 10.1371/journal.pone.0124387.
32. Greenhalgh T, Koh GCH, Car J. COVID-19: A remote assessment in primary care. *BMJ.* 2020 Mar 25;368:m1182. doi: 10.1136/bmj.m1182.
33. Hewitt H, Gafaranga J, McKinstry B. Comparison of face-to-face and telephone consultations in primary care: Qualitative analysis. *British Journal of General Practice.* 2010 May 1;60(574):e201–e212.
34. Car J, Koh GC, Foong PS, Wang CJ. Video consultations in primary and specialist care during the covid-19 pandemic and beyond. *BMJ.* 2020 Oct 20;371:m3945. doi: 10.1136/bmj.m3945.
35. *Virtual Health Handbook for PHSA Staff.* Provincial Health Services Authority. 2021. www.phsa.ca/health-professionals-site/Documents/Office%20of%20Virtual%20Health/Virtual%20Health%20Handbook.pdf.
36. Car J, Koh GC, Foong PS, Wang CJ. Video consultations in primary and specialist care during the COVID-19 pandemic and beyond. *BMJ.* 2020 Oct 20;371:m3945. doi: 10.1136/bmj.m3945. In Section *Getting Started.*
37. Freeman KA, Duke DC, Harris MA. Behavioral health care for adolescents with poorly controlled diabetes via Skype: Does working alliance remain intact? *Journal of Diabetes Science and Technology.* 2013 May 1;7(3):727–735. doi: 10.1177/193229681300700318.

38. Sucala M, Schnur JB, Constantino MJ, Miller SJ, Brackman EH, Montgomery GH. The therapeutic relationship in e-therapy for mental health: A systematic review. *Journal of Medical Internet Research*. 2012 Aug 2;14(4):e110. doi: 10.2196/jmir.2084.
39. Starfield B, Steinwachs D, Morris I, et al. Patient-provider agreement about problems. Influence on outcome of care. *JAMA*. 1979;242:344–346.
40. Donaghy E, Atherton H, Hammersley V, McNeilly H, Bikker A, Robbins L, Campbell J, McKinstry B. Acceptability, benefits, and challenges of video consulting: A qualitative study in primary care. *British Journal of General Practice*. 2019 Aug 29;69(686):e586–e594. doi: 10.3399/bjgp19X704141.
41. Powell RE, Henstenburg JM, Cooper G, Hollander JE, Rising KL. Patient perceptions of telehealth primary care video visits. *Annals of Family Medicine*. 2017 May;15(3):225–229. doi: 10.1370/afm.2095.

PART FOUR

Learning and Teaching the Patient-Centered Clinical Method

INTRODUCTION

JUDITH BELLE BROWN AND W WAYNE WESTON

In this part of the book, we examine how to learn about and teach the patient-centered clinical method, illustrating each chapter with relevant examples. Chapter 10 describes three goals of health professional education: learning how to deal with disease, developing a professional identity, and learning to heal. Chapter 11 explores the parallel process between being patient- and learner-centered, with a matching of each of the four components. Chapter 12 describes many challenges (and solutions) in teaching and learning the patient-centered clinical method including the complexity of clinical practice, teacher inexperience, and the competing demands on their time. Chapter 13 suggests a powerful teaching tool, the patient-centered case presentation.

DOI: 10.1201/9781003394679-13

10

Becoming a Physician: The Human Experience of Medical Education

W WAYNE WESTON AND JUDITH BELLE BROWN

THREE FUNDAMENTAL GOALS OF MEDICAL EDUCATION

"To be a physician requires a transformation of the individual – one does not simply learn to be a physician, one becomes a physician".[1]

In becoming physicians, students must develop in three areas: (1) gaining medical knowledge and technical competence in dealing with disease, (2) developing a professional identity, and (3) learning to heal.

Gaining Medical Knowledge and Technical Competence in Dealing with Disease

"The medical care of patients requires in-depth comprehension of pathophysiology and the behavior of diseases. Clinicians must also know and understand persons sick and well and be aware of the multiplicity of influences on their lives and actions".[2]

Physicians are set apart from other healthcare professionals "by their superior clinical expertise based on a deep grounding in biomedical science and understanding of the pathobiology of disease".[3] But so many other topics have been added to the curricula in recent years that some have expressed concern about the competence of the new graduates. Other critics,[4] however, applaud the introduction arguing that it produces better-rounded complete physicians. Jones provides a powerful argument for including the arts and humanities in medical education:

> Much of the value that the arts and humanities offer to medicine cannot be reduced to simple measures. Literature, for instance, provides a mode of practice for difficult aspects of medical care. Medical students and physicians inevitably face difficult moral choices and other dilemmas in patient–doctor relationships. Would you, as a clinician, ever withhold a diagnosis from a patient if a family asked? Would you be willing to implement an advanced directive and withdraw life support from a dying patient? Bioethicists can teach arguments,

DOI: 10.1201/9781003394679-14

rules, and expectations, but literature can often be more valuable. Students can encounter these dilemmas, in advance, through reading, whether fiction (e.g., Alberto Tyszka *The Sickness*) or memoir (e.g., Phillip Roth, *Patrimony*). When encountering difficult situations in reading, students have the chance for sustained, thoughtful reflection, as well as a chance to appreciate and reconcile multiple perspectives. They will then be better prepared to respond well when they encounter these dilemmas on the wards.[5]

However, the "basic sciences" are frequently perceived to be the principal preoccupation of medical school, especially in the preclinical years.[6] Most schools have introduced courses in communication during the preclinical years but usually fail to reinforce what was learned during the clerkship and residency.[7] Throughout medical education, students are immersed in the biological sciences and quickly learn the value system of the medical establishment – the primary task of medicine is the recognition and treatment of disease. Consequently, everything else – communication skills as well as psychological, social, and environmental factors – may appear peripheral. As a result, when students' progress through medical school, their ability to communicate effectively and empathize with patients deteriorates. This decline has been noted for decades and is a continuing problem today.[8-11] Remen describes how medical education can result in a loss of idealism and increased cynicism:

> The first-year class enters filled with a sense of privilege and excitement about becoming doctors. Four years later, this excitement has given way to cynicism and numbness. By graduation, students seem to have learned what they have come to do but forgotten why they have come.[12]

Developing a Professional Identity

Becoming a physician is more than simply learning a set of knowledge, skills, and attitudes; medical training not only teaches a body of knowledge but also changes the person. In this sense, medical education is as much about the acquisition of values and character development as it is about learning a discipline.[13-15] Unfortunately, although these issues have been acknowledged for decades, medical education is often inimical to healthy personal development.[16, 17]

Research on identity formation is dominated by a Western cultural perspective. In a scoping review of the literature on professional identity formation in medicine, nursing, and counseling/psychology, the authors found only a minority of articles

> examined trainee's sociocultural data, such as race, ethnicity, gender, sexual orientation, age, and socioeconomic status in a robust way . . . thereby disadvantaging trainees from diverse populations and preserving the status quo of an historically white, male medical culture.[18]

Students from these diverse populations struggle with the pressure to conform to the dominant culture which denies their individuality. Frost and Regehr argue that teachers need to find ways to help students negotiate their struggles:

> Rather than insisting that students become like "us," we should help to inform and structure their negotiations in a more sophisticated way so that all students are able to construct identities as physicians that will allow them to retain and

take advantage of their individuality while respecting and honoring professional values and norms.[19]

The dominant Western perspective on professional identity formation is being challenged by those from other cultures.[20-22] Mokhachane et al.[23] describe the use of an African metaphor to reorient professional identity formation (PIF) to reflect the influence of an Ubuntu-based value system:

> There are pitfalls in the PIF discourse which seem to result from notions originating in Western contexts of what a professional identity is and how it is created. The calabash represents something that is different from the Western perspective. It is a metaphor and a space to think about what ingredients are needed to create something that everybody can participate in and partake in. On the other hand, the Western ways of thinking about PIF are rigid or militant. They focus on the individual, not the context and not on the interrelationships. From the Ubuntu perspective, these theories do not fit and PIF needs something that thinks about the relationship among these different things. By expanding studies to include non-Western settings, the field may begin to unearth the nuances of how identities unfold rather than forcing them to conform to Western understanding.[23]

Becoming a physician involves joining a community of practice – learning its norms and committing to the societal expectations of physicians.[24] For generations, these demands were expected but unspoken and learned primarily by observing the behavior of more senior members of the medical school and participating in the care of patients. "Formal knowledge is transmitted, but because of the social nature of the learning, much knowledge transfer is informal, leading to the acquisition of both explicit and tacit knowledge".[25] At first, the expectations of the profession were learned as ethical requirements and later as demands of professionalism and more recently as attributes of professional identity – "a representation of self, achieved in stages over time during which the characteristics, values, and norms of the medical profession are internalized, resulting in an individual thinking, acting, and feeling like a physician".[26] This begins from day one of medical school; in fact, it may even begin from the time a student decides on medicine as a career.[27] The study of anatomy by cadaveric dissection in the first year of medical school is often mentioned by students as a turning point in their transition from laypersons to professionals. In addition to learning about the detailed structure of the human body, students learn technical skills of dissection, coping strategies to deal with their emotional reactions to working with cadavers, and skills in working in teams.[28] However, it is through experiences with patients, especially during the clinical clerkship when students work as part of the clinical team and have responsibility for patient care, that they begin to feel like doctors.[29] The metamorphosis is dramatic:

> Students arrive in medical school as twenty-one-year-old college graduates or as thirty-year-old career changers, many with little exposure to illness, care of patients, or the work of the physician. Four years later they graduate, having done about five hundred complete physical examinations, made three hundred clinical notes on patients with health problems requiring hospitalization, assisted at the delivery of ten to thirty babies, and sat, perhaps three times, at a bedside as someone they had cared for died. The transformative power of these experiences must not be underestimated.[30]

Learning to Heal

The patient, though conscious that his condition is perilous, may recover his health through his contentment with the goodness of the physician.[31]

(Hippocrates quoted in Huth and Murray)

Scant attention has been paid to healing in medical education, except for wound healing.[32-35] Consequently, not all physicians become healers. Those who do learn by reflecting on their experiences with patients or from their own personal encounters with illness. They discover the limitations of a narrow biomedical model and recognize that patients need more than evidence-based therapies.[36-40] "To be a healer is to help patients find their own way through the ordeal of their illness to a new wholeness".[41]

Cassell describes an approach to patients that reflects a different idea of what constitutes sickness: "A person is sick who cannot achieve his or her purposes and goals because of impairments of function that are believed to be in the domain of medicine".[42] Compared to the usual approach to the medical history, the focus is wider. Knowing the disease, the healer is concerned with establishing the functional status of the patient – what the patient can and cannot do. What is interfering with the accomplishment of the patient's goals? How does the patient attempt to surmount these impairments? These questions apply not only to the initial contact with the patient. They are important in visits to hospitalized patients, to those coming for an office visit or for a consultation, and for (the increasingly common) telephone or email contacts.[43]

Consistent with Cassell's focus on the functional status of the patient and recognizing that aging with chronic disease has become the norm, Huber et al. (2011) proposed a reformulation of the WHO definition of health as "the ability to adapt and to self manage".[44]

It is important to note that learning to be a healer continues after formal education is completed. The seeds may be planted during the training period but only grow and develop as physicians experience the power of the healing relationship in practice. When teachers introduce the concept of healing, they need to be cautious about the expectations they place on their students.

These young physicians often find the tasks of diagnosing and treating the biological dimensions of their patients' problems challenging enough; pushing them to become therapeutic instruments of healing may leave them overwhelmed. They need frequent encouragement, support, effective role modeling, and opportunities to discuss their feelings and internal struggles to adopt the healer's mantle.

In a scoping review into the origins of cynicism among medical trainees, Hershey and Stoddard (2021) describe the possible sources of cynicism.[45] The environment and culture of medical education is arduous with a vast and demanding curricular content, coming face-to-face with suffering and death, grueling work hours, and separation from their usual supports. The ethics and morals taught in class are too often at odds with the hidden curriculum taught through the students' interactions with faculty and senior trainees. In a study of shame in medical clerkship, Whelen et al. describe how medical students are in a vulnerable position because of their lack of experience, expected to learn and adapt quickly in unfamiliar settings characterized by high-stakes activities and time pressure where their grades and future will depend on their teacher's appraisal. Students are often unable to assess their own abilities and depend on their supervisors for helpful feedback. But supervisors are too often overwhelmed with their own demands to attend to the needs of their students. Even basic courtesies may be ignored:

Clinicians' shame-inducing social behaviour consisted of breaches of social norms for respectful conduct, e.g., not acknowledging students' presence, not making eye contact, not using their names or not shaking hands when meeting for the first time . . . One student entered a physician's office at the start of a two-week hospital rotation: *I said, "Hi I'm a medical student." This doctor turned around and looked at me and said "Congratulations!" Then he continued working. My heart was in my head, it was pounding, I was sweaty, and I thought "Sorry for existing".*[46]

Such experiences may have lasting harmful effects on student's confidence and professional identity formation as well as their capacity and willingness to be a healer.

In recent years, many schools have introduced courses on healing.[38] Boudreau and colleagues have modified the whole curriculum based on a "coherent framework for a scientifically guided and humanistic medicine . . . based on the fundamental premise that healing is the doctor's primary obligation".[47, 48] Buck et al. describe their development of a popular physician healer track in medical school – "a 500-contact-hour curricula integrated over 4 years, focusing on self-awareness, reflection, being-with-suffering, communication and professional identity development".[49]

In a study of healing, Churchill and Schenck interviewed 50 practitioners identified by their peers as "healers". "Eight skills emerged as pivotal from the transcripts of these interviews: do the little things; take time; be open and listen; find something to like, to love; remove barriers; let the patient explain; share authority, and be committed".[50] In an in-depth exploration of these eight skills,[51] Schenck and Churchill discuss the privileged nature of healing relationships and the importance of presence:

The greatest gift you give anybody is your presence, not in the verbal sense [talking], but just being present . . . to sit down on their level and be quiet. That is a gift. It is the greatest gift I can give them. My expertise is not what my gift is. My gift is to be present; and then I help people. But it is a challenge to remember. And it is a beautiful thing, because it is such a privilege. Not many people get to do that. The privilege of being given the gift of another person to you. I get the gift of their lives to me. And you never cease to be amazed by that gift that you get by being there for somebody. They give me the gift of healing and I give them back my presence. It is amazing how patients really understand that.[51]

UNDERSTANDING THE ROLE OF TEACHERS IN MEDICAL EDUCATION

To help their students negotiate these three facets of development, teachers need a conceptual framework that will guide their understanding of the human experience of medical education. A confluence of writings from several streams provides us with valuable insights.

We begin with a brief overview of four streams of writings:

- **Personal narratives:** These are first-hand accounts of the journey through medical school and residency that provide valuable insights about issues their teachers might need to consider. A remarkable number of students and physicians have written about their personal experiences and struggles during their medical education and the early years of practice.[52-65] And there are many more. Some were written in scarce moments during training;

others were written after graduation when students had time to reflect on their experiences of training. Poirier, a professor emeritus of literature and medical education[66] surveyed 40 memoires like this published in the United States between 1965 and 2005. Despite the number of different authors and the 40-year time differences, the issues identified by students were similar – excessive curricular demands, sleeplessness, emotional exhaustion, challenges in relationships with teachers, and concerns about the loss of idealism that led them to choose a medical career. In addition, a number of self-help books provide useful insights into the struggles of student doctors.[16, 67]

- **Developmental theory:** Research by psychologists, sociologists, and medical educators on adult learning and development provide valuable frameworks for understanding the personal and professional development of physicians.[68–75]

It is important to recognize that professional identity formation is taking place in the complex context of ongoing personal identity formation and is influenced by each student's unique racial, ethnic, cultural, educational, and family background. In a scoping review of professional identity formation (PIF), Sarraf-Yazdi et al. explored these complex interrelationships: "PIF is a complex, nonlinear and fluid process through which medical students navigate competing influences between their professional roles and personal lives, and iteratively construct and deconstruct evolving views of the self".[14] Sanders et al.[76] provide a valuable comprehensive commentary on the importance of developmental student support during medical education:

> Developmental student support in undergraduate medical education is an integral aspect of the function of all medical schools. It is not limited to students who struggle but recognizes that all students will have times where their understanding of the world, self and others will be challenged. These moments are opportunities for personal growth and development. The time at medical school, from entering to departure, is only a part of the lifelong journey of becoming and being a doctor, but it is a highly significant time for personal development, as well as developing the required academic and clinical competences.[76]

- **Mentoring:** According to Henry-Noel et al.

> Mentors are role models who also act as guides for students' personal and professional development over time. Mentors can be instrumental in conveying explicit academic knowledge required to master curriculum content. Importantly, they can enhance implicit knowledge about the 'hidden curriculum' of professionalism, ethics, values, and the art of medicine not learned from texts. In many cases, mentors also provide emotional support and encouragement. It must be noted that to be an effective mentor, one must engage in ongoing learning in order to strengthen and further mentoring skills.[77]

Several authors[42, 78–80] describe the learner–teacher relationship as a mentoring relationship. This concept leads to a number of practical suggestions for improving one-to-one teaching. Mentoring is also important for teachers. It impacts career selection, improves job satisfaction and compensation, and optimizes research productivity. Mentorship promotes career success in numerous ways. Physicians with mentors are twice as likely to be promoted as compared to physicians without mentors.[81]

- **Professionalism and professional identity formation:** Interest in professionalism, as reflected in increased publication of journal articles and books, has grown rapidly in the past two decades.[82-87] Cooke et al. call for professional formation to be the fundamental goal of medical education. They prefer the term "professional formation" rather than "professionalism".

> To emphasize the developmental and multifaceted nature of the construct . . . The physician we envision has, first and foremost, a deep sense of commitment and responsibility to patients, colleagues, institutions, society, and self and an unfailing aspiration to perform better and achieve more. Such commitment and responsibility involves habitual searching for improvement in all domains – however small they may seem – and willingness to invest the effort to strategize and enact such improvements.[30]

In the remainder of this chapter, we will elaborate on each of these four areas.

Personal Narratives

A central task of development is to find meaning in our lives and in our work. One way to do this is by telling stories.

> Narrative learning . . . offers us a new way to think about how learning occurs. . . . When we're learning something, what we're essentially doing is trying to make sense of it, discern its internal logic, and figure out how it's related to what we know already. The way we do this is by creating a narrative about what we're learning; in other words, we work to story it, to make the elements of what we do not yet fully understand hang together. We work to achieve coherence.[88]

Common to hundreds of myths and legends across numerous cultures and times is the tale of the heroic quest:

> The hero ventures forth from the world of common day into a region of supernatural wonder: fabulous forces are there encountered and a decisive victory is won: the hero comes back from this mysterious adventure with the power to bestow boons on his fellow man.[78]

Through the "heroic quest" of medical school, the student conquers many "fabulous forces" and becomes a physician: they are transformed.

Klass describes her experience at Harvard Medical School in these terms:

> The general pressure of medical school is to push yourself ahead into professionalism, to start feeling at home in the hospital, in the operating room, to make medical jargon your native tongue; it's all part of becoming efficient, knowledgeable, competent. You want to leave behind that green, terrified medical student who stood awkwardly on the edge of the action, terrified of revealing limitless ignorance, terrified of killing a patient. You want to identify with the people ahead of you, the ones who know what they are doing . . . One of the sad effects of my clinical training was that I think I generally became a more

impatient, unpleasant person. Time was precious, sleep was often insufficient, and in the interest of my evaluations, I had to treat all kinds of turkeys with profound respect.[89]

Cohen describes his experience as a mature sophomore medical student after doctoral training as an educational psychologist and serving as Director of Research in Education for the Department of Medicine. One day in his physical diagnosis course, he was given one hour to conduct a history and physical examination on a new patient and write up his findings. His reflections on this experience illustrate how the curriculum was at odds with his learning goals:

> I was astonished by my behavior with that patient. Intensive training in interpersonal communications would not have altered how I behaved. Given the time constraint, I dispensed with small talk, barely retaining a semblance of amenity. I omitted my usual preventive medicine questions about seat-belt usage and my chronic disease questions such as problems in complying with his therapeutic regimen. The focus of my thinking was on the patient's physical signs and symptoms and the physiological reasons for them.[90]

Another medical student, Melvin Konner, had been a professor of anthropology prior to medical school. He describes his experiences in the clerkship as follows:

> And of course, last but hardly least, I now tend to see people as patients. I noticed this especially with women. It is often asked whether male medical students become desexualized by all those women disrobing, all those breast examinations, and all those manual invasions of the most intimate cavities. I found that to be a rather trivial effect. What I found more impressive was the general tendency to see women as patients. This clinical detachment comes not from gynaecology but from all the experiences of medicine. During my medicine rotation when, on a bus, I noticed the veins on a woman's hand – how easily they could be punctured for the insertion of a line – before noticing that she happened to be beautiful.[91]

All three examples illustrate how the journey through medical school may desensitize students to human suffering – they become more impatient and detached. The experience of postgraduate training may be even more brutalizing, leaving young physicians feeling abused. Mistreatment of medical students has been documented since the 1960s[92] and remains a serious problem in medical schools worldwide.[93] "Medical students who report mistreatment were more likely to experience depression, alcohol abuse, low career satisfaction, low opinion of the physician profession, increased desire to drop out of school, and even suicidality".[94] In addition, there is evidence that students who feel abused by their teachers are more likely to abuse their patients.[95, 96] Such an environment is inimical to learning to be patient-centered.

In a beautifully crafted account, we read about the experiences of a young physician as he enters practice on his own. Mikhail Bulgakov, a newly graduated Russian physician was posted to an isolated rural community from 1916–1918. A few years later he wrote about his experiences in a series of articles that were combined into a highly praised narrative after his death. In one excerpt, he describes his terrifying experience of managing a young pregnant woman with a transverse lie:

And there was I, all on my own, with a woman in agony on my hands and I was responsible for her. I had no idea, however, what I was supposed to do to help her, because I had seen childbirth at close quarters only twice in my life in a hospital, and both occasions were completely normal. The fact that I was conducting an examination was of no value to me or to the woman; I understood absolutely nothing and could feel nothing of what was inside of her.

It was time to make some sort of decision.

"Transverse lie . . . since it's a transverse lie I must . . . I must . . ."

"Turn it round by the foot," muttered Anna Nikolaevna as though thinking aloud, unable to restrain herself.

An older, more experienced doctor would have looked askance at her for butting in, but I am not the kind to take offence.

"Yes," I concurred gravely, "a podalic version."

The pages of Döderlein flickered before my eyes. Internal method . . . Combined method . . . External method . . . Page after page, covered in illustrations. A pelvis; twisted, crushed babies with enormous heads . . . a little dangling arm with a loop on it.

Indeed I had read it not long ago and had underlined it, soaking up every word, mentally picturing the interrelationship of every part of the whole and every method. And as I read it I imagined that the entire text was being imprinted on my brain forever.

Yet now only one sentence of it floated back into my memory: "A transverse lie is a wholly unfavorable position".[97, 98]

Using the excuse of needing a cigarette, he rushed home to read Döderlein's *Operative Obstetrics* to refresh his memory and then returned to the hospital where he successfully delivered the baby. It is a vivid reminder for young physicians encountering conditions in practice for which they had not been prepared. Because medicine is so vast, it is not possible to prepare students for every possible condition they might face, but they need to be guided to develop strategies to safely and effectively manage such situations.

Conrad provides a valuable analysis of four book-length memoires of medical education from the viewpoint of those who experienced it:

In *Gentle Vengeance* LeBaron asks, "What's the hamburger machine that chops up nice kids and turns them into the doctors that I know?" LeBaron[99] examining these four accounts gives us some insight into the meat-grinding process. Medical school does an excellent job of imparting medical knowledge and technique, but is inadequate in conveying humane and caring values. There is precious little in medical education that facilitates humanistic medical care. Technological medicine, with its disease orientation, myriad lab tests, complex interventions, and "fix-it" mentality, pays scant attention to teaching about doctor–patient relations. The medical student's life of long hours, sleep deprivation, excessive responsibility, and dealing with unreflective and arrogant superiors inhibits the growth of compassion and empathy. Our medical training system, with this emphasis on facts and technical interventions, produces competent and knowledgeable physicians but not caring doctors.[100]

In a powerful and moving story of her internal medicine residency at New York's Bellevue Hospital, the oldest public hospital in the United States, Danielle Ofri describes how her experiences as a resident shaped her development as a physician and healer. In caring for Mercedes, a young woman with headache, Ofri was horrified to learn that 3 days after examining her in the outpatient department, Mercedes was in the intensive care unit, brain-dead from an illness that never was explained. Although she was off duty and not the attending physician, Ofri felt compelled to see the patient and arrived shortly after the family had been informed of the hopelessness of Mercedes' condition and was being consoled by the chaplain.

> He (the chaplain) glanced at me from across the bed where he was standing with one of the sisters and he must have seen a tear welling up in my eye. He circled back to where I stood and silently reached out his arm, resting it on my shoulder. The gentle weight settled onto my shoulder blades. It absorbed into the strain of my back, melting the muscles that were clenching and smothering me. My stethoscope twisted off my neck onto the floor as I leaned into his black tunic and began to cry. His arms circled around me . . . I collapsed deeper into his chest, sobbing and sobbing. The family stared with quiet amazement as I cried uncontrollably in the arms of a strange priest. One of the sisters left Mercedes' side and came to me. She stroked my back, her fingers running along my hair. I cried for Mercedes. I cried for her family and her two little children . . . I cried for the death of my belief that intellect conquers all.[59]

Ofri goes on to describe how this experience changed her:

> And while I was intellectually frustrated, I felt strangely emotionally complete. That night in the ICU with Mercedes was excruciatingly painful, but it was also perhaps my most authentic experience as a doctor. Something was sad. And I cried. Simple logic, but so rarely adhered to in the high-octane world of academic medicine. Standing in the ICU, the chaplain's arms around me, surrounded by Mercedes's family, I felt like a person. Not like a physician or a scientist or an emissary from the world of rational logic, but just a person . . . I still didn't know why I had initially entered the field of medicine ten years ago, but I now knew why I wanted to stay.[59]

Developmental Theory

Developmental theory provides a way of understanding learning, not simply as the accumulation of knowledge but as a transformational experience. Klass[94], Konner,[96] and Ofri[59] describe their own experiences of being changed, of no longer being able to see the world "through preclinical eyes." Foster reminds us that

> Becoming a medical professional is a complex and multifaceted process. It is also an irreversible transformation, one which cannot be undone. In becoming a doctor, the way that one feels about oneself and the way in which one interacts with the world are forever influenced by assuming the identity of "doctor".[101]

Perry[70, 71] provides a theory of intellectual and ethical development in adults that is helpful to make sense of these changes in thinking and perceiving.[102] According to Perry,[71] students' progress from thinking that is simplistic and "black and white" to where they recognize and can accept different points of view. In the first stage, students view knowledge as dualistic – there is one right answer, determined by the authorities. Excessive reliance on lectures and multiple-choice examinations may reinforce the dualistic stage. Students at this stage may resent teachers who use small group facilitation and learner-centered approaches because they seem to take too long to get to the one right answer; they prefer simply to be told. Next, students recognize different perspectives on issues but lack skills to evaluate them. At this stage, they may conclude that everyone is entitled to their own opinion and all answers are equally valid. They may become cynical and nihilistic, thinking that no one knows anything for sure. Then students develop the ability to critically compare different viewpoints but may be frozen in indecision because they can see the merits of each opinion. Finally, a stage of commitment is attained in which the learners are able to tolerate ambiguity and uncertainty and are willing to act according to their values and beliefs, even when plausible alternatives are recognized. Students recognize that they must take the risk of making their own choices. Until students reach this stage, they will have difficulty taking charge of their own learning.

> Perry described three alternatives to the progression from dualism to commitment in relativism. One was "temporizing", where students' development appeared to be delayed with an explicit hesitation to proceed with the next step. Another alternative was "escape" whereby students avoided the responsibility of commitment and sought refuge in relativism. And the last one was a "retreat" to a dualistic orientation, in order to find security and avoid coping with a too challenging environment.[103]

Teachers can help their students' progress by addressing the special needs at each stage. Dualistic students benefit from being exposed to alternative viewpoints to help them realize the complexity of the concepts being learned. Students in relativism benefit from learning critical appraisal skills so that they can weigh the evidence for different opinions. Teachers need to be supportive and encouraging of student development, avoid being judgmental and model a capacity "to be both wholehearted and tentative"[71] – the willingness to make firm commitments in the face of uncertainty and opposing opinions, while remaining open to new information.

Perry's (1981) approach, consistent with constructivist theory, emphasizes the importance of students finding meaning in their own experiences. As students grow and develop, they discover new and complex ways of thinking and seeing. Perry argues that this often demands a "loss of innocence" that may be painful and difficult.

> It may be a great joy to discover a new and complex way of thinking and seeing; but yesterday one thought in simple ways, and hope and aspiration were embedded in those ways. Now that those ways are left behind, must hope be abandoned too?[71]

He cautions us that it takes time for students to come to terms with their new insights – "for the guts to catch up with such leaps of the mind".[70] Time is needed to mourn the loss of simpler ways of thought. This may explain why development is stepwise, with occasional retreats to older and more familiar ideas, rather than steady progress.

Although Perry's studies are now over 50 years old, they form the basis of continuing study of cognitive development. Researchers such as Belenky et al.,[104] Baxter Magolda,[105] and King and Kitchener[106] have enriched our understanding of the epistemological changes that Perry described by incorporating the unique perspective of women. "Their research strongly suggests that college students' knowledge structures . . . can progress from a state of simple, absolute certainty into complex, evaluative symptoms".[107] West goes on to argue "because these authors did not all study epistemological development in exactly the same manner, the strong correspondence in the ways of knowing that were demonstrated by the participants in these disparate studies suggests that the observed phenomenon is robust".[109] Another criticism of Perry's schema is its limited focus on Ivy League, White male college students which might not apply to students from other cultural groups. Thomas addresses this concern in a study referencing Knefelkamp who argues that Perry's model is sufficiently descriptive and adaptable to accommodate increasingly diverse student populations. According to Knefelkamp,[108] Perry's original scheme itself has been validated through instruments that take into account the variety of cultures and experiences that students bring to college[109] Decker[110] reflects on how the student development theories of William Perry[70, 71] and Robert Kegan[111] help teachers to understand how students change the way they make sense of the world during their college years. Kegan's theory has been used in many studies of the developmental stages of medical students.[112]

Mentoring

"An old African proverb says 'If you want to travel fast, travel alone; if you want to travel far, travel together.' At its core, that is what mentoring is: traveling far, together, in a relationship of mutual learning".[42]

Mentoring is an important, perhaps essential, component of medical education. In a qualitative study of medical students, Kalén et al. describe medical students' experiences of mentoring:

> Having a mentor gave a sense of security and constituted a "free zone" alongside the undergraduate programme. It gave hope about the future and increased motivation. The students were introduced to a new community and began to identify themselves as doctors. We would argue that one-to-one mentoring can create conditions for medical students to start to develop some parts of the professional competences that are more elusive in medical education programmes, such as reflective capacity, emotional competence and the feeling of belonging to a community.[113]

Mentors guide students along the journeys of their lives. They are trusted because they have already made the journey. According to Levinson,[114] mentors are especially important at the beginning of people's careers or at crucial turning points in their professional lives. Mentors are people who have already accomplished the goals sought by the students. A mentor is typically an older, more experienced member of the profession who takes the student "under his or her wing". The role of the university as a parent-substitute is reflected in our reference to the university as our "alma mater" and in the term *in loco parentis* – in the place of the parent.

Zachary and Fain[42] describe the importance of preparation for a mentoring relationship:

> Just as a good gardener always prepares the ground before planting a tender seedling, a mentor should prepare for the important work that lies ahead. Self-awareness – understanding our own motivations, our strengths and challenges – is the key to getting ready to mentor and getting to know your mentee engenders respect, trust, and understanding – all necessary ingredients for a productive relationship. Taking time to prepare for a new mentoring relationship nurtures the meaningful connections that build a productive mentoring relationship and sustains it over time.[42]

In the beginning, the student often experiences the mentor as a powerful authority – a parental figure with almost magical skill. This is also a potential source of trouble in the relationship, especially with students who have a previous history of problems with authority figures. It is in the context of this relationship that students grow into their professional identity. In the early stages of their intellectual and personal development, students look to the mentor as all-knowing and expect to be given the right answers to questions. They are not ready to see the mentor's clay feet. The mismatch between what students were taught in the preclinical years and what they see their clinical teachers doing is one of the explanations for the increase in cynicism during the clerkship year.[86, 115, 116] This common phenomenon led one author to describe the curriculum as divided into two halves – the pre-cynical and the cynical years.[117] As the students learn and develop, they recognize that authorities are not always right and that even their mentor is human. Eventually, with a growing sense of their own professional identity, students recognize mentors as colleagues. In a study of medical students and residents, Brown et al.[118] found that the mentoring relationship was evolutionary and fluid in nature. Participants reported that they sought out different mentors for different personal and professional needs and at different stages of their education.

Daloz[78] provides a valuable framework for understanding the tasks of mentors. Effective mentors provide a balance of support and challenge and, at the same time, provide vision (see Figure 10.1).

SUPPORT

"Be with" the students. Let them know that they are understood and cared for. Such support promotes the basic trust needed to summon the courage to move ahead. The mentor is tangible proof that the journey can be made. Listen empathically – what is it like in the students' world; what gives it meaning; how do they view themselves; how do they decide among conflicting ideas; what do they expect from their teachers? Note the similarities between these learner-centered questions and those we suggest that doctors ask of their patients to explore the illness experience (see Chapter 3).

Zachary and Fain remind us of the importance of listening:

> Most mentees will tell you that the most important way their mentor can support them is to listen. When you genuinely listen to what your mentee is saying, and prove it by reflecting that understanding back to your mentee, your mentee will feel heard and cared for.[42]

Figure 10.1 Framework of the Tasks of Mentors[81]

Setting aside time indicates that students' ideas matter and that they are important as people. Preparatory empathy is helpful. Before the student arrives, remind yourself what it was like to be a student starting a new rotation. Prepare yourself to respond to indirect cues. Students are generally wary at first and may not be direct with authority figures. Express positive expectations. Whenever possible, build self-esteem and confidence.

CHALLENGE

Mentors toss little bits of disturbing information in their students' paths, little facts and observations, insights and perceptions, theories and interpretations – cow plops on the road to truth – that raise questions about their students' current worldviews and invites them to entertain alternatives to close the dissonance, accommodate their structures, think afresh.[81]

(italics in the original)

Daloz justifies this approach by reference to the work of Festinger[119] on cognitive dissonance – a gap between one's perceptions and one's expectations – which creates an inner need to harmonize the apparent conflict and thus motivates new learning. "According to Piaget, individuals seek a steady state or equilibrium between themselves and their environment. When that equilibrium is disrupted, the resulting state of disequilibrium triggers the need for a shift in one's current conceptualization"[120] (Piaget quoted in Kay et al.).

Medical school may teach a narrow approach to practice focused on the conventional medical model – "find the problem and fix it". When it works, this approach is impressive. However, it often fails, leading to frustration and sometimes to blaming the victim for being "difficult". In such situations, the mentor could challenge the student to reconsider their underlying assumptions about medical practice. Directly confronting the learner might sound judgmental and provoke defensiveness; instead, consider other strategies:

- Share a story of your own struggles to find a more effective approach to such patients.
- Discuss seminal readings on clinical practice – for example.[41, 121–128] Additional examples are available in a book consisting of a collection of the classic publications on family medicine selected by family physicians from around the world demonstrating the broad scope of primary health care delivered by family doctors and serving as an inspiration to current family doctors as well as to doctors in training and medical students.[129]
- Encourage students to write about their reflections on difficult interactions and regularly discuss their ideas.[130]
- Provide frequent, thoughtful, candid, and constructive feedback focused on the learning needs of the mentee. Zachary and Fain describe the importance of creating a safe context for sharing feedback: "A safe context for giving and receiving feedback is built on a foundation of trust and within a framework of readiness and expectation. When your mentee trusts that your intention is aligned with their best interest, and you trust that their intention in feedback is to make the most of your mentoring relationship, you pave the way for ongoing feedback".[42]
- Ask questions that require thoughtful answers e.g., "Could you tell me a little more about what you mean by . . . ?" "Is there another way to look at this?" Other examples: "That seems logical but let's take a moment to brainstorm some other possibilities." "It sounds like you have a lot of good options! Is there one that you really resonate with?" "That's a great idea. How do you think we might put it into action?".[42]
- Offer opportunities to try out different approaches with you role-playing a patient who they struggled with.

- In our increasingly diverse culture, it is important to help students recognize that their strongly held ideas may not be the only way to see things. Patients and colleagues may be doing their best to make sense of their situation from a culturally different context from the student. "Our ways make sense to us, there's to them; we differ because our worlds differ".[81] Mentors can help students to be more compassionate of other viewpoints by challenging students to consider each side, to give each its due before they take a stand.
- Asking pointed questions, pointing out contradictions, or offering alternative points of view may help push students past the stage of dualism; encouraging them to take a stand on a difficult issue or to criticize an expert may help them to develop a commitment. Professional learning involves the construction of new frames of meaning; therefore, students need the opportunity to try out their understandings and clarify contradictions. Hearing the views of their peers is often helpful. Pushing different points of view and challenging students to not only comprehend the differences but also deeply appreciate contrasting points of view stimulates personal development.

VISION

Inspire learners to see new meaning in their work and to keep struggling despite confusion and discouragement. Vision sustains learners in their attempts to apprehend a fuller, more comprehensive image of the world. One way of providing vision is through being a role model for the student. Palmer presents a view of the importance of inner strength and courage in teaching:

> Teaching, like any truly human activity, emerges from one's inwardness, for better or worse. As I teach, I project the condition of my soul onto my students, my subject, and our way of being together. The entanglements I experience in the classroom are often no more or less than the convolutions of my inner life. Viewed from this angle, teaching holds a mirror to the soul. If I am willing to look in that mirror and not run from what I see, I have a chance to gain self-knowledge – and knowing myself is as crucial to good teaching as knowing my students and my subject.[131]

Provide a framework for understanding the developmental tasks facing the individual student. Offer a vision of the role of the physician that goes beyond the enumeration of skills to be learned and which acknowledges the personal and spiritual qualities inherent in becoming a healer. Suggest a new language. According to Fowler,[132] a mentor's primary function is to "nurturize into new metaphors". They give learners new ways to think about the world. The good teacher helps students not so much to solve problems as to see them anew. To think in new ways requires learners to learn a new vocabulary and especially to develop new metaphors. Physicians may be constrained by the dominant military metaphor in medicine that implies we are always "doing battle" with disease and must adopt an aggressive, interventionist approach.

Bleakley challenges us to recognize the potential harms of this metaphor:

> Contemporary descriptions of cancer and AIDS can move beyond the literal illness to offer accusatory metaphors. These metaphors bring about shame and guilt in those suffering from illness and may prevent them from seeking appropriate treatment. This resonates with cultures of shaming and scapegoating rather than support and understanding. Medicine may not help patients to deal with illness where it typically employs martial metaphors to describe its work, such as "fighting cancer". The already exhausted patient may feel that he or she

is not up for the "fight" or does not characteristically frame illness through such metaphors of direct enemy engagement.[133]

To see physicians as "witnesses" to their patients' illnesses, who help give that suffering some meaning, frees physicians to be more imaginative in their approaches to healing. For example, in *A Fortunate Man*, Berger describes John Sassall, a country doctor working in a remote and impoverished English rural community:

> He does more than treat them when they are ill; he is the objective witness of their lives . . . He keeps the records so that, from time to time, they can consult them themselves. The most frequent opening to a conversation with him, if it is not a professional conversation, are the words "Do you remember when . . . ?" He represents them, becomes their objective (as opposed to subjective) memory, because he represents their lost possibility of understanding and relating to the outside world, and because he also represents some of what they know but cannot think.[134]

It is the doctor's acceptance of what the patient tells him and the accuracy of his appreciation as he suggests how different parts of his life may fit together, it is this which then persuades the patient that he and the doctor and other men are comparable because whatever he says of himself or his fears or his fantasies seem to be at least as familiar to the doctor as to him. He is no longer an exception. He can be recognized.[134]

Professional Identity Formation

Medical education borrowed the concept of professional identity formation from the education of clergy.

> A distinguishing feature of professional education is the emphasis on forming in students the dispositions, habits, knowledge, and skills that cohere in professional identity and practice, commitments and integrity. The pedagogies that clergy educators use toward this purpose – formation – originate in the deepest intentions for professional service: for doctors and nurses, healing; for lawyers, social order and justice; for teachers, learning; and for clergy, engaging the mystery of human existence.[135]
>
> Professional identity formation as an educational movement evolved as it became apparent that an approach to improving physicians' professional performance based on teaching professionalism, while a step forward, had inherent contradictions that were difficult to overcome. A feeling developed that producing graduates who merely acted like physicians somehow lacked authenticity. The behavior of the "good physician" should spring from within, being based on "who they are".[136]

Coulehan and Williams describe how the curriculum may lead some students to abandon the idealism that brought them into medicine. They illustrate their thesis, that "the culture of clinical training is often hostile to professional virtue",[86] by quoting from a short narrative written by a particularly gifted and socially aware student who was so worn down by the curriculum that she opted for peace as a survival strategy, putting off her idealism until some undefined future date.

When I arrived in medical school, I was eager to get involved . . . as medical students, I was sure that we would have some clout and certainly a commitment to the well-being of others. . . . However, medical school is an utter drain. For two years lecturers parade up and down describing their own particular niche as if it were the most important thing for a student to learn. And then during the clinical years, life is brutal. People are rude, the hours are long, and there is always a test at the end of the rotation. . . . After a while I reasoned that the most important thing I could do for my patient, for my fellow human beings, for the future of medicine, as well as for me, was to assure myself some peaceful time. . . . And rather than try to change everything that I consider wrong in the hospital or the community at large, I just try to get through school in the hope that I will move on to bigger and better things when I have more control over my circumstances. On the other hand, I do believe that habits formed now will rarely be overcome in the future. So I regret not having spoken up on more issues. But I was often too tired.[86]

Some students choose to narrow their responsibilities to developing technical competence as the best way to serve their patients. Others adopt a "non-reflective professionalism" by treating their patients as objects of technical services.

Dall'Alba cautions us to be wary of the dominant model of education that "generally appears to take for granted that the purpose of higher education is primarily the development of knowledge and skills".[88] She suggests, instead, that education should begin with a concept of care "highlighting the ontological dimension of education and its role in contributing to who students are becoming".[88] She elaborates on the central role of caring in the curriculum:

Reducing the practice of medicine, social work or engineering to "skills" or "competencies" overlooks the engagement, commitment and risk involved. . . . For instance, in order to skillfully engage in professional practice, health of patients must matter to medical practitioners, social workers must be concerned about the well-being of their clients and it must matter to engineers that a bridge they build will support the weight of vehicles travelling over it. . . . A focus on narrowly defined skills or competencies overlooks and undervalues the ontological dimension of professional practice and of learning to be professionals. It thereby undermines the relationships among what we know, how we act and who we are.[88]

Critics of the modern professionalism movement decry the hankering for a nostalgic concept of physicians willing to sacrifice everything for the benefit of their patients and argue for more attention to the academic environment in which students are educated.[30, 137–139]

GUIDELINES FOR TEACHERS

- Get to know your learners, not just as students or residents but as persons. Find out what is important to them – their family, close friends, interests outside of medicine. Do they have any major obligations or commitments (e.g., a sick parent)? What do they like to do when they are not working? What are their future plans? Share aspects of your own life. "Within the learning environment, importance needs to be placed on the development of positive teacher–student relationships, as these relationships have immeasurable effects on students' academic outcomes and behaviour".[140]

- As a mentor, challenge your learners to go further, while also providing the support they need for their learning and development. Help them clarify their vision of the kind of doctor they strive to become. It is important for mentors and mentees to co-create clear, realistic measurable goals of the mentoring relationship and a game plan for how they will be accomplished.[42]
- Remember that students sometimes feel overwhelmed with the biomedical curriculum and may discount communication issues as a strategy to survive medical school. Help them develop their skills and comfort with the conventional clinical method so that they will not be so preoccupied with their biomedical competencies that they have no time or energy for a more comprehensive patient-centered approach. Create a learning environment where students can disclose their areas of ignorance, their errors, and their personal struggles without fear of judgment.
- Teach by example. The power of role modeling is emphasized in the following quotation attributed to Albert Einstein and to Albert Schweitzer: "Setting an example is not the main means of influencing others, it is the only means". According to social learning theory,[141, 142] we often learn more by observation than from verbal instruction. In fact, many of the skills acquired in medical education are too complex to describe in words; such tacit abilities, such as clinical reasoning, must be demonstrated by a teacher or skilled peer. Additionally, the commitment to patient-centered care, modelled by a respected teacher, powerfully motivates learners to do the same.
- Help them learn how to attend to what the patient wants to talk about and to realize that listening may be more therapeutic than any biomedical intervention.
- Help them develop survival strategies to avoid becoming overwhelmed. For example, physicians need colleagues or mentors with whom they can discuss difficult or emotionally draining encounters with patients.
- Help students to reflect on their experiences and how to learn from them. This provides the tools for a lifetime of learning.
- Use the parallels in the relationship between teacher and learner to demonstrate aspects of the patient–doctor relationship. There should be the same caring and attention to the humanity of the learner that we expect the learner to demonstrate with patients. Cavanaugh summarized the research on the importance of creating a caring environment for medical education and concluded: "Role modelling, mentoring and coaching can effectively incorporate caring principles and practices to facilitate the transmission of caring attitudes and behaviors in aspiring physician".[143]
- Remember how stressful medical education can be and attend to the personal struggles of students as well as to their learning needs. Learning to be a doctor involves a profound change in identity, which may be difficult for some students. Watch for signs of unhealthy coping strategies, or frank mental illness, and be prepared to intervene. Faculty, like students, have a tendency to deny the seriousness of these problems and may assume the student is "just having a bad day". Don't procrastinate; explore the problem promptly and sensitively and be prepared to provide modified work responsibilities or sick leave and the appropriate professional help.

CONCLUSION

Learning to be a patient-centered clinician challenges students to develop their skills and, more importantly, themselves. The task can feel overwhelming at times and may awaken feelings of vulnerability and inadequacy as students grapple at the growing edges of their abilities. Their teachers must be responsive to their struggles and address the learners' needs and concerns. Teachers must model, in their behavior with students, the quality of interaction they expect students to demonstrate with patients.

We have woven several strands of educational thought that provide the fabric of a comprehensive approach to health professions education. Health professional education is a journey guided by wise mentors who are sensitive to the issues involved in human development and the unique challenges of becoming a clinician. At the same time, teachers must be skilled in the use of a variety of teaching strategies for teaching procedural skills[144] and specific interviewing and history taking skills.[145] Combining this repertoire of teaching methods into a seamless whole will help provide the learning environment needed to foster the human dimensions of health professions education. It is only in such a setting that the patient-centered clinical method can be mastered.

A MESSENGER: CASE ILLUSTRATING BECOMING A PHYSICIAN

Barry Lavallee and Judith Belle Brown

The silence of Doris' inner suffering still haunts me. It reaches into a place I thought was well concealed, and I am shocked at the occasional eruption within me as I encounter patients such as Doris. Intuitively, I always knew that working with my own people was right. I understood many things that others might find repulsive. I was not afraid of scabies, snotty noses, an unclean elder, and I was not shocked to hear that Mrs Wolf's children were all in care. Looking beyond the physical appearance and understanding the origin of social chaos requires patience, compassion, and empathy.

As a third-year medical student, I became friends with a physician who attended our local Indigenous church. Cliff was unlike my regular supervisors; he understood Indigenous people, and he had faith in their spiritual strength. I accepted his offer to do clinical work and study at the inner-city clinic where he worked. After all, this was the area where I had spent most of my childhood. Classic epidemiological parameters defined this patient population; most were Indigenous, economically disadvantaged, uneducated, and most times were in a survival mode.

In Cliff, I had finally found a teacher with whom I could explore all my fears, worries, anxieties, and triumphs. No longer did I have to pretend that I was not one of them. I could be myself, although I was unsure what that meant. I bathed or showered every day, I knew who my parents were, and I had a connection to a community. I had a past, present, and a future. I saw a variety of patients, many of whom, as I found out in time, were related to me. Cliff and I looked beyond the physical scars marking a violent life and searched for meaning, truth, and dignity in those we treated.

Sniffing solvents to induce an emotional coma was common in that inner-city community. I saw many patients whose reality was permanently affected by such organic elixirs. No problem, I thought. As children, my siblings and I saw many of our friends turn to sniff to escape their painful worlds. "Sure, I can handle these patients", I reassured myself. One afternoon, I was called into the treatment room to see a patient with multiple ulcers to her legs and arms. I walked into the room and there sat Doris, a young Indigenous woman engulfed with the all-too-familiar sweet and caustic smell of sniff.

I approached her as I have been taught in medical school. "Hi, my name is Barry, and I am a medical student. How are you?" There was no response. Perhaps she was still high or maybe she didn't hear me, I wondered. Her eyes remained fixed on the floor, locked in a world known only to her. I moved closer and repeated myself. Again, there was no reply. I looked over at the nurse, and she just raised her eyebrows and shrugged her shoulders as if to say, "I don't know". I was uncomfortable. "Where do you live . . . where is your family . . . when did you first notice the sores . . . have you seen someone else for this problem?" She didn't answer any of the questions. I left the room to speak with the nurse. "She comes here occasionally and all we know is that she lives on the streets and hangs around Main Street", she replied.

I quickly examined her, ordered a few tests and realized that I felt just as helpless as she looked. Her acquiescence to my examination, as I understand today, mirrored that to "her station in life". Perhaps, she thought of herself as just another "dirty Indian". How often had she been beaten down? She breathes, moves her limbs, and I know the nurse obtained a blood pressure, but something is missing. I thought to myself. What happened to you? What set of circumstances makes you express your pain with such cruelty? My heart raced and fear began to overwhelm me.

Cliff walked into the room. I started to tell him her story and then, suddenly stopped as the burning tears raced down my cheeks. I swallowed with difficulty and as if to challenge the reality of the situation, I gazed upon her again. A physical form resembling a young woman sat on that examining table, yet this human was devoid of emotion, spirit . . . but the most painful reality was to witness the lack of hope in her eyes.

"I don't understand", I said to my supervisor. Cliff looked at me and seeing how powerless I felt in the face of such suffering and indignity quietly said, "Sometimes, all you can do is just pray for understanding".

Today, I recognize what transpired during that important moment in my life. Doris helped me recognize the very demons I had lived with for so long. My journey had begun. I knew the pain one feels when all your life you wish your skin was a different color. The confusion one feels upon hearing the ancient and melodic language of your loving grandparents and then to have the same relatives call it the language of the "savages". I remember having my skin scrubbed so hard that it bled. As if, somehow, the daily cleansing removed me from that shameful category of "dirty Indians". The heartache my siblings and I felt when we were told to stay away from "those Indians" . . . the words conveyed with disgust and hate by my mother as she picked the nits from our hair. My parents never really understood the attraction we had for children of our own race, in that white world of our childhood. Mostly, I knew the confusion it created in my soul as I attempted to balance the love I felt for my family with the hate I had for who we were. Doris spoke to me back then, as she does today, and the power of her message will reverberate within my spirit forever.

In your silence and through your suffering Doris, I have found hope. I am left with a vision . . . and, in that vision, I see our ancestors. Their beckoning leads me toward the future. The wall of silence is broken, and a dignity made of truth, faith, and respect takes its place. I am free . . . and I stand firm. Doris, as a sign of my gratitude, I will burn sweet-grass in your honor and keep you in my heart.

REFERENCES

1. Fuks A, Brawer J, Boudreau JD: The foundation of physicianship. *Perspectives in Biology and Medicine*. 2012;55:114–126.
2. Cassell EJ: *The Nature of Clinical Medicine – The Return of the Clinician*. Oxford: Oxford University Press, 2015: 24.
3. Buja LM: Medical education today: all that glitters is not gold. *BMC Medical Education*. 2019;19:110.
4. Chiavaroli N, Huang C-D, Monrouxe L: Learning medicine with, from, and through the humanities. In: Swanwick T, Forrest K, O'Brien BC (Editors): *Understanding Medical Education – Evidence, Theory, and Practice*. Oxford: Wiley Blackwell, 2019: 223–237.
5. Jones DS: A complete medical education includes the arts and humanities. *American Medical Association Journal of Ethics*. 2014;16(8):636–641, 638–639.
6. Brown JB, Noble LM, Papageorgiou A, Kidd J (Editors): *Clinical Communication in Medicine*. Oxford: Wiley Blackwell, 2016.
7. Rosenbaum ME: Dis-integration of communication in healthcare education: workplace learning challenges and opportunities. *Patient Education and Counseling*. 2017;100:2054–2061.
8. Haidet P: Patient-centeredness and its challenge of prevailing professional norms. *Medical Education*. 2010;44:643–644.
9. Taveira-Gomes I, Mota-Cordoso R, Figueiredo-Braga M: Communication skills in medical students – an exploratory study before and after clerkships. *Porto Biomedical Journal*. 2016;1(5):173–180.
10. Wilcox MV, Orlando MS, Rand CS, et al.: Medical students' perceptions of the patient-centeredness of the learning environment. *Perspectives on Medical Education*. 2017;6(1):44–50.
11. Suciu N, Melit LE, Marginean CO: Teaching communication in medical students – a cornerstone for patient's outcome. *Romanian Journal of Medical Practice*. 2021;16(2):143–147.
12. Remen RN: Recapturing the soul of medicine – physicians need to reclaim meaning in their working lives. *Western Journal of Medicine*. 2001;174:4–5.
13. Cruess RL, Cruess SR, Boudreau JD: A schematic representation of the professional identity formation and socialization of medical students and residents: a guide for medical educators. *Academic Medicine*. 2015;90:718–725.
14. Sarrof-Yazdi S, Teo YN, How AEH, et al.: A scoping review of professional identity formation in undergraduate medical education. *Journal of General Internal Medicine*. 2021;36(11):3511–3521.
15. Park GM, Hong AJ: "Not yet a doctor": medical student learning experiences and development of professional identity. *BMC Medical Education*. 2022;22:146.
16. Peterkin AD: *Staying Human during Residency Training: How to Survive and Thrive after Medical School*, 6th edition. Toronto: University of Toronto Press, 2016.
17. Pagnin D, de Queiroz V: Comparison of quality of life between medical students and young general populations. *Education for Health*. 2015;28:209–212.
18. Volpe RL, Hopkins M, Haidet P, et al.: Is research on professional identity formation biased? Early insights from a scoping review and metasynthesis. *Medical Education*. 2019;53:119–132, 119.
19. Frost HD, Regehr G: "I am a Doctor": negotiating the discourses of standardization and diversity in professional identity construction. *Academic Medicine*. 2013;88(10):1570–1577, 1574.

20. Wyatt TR, Rockich-Winston N, Taylor T, White D: What does context have to do with anything? A study of professional identity formation in physician-trainees considered underrepresented in medicine. *Academic Medicine.* 2020;95(10):1587–1593.

21. Helmich E, Yeh H-M, Kalet A: Becoming a doctor in different cultures: toward a cross-cultural approach to supporting professional identity formation in medicine. *Academic Medicine.* 2017;92(1):58–62.

22. Nuttman-Shwartz O: Rethinking professional identity in a globalized world. *Clinical Social Work Journal.* 2017;45:1–9.

23. Mokhachane M, George A, Wyatt T, et al.: Rethinking professional identity formation amidst protests and upheaval: a journey in Africa. *Advances in Health Sciences Education.* 2023;28:427–452.

24. Buckley H, Steinert Y, Regehr G, Nimmon L: When I say . . . community of practice. *Medical Education.* 2019;53:763–765.

25. Cruess R, Cruess SR, Steinert Y: Medicine as a community of practice: implications for medical education. *Academic Medicine.* 2018;93(2):185–191, 187–188. https://doi.org/10.1097/ACM.0000000000001826.

26. Cruess RL, Cruess SR, Boudreau JD, et al.: Reframing medical education to support professional identity formation. *Academic Medicine.* 2014;89:1446–1451.

27. Yakov G, Riskin A, Flugelman AA: Mechanisms involved in the formation of professional identity by medical students. *Medical Teacher.* 2021;43(4):428–438.

28. Parker E, Randall V: Learning beyond the basics of cadaveric dissection: a qualitative analysis of non-academic learning in anatomy education. *Medical Science Educator.* 2021;31:147–153.

29. Brennan N, Corrigan O, Allard J, Archer J, Barnes R, Bleakley A, Collett T, De Bere SR: The transition from medical student to junior doctor: today's experiences of tomorrow's Doctors. *Medical Education.* May 2010;44(5):449–458.

30. Cooke M, Irby DM, O'Brien BC: *Educating Physicians: A Call for Reform of Medical School and Residency.* San Francisco, CA: Jossey-Bass, 2010: 41, 66.

31. Huth EJ, Murray J: *Medicine in Quotations: Views of Health and Disease through the Ages,* 2nd edition. Philadelphia: American College of Physicians, 2006.

32. Weston WW: The person: a missing dimension in medical care and medical education. *Canadian Family Physician.* 1988;34:1705–1803.

33. Novack DH, Epstein RM, Paulsen RH: Toward creating physician-healers: fostering medical students' self-awareness, personal growth, and well-being. *Academic Medicine.* 1999;74(5):516–520.

34. Sajja A, Puchalski C: Healing in modern medicine. *Annals of Modern Medicine.* 2017;6(3):206–210.

35. Sternszus R, Regehr G: When I say . . . healing. *Medical Education.* 2018;52(2):148–149.

36. Street Jr RL, Makoul G, Arora NJ, Epstein RM: How does communication heal? Pathways linking clinician-patient communication to health outcomes. *Patient Education and Counseling.* 2009;74:295–301.

37. Pulchalski CM, Blatt B, Kogan M: Spirituality and health: the development of a field. *Academic Medicine.* 2014;89(1):10–16.

38. Kearsley JH: Transformative learning as the basis for teaching healing in the development of physician-healers. *International Journal of Whole Person Care.* 2015;2(1):21–37.

39. Szawarska D: Curing and healing: two goals of medicine. In: Schramme T, Edwards S (Editors): *Handbook of the Philosophy of Medicine.* Dordrecht: Springer, 2015. https://doi.org/10.1007/978-94-017-8706-2_59-1.

40. Sajja A, Pulchalski C: Training physicians as healers. *AMA Journal of Ethics*. 2018;20(7):E655– E663.
41. McWhinney IR, Freeman TR: *McWhinney's Textbook of Family Medicine*, 4th edition. Oxford: Oxford University Press, 2016: 160.
42. Zachary LJ, Fain LZ: *The Mentor's Guide – Facilitating Effective Learning Relationships*, 3rd edition. San Francisco: Jossey-Bass, 2022: xvii, 101, 138, 170, 185, 192.
43. Cassell EJ: *The Nature of Healing – The Modern Practice of Medicine*. Oxford: Oxford University Press, 2013: 126.
44. Huber M, Knottnerus JA, Green L, et al.: How should we define health? *BMJ*. 2011;343. https://doi.org/10.1136/bmj.d4163.
45. Hershey MS, Stoddard HA: A scoping review of research into the origins of cynicism among medical trainees. *Medical Science Educator*. 2021;31:1511–1517.
46. Whelen B, Hjorleifsson S, Schei E: Shame in medical clerkship: "You just feel like dirt under someone's shoe". *Perspectives on Medical Education*. 2021;10:265–271.
47. Boudreau JD, Cassell EJ, Fuks A: *Physicianship and the Rebirth of Medical Education*. Oxford: Oxford University Press, 2018: 195.
48. Boudreau JD, Cassell EJ, Fuks A: A healing curriculum. *Medical Education*. 2007;41:1193–1201.
49. Buck E, Billingsley T, McKee J, et al.: The physician healer track: educating the hearts and minds of future physicians. *Medical Education Online*. 2020;26:1844394. https://doi.org/10.1080/10872981.2020.
50. Churchill LR, Schenck D: Healing skills for medical practice. *Annals of Internal Medicine*. 2008;149:720–724.
51. Schenck D, Churchill LR: *Healers – Extraordinary Clinicians at Work*. Oxford: Oxford University Press, 2012: 209.
52. Doctor X: *Intern*. New York: Harper & Row, 1965.
53. Bulgakov M: *A Country Doctor's Notebook*. London: Vintage Books, 2010. (From the English translation by Collins and Harvill Press in 1975)
54. Rothman EL: *White Coat: Becoming a Doctor at Harvard Medical School*. New York: Perennial, 1999.
55. Marion R: *Intern Blues: The Timeless Classic about the Making of a Doctor*. New York: Perennial, 2001.
56. Gutkind L (Editor): *Becoming a Doctor: From Student to Specialist, Doctor-Writers Share Their Experiences*. New York, NY: WW Norton, 2010.
57. Gutkind L: *Becoming a Doctor: From Student to Specialist*. New York: WW Norton, 2011.
58. Ofri D: *Singular Intimacies – Becoming a Doctor at Bellevue*. Boston: Beacon Press, 2003, 233, 236.
59. Ofri D: *Incidental Findings – Lessons from My Patients in the Art of Medicine*. Boston: Beacon Press, 2005.
60. Ofri D: *Medicine in Translation – Journeys with My Patients*. Boston: Beacon Press, 2010.
61. Ofri D: *What Doctors Feel: How Emotions Affect the Practice of Medicine*. Boston: Beacon Press, 2013.
62. Ofri D: *What Patients Say, What Doctors Hear*. Boston: Beacon Press, 2017.
63. Kay A: *This Is Going to Hurt: Secret Diaries of a Young Doctor*. London, UK: Pan MacMillan, 2017.
64. Klein M: *Dissident Doctor – Catching Babies and Challenging the Status Quo*. Madeira Park, BC: Douglas and McIntyre, 2018.
65. Weiner SJ: *On Becoming a Healer: The Journey from Patient Care to Caring about Your Patients*. Baltimore: Johns Hopkins University Press, 2020.

66. Poirier S: *Doctors in the Making: Memoirs and Medical Education*. Iowa City: University of Iowa Press, 2009.

67. Kelly IV JD: *The Resilient Physician: A Pocket Guide to Stress Management*. New York: Springer, 2018.

68. Perry Jr WG: *Forms of Intellectual and Ethical Development in the College Years: A Scheme*. Jossey-Bass Higher and Adult Education Series. San Francisco, CA: Jossey-Bass Publishers, 1999, 108.

69. Perry WG: Cognitive and ethical growth: the making of meaning. In: Chickering AW, Associates (Editors): *The Modern American College*. San Francisco, CA: Jossey-Bass, 1981: 96, 108.

70. Zabarenko RN, Zabarenko LM: *The Doctor Tree – Developmental Stages in the Growth of Physicians*. Pittsburgh, PA: University of Pittsburgh Press, 1978.

71. Knowles MS, Holton III EF, Swanson RA, Robinson PA: *The Adult Learner: The Definitive Classic in Adult Education and Human Resource Development*, 9th edition. London: Routledge; Taylor & Francis, 2020.

72. Cranton P: *Understanding and Promoting Transformative Learning: A Guide to Theory and Practice*. Sterling, VA: Stylus Publishing, 2016.

73. Kegan R: What "form" transforms? A constructive-developmental approach to transformative learning. In: Illeris, E (Editor): *Contemporary Theories of Learning. Learning Theorists in Their Own Words*, 2nd edition. London: Routledge, 2018.

74. Merriam S, Baumgartner LM: *Learning in Adulthood: A Comprehensive Guide*, 4th edition. San Francisco: Jossey-Bass, 2020.

75. Newman BM, Newman PR: *Theories of Human Development*, 3rd edition. New York: Routledge, 2022.

76. Sanders J, Patel ZR, Steele H, McAreavey M: Developmental student support in undergraduate medical education: AMEE Guide No. 92. *Medical Teacher*. 2014;36:1015–1026.

77. Henry-Noel N, Bishop M, Gwede CK, et al.: Mentorship in medicine and other health professions. *Journal of Cancer Education*. 2019;34:629–637.

78. Daloz LA: *Mentor: Guiding the Journey of Adult Learners*, 2nd edition. San Francisco, CA: Jossey-Bass, 2012: 26, 208, 217, 221.

79. Chua WJ, Cheong CWS, Lee FQH, et al.: Structuring mentoring in medicine and surgery. A systematic scoping review of mentoring programs between 2000 and 2019. *Journal of Continuing Education in the Health Professions*. 2022;42(3):153–158.

80. Fornari A (Author), Shaw DT (Editor): *Mentoring in Health Professions Education: Evidence-Informed Strategies across the Continuum*. New York: Springer, 2022.

81. Bhatnagar V, Diaz S, Bucur PA: The need for more mentorship in medical school. *Cureus*. 2020;12(5). https://doi.org/10.7759/cureus.7984.

82. Coulehan J, Williams PC: Vanquishing virtue: the impact of medical education. *Academic Medicine*. 2001;76(6):598–605.

83. Inui TS: *A Flag in the Wind: Educating for Professionalism in Medicine*. Washington, DC: Association of American Medical Colleges, 2003.

84. Dall'Alba G: *Learning to be Professionals*. New York, NY: Springer, 2009: 64, 65.

85. Scanlon L (Editor): *"Becoming" a Professional – An Interdisciplinary Analysis of Professional Learning*. New York: Springer, 2011.

86. McKee A, Eraut M (Editors): *Learning Trajectories, Innovation and Identity for Professional Development*. New York: Springer, 2012.

87. Cruess RL, Cruess SR, Steinert Y: *Teaching Medical Professionalism – Supporting the Development of a Professional Identity*, 2nd edition. Cambridge: Cambridge University Press, 2016.

88. Clark MC, Rossiter M: Narrative learning in adulthood. *New Directions for Adult and Continuing Education.* 2008(119):61–70.

89. Klass P: *A Not Entirely Benign Procedure: Four Years as a Medical Student.* New York, NY: GP Putman, 1987: 18, 107.

90. Cohen SJ: An educational psychologist goes to medical school. In: Eisner EW (Editor): *The Educational Imagination: On the Design and Evaluation of School Programs,* 2nd edition. New York, NY: Macmillan, 1985: 332.

91. Konner M: *Becoming a Doctor: A Journey of Initiation in Medical School.* New York, NY; London, UK: Viking-Penguin Press, 1988: 106, 366.

92. Becker HS, Geer B, Hughes EC, Strauss AL: *Boys in White: Student Culture in Medical School.* Chicago: University of Chicago Press, 1961.

93. Makowska M, Wylezalek J: A qualitative study of the mistreatment of medical students by their lecturers in Polish medical schools. *International Journal of Environmental Research and Public Health.* 2021;18:12271.

94. Major A (Editor): To bully and be bullied: harassment and mistreatment in medical education. *American Medical Association Journal of Ethics.* 2014;16(3):155–160.

95. Silver HK, Glicken AD: Medical student abuse: incidence, severity, and significance. *JAMA.* 26 January 1990;263(4):527–532.

96. Baldwin Jr DC, Daugherty SR, Eckenfels EJ: Student perceptions of mistreatment and harassment during medical school – a survey of ten United States schools. *Western Journal of Medicine.* 1991;155:140–145.

97. Bulgakov M: Baptism by rotation (excerpt). *Academic Medicine.* 2015;90(5):622.

98. Bulgakov M: *A Country Doctor's Notebook.* Translated from the Russian by Michael Glenny. London, UK: Vintage Books, 2010. (First published in Great Britain by Collins and Harvill Press in 1975;3020: 56–57.)

99. LeBaron C: *Gentle Vengeance.* New York, NY: Penguin Press, 1982: 58.

100. Conrad P: Learning to Doctor: reflections on recent accounts of the medical school years. *Journal of Health and Human Behavior.* 1988;29:323–332.

101. Foster K: Becoming a professional Doctor. In: Scanlon L (Editor): *"Becoming" a Professional – An Interdisciplinary Analysis of Professional Learning.* New York, NY: Springer, 2011: 171.

102. Moore WS: Student and faculty epistemology in the college classroom: the Perry schema of intellectual and ethical development. In: Prichard KW, Sawyer RM (Editors): *Handbook of College Teaching: Theory and Applications.* Westport, CT: Greenwood Press, 1994.

103. Friedman M, Prywes M, Benbassat J: Hypothesis: cognitive development of medical students is relevant for medical education. *Medical Teacher.* 1987;9(1):91–96.

104. Belenky MF, Clinchy BM, Goldberger NR, Tarule JM: *Women's Ways of Knowing: The Development of Self, Voice, and Mind.* New York: Basic Books, 1986.

105. Baxter Magolda MB: *Knowing and Reasoning in College: Gender-Related Patterns in Students' Intellectual Development.* San Francisco: Jossey-Bass, 1992.

106. King PM, Kitchener KS: *Developing Reflective Judgment.* San Francisco: Jossey-Bass, 1994.

107. West EJ: Perry's legacy: models of epistemological development. *Journal of Adult Development.* 2004;11(2):61–70.

108. Knefelkamp LL: The influence of a classic. *Liberal Education.* 2003;89:10–15.

109. Thomas JA: An analysis of epistemological change by gender and ethnicity among gifted high school students. *Gifted Child Quarterly.* 2008;52(1):87–98.

110. Decker A: Student-centered practice in the 21st century community college. *Community College Journal of Research and Practice.* 2013;37:561–565.

111. Kegan R: *The Evolving Self: Problem and Process in Human Development.* Cambridge, MA: Harvard University Press, 1982.

112. Lewin LO, McManamon A, Stein MTO, Chen DT: Minding the form that transforms: using Kegan's model of adult development to understand personal and professional identity formation in medicine. *Academic Medicine.* 2019;94(9):10299–10304.

113. Kalén S, Ponzer S, Silén C: The core of mentorship: medical students' experiences of one-to-one mentoring in a clinical environment. *Advances in Health Sciences Education Theory and Practice.* 2012;17(3):389–401.

114. Levinson DJ: *Seasons of a Man's Life.* New York, NY: Knopf, 1978.

115. Billings ME, Lazarus ME, Wenrich M, et al.: The effect of the hidden curriculum on resident burnout and cynicism. *Journal of Graduate Medical Education.* 2011;3(4):503–510.

116. Peng J, Clarkin C, Doja A: Uncovering cynicism in medical training: a qualitative analysis of medical online discussion forums. *BMJ Open.* 2018;8:e022883. https://doi.org/10.1136/bmjopen-2018-022883.

117. Simpson MA: *Medical Education: A Critical Approach.* London: Butterworths, 1972: 64.

118. Brown JB, Thorpe C, Paquette-Warren J, et al.: The mentoring needs of trainees in family practice. *Education for Primary Care.* 2012;23(3):196–203.

119. Festinger L: A theory of cognitive dissonance. In: Daloz LA (Editor): *Mentor: Guiding the Journey of Adult Learners,* 2nd edition. San Francisco, CA: Jossey-Bass, 1999. (First published in 1957.)

120. Kay D, Berry A, Coles NA: What experiences in medical school trigger professional identity development? *Teaching and Learning in Medicine.* 2019;31(1):17–25.

121. Selzer R: *Mortal Lessons: Notes on the Art of Surgery.* New York: Harper & Row, 1996.

122. Morland P: *A Fortunate Woman – A Country Doctor's Story.* London, UK: Pan Macmillan, 2022.

123. LaCombe MA (Editor): *On Being a Doctor 2 – Voices of Physicians and Patients.* Philadelphia, PA: American College of Physicians, 2000.

124. Loxterkamp D: *What Matters in Medicine – Lessons from a Life in Primary Care.* Ann Arbor: The University of Michigan Press, 2013.

125. Cassell EJ: *The Nature of Suffering and the Goals of Medicine,* 2nd edition. Oxford: Oxford University Press, 2004.

126. McWhinney IR: Medicine as an art form. *CMA Journal.* 1976;114:98–101.

127. Berger J, Mohr J: *A Fortunate Man: The Story of a Country Doctor.* London: Penguin Press, 1967.

128. Gawande A: *Being Mortal: Medicine and What Matters in the End.* New York: Picador, 2017.

129. Kidd M, Heath I, Howe A: *Family Medicine – The Classic Papers.* London: CRC Press; Taylor & Francis, 2017.

130. Hamshire C, Forsyth R, Bell A, et al.: The potential of student narratives to enhance quality in higher education. *Quality in Higher Education.* 2017;23(1):50–64.

131. Palmer PJ: *The Courage to Teach: Exploring the Inner Landscape of a Teacher's Life.* 10th anniversary edition. San Francisco, CA: Jossey-Bass, 2007: 2–3.

132. Fowler JW: *Stages of Faith: The Psychology of Human Development and the Quest for Meaning.* San Francisco, CA: Harper & Row, 1981.

133. Bleakley A: *Patient-Centered Medicine in Transition – The Heart of the Matter.* New York: Springer, 2014: 124.

134. Berger J, Mohr J: *A Fortunate Man: The Story of a Country Doctor.* New York, NY: Pantheon Books, 1967: 76, 109.

135. Foster CR, Dahill LE, Golemon LA, et al.: *Educating Clergy: Teaching Practices and Pastoral Imagination*. San Francisco, CA: Jossey-Bass, 2006: 100.

136. Cruess SR, Cruess RL: The development of professional identity. In: Swanwick T, Forrest K, O'Brien BC (Editors): *Understanding Medical Education: Evidence, Theory, and Practice*. Hoboken, NJ: Wiley Blackwell, 2019: 250–251.

137. Wear D, Kuczewski MG: The professionalism movement: can we pause? *American Journal of Bioethics*. 2004;4(2):1–10.

138. Hafferty FW, Levinson D: Moving beyond nostalgia and motives: towards a complexity science view of medical professionalism. *Perspectives in Biology and Medicine*. 2008;51(4):599–615.

139. Hafferty FW: Professionalism and the socialization of medical students. In: Cruess RL, Cruess SR, Steinert Y (Editors): *Teaching Medical Professionalism*. Cambridge: Cambridge University Press, 2009.

140. Liberante L: The importance of teacher-student relationships, as explored through the lens of the NSW quality teaching model. *Journal of Student Engagement: Education Matters*. 2012;2(1):2–9.

141. Bandura A: *Social Learning Theory*. Englewood Cliffs, NJ: Prentice Hall, 1977.

142. Horsburgh J, Ippolito K: A skill to be worked at: using social learning theory to explore the process of learning from role models in clinical settings. *BMC Medical Education*. 2018;18:156.

143. Cavanaugh SH: Professional caring in the curriculum. In: Norman GR, van der Vleuten CPM, Newble DI (Editors): *International Handbook of Research in Medical Education*. Dordrecht: Kluwer Academic Publishers, 2002: 992.

144. Sawyer T, White M, Zaveri P, et al.: Learn, see, practice, prove, do, maintain: an evidence-based pedagogical framework for procedural skill training in medicine. *Academic Medicine*. 2015;90(8):1025–1033.

145. Sfard A: *Thinking as Communicating: Human Development, the Growth of Discourses, and Mathematizing*. Cambridge, UK: Cambridge University Press, 2008.

11

Learner-Centered Teaching

W WAYNE WESTON AND JUDITH BELLE BROWN

I am a little embarrassed to tell you that I used to want credit for having all the intelligent insights in my classroom. I worked hard to learn these facts . . . I secretly wanted my students to look at me with reverence. I now believe that the opposite effect should occur – that the oracle, the locus and ownership of knowledge, should reside in each student and our principal goal as teachers must be to help our students discover the most important and enduring answers to life's problems within themselves. Only then can they truly possess the knowledge that we are paid to teach them.[1]

In this chapter we describe a learner-centered approach to medical education, a conceptual model for teaching that parallels the patient-centered clinical method. In the same way that patient–practitioner relationships have changed, so have the relationships between learners and teachers. These parallels provide a framework to understand the changing roles of teachers and learners in health sciences education. This framework also serves as a tool – learners' experiences of their relationships with their teachers help them understand their relationships with patients. For example, when teachers interact with learners as autonomous adults with a key role in important decisions about their education, they illustrate the kind of relationship teachers expect learners to develop with patients. Analogous to the patient-centered clinical method, the learner-cantered method comprises four interactive components (see Box 11.1 and Figure 11.1).

1 Needs assessment: exploring both gaps and goals
2 Understanding the learner as a whole person
3 Finding common ground
4 Enhancing the learner–teacher relationship

This approach to teaching is consistent with a number of current concepts of learning. One popular theory of learning in adults, andragogy, was first described by Alexander Kapp, a German high school teacher in 1833[2] and described in a history of andragogy by Henschke.[3] The term was brought to America in 1926 by Lindeman[4] where it was later popularized by Knowles and colleagues (2020)[5] and elaborated by other authors.[6, 7]

DOI: 10.1201/9781003394679-15

BOX 11.1: The Learner-Centered Method of Education – The Four Interactive Components of the Learning/Teaching Process

1 Needs assessment: exploring both gaps and goals:
   - *gaps* – requirements for completion of training
   - *goals* – special interests and areas of discomfort.

2 Understanding the learner as a whole person:
   - *the learner* – personal background, current situation, and developmental issues
   - *the context* – opportunities and constraints of the learning environment.

3 Finding common ground:
   - priorities
   - teaching/learning methods
   - roles for teacher and learner.

4 Enhancing the learner–teacher relationship:
   - empathy, respect, genuineness
   - sharing power
   - self-awareness
   - transference and countertransference.

The writings on andragogy often focus on several principles of adult learning that distinguish it from pedagogy and suggest approaches teachers could use to promote learning:

- With age, learners become more self-directed and actively involved in their own learning.
- Learning builds on students' previous experiences.
- Readiness to learn is closely related to the developmental tasks inherent in the learner's social or work-related roles.
- Adult learners are more concerned about learning for immediate application rather than for future use.
- Internal motivation is more important than external reward.
- Adults want to know why they need to learn something.

Although adult learning theory has been criticized for lack of empirical support[8] and for focusing too much on the individual and downplaying the powerful influence of the sociocultural environment, it has reminded us to pay more attention to the learner's experiences and their aspirations. Other theories of learning – social cognitive theory, transformative learning, self-directed learning, and experiential learning – address the complexities of learning in the health sciences and the central role of the learner:

> The learner actively interacts with a changing, complex environment. The curriculum can no longer be viewed as something which is transmitted to or acts upon the students, be they undergraduate, postgraduate or practicing physicians. There is an important element of human agency. Moreover, in practice, the physician-learner is stimulated to learn through interactions in the practice environment.[8]

This "human agency" is well described by constructivist learning theory[9] that emphasizes the central role of students in learning. Everything humans learn is strongly influenced by what they know already, and their prior knowledge shapes how they construct new understandings. Consequently, a teacher's first task is to find out what their students already know. One common misunderstanding of constructivism and self-directed learning is that the teacher's role is reduced to that of a facilitator who provides encouragement and indirect guidance but does not offer any direct instruction. This fails to recognize that students often misunderstand aspects of the complex disciplines basic to medicine. Some threshold concepts are particularly troublesome for students. Threshold concepts are inherently difficult to learn – concepts that appear counterintuitive or at odds with their prior learning but must be understood before a student can move on in their studies. Healthcare students might need help from their teachers to achieve a full understanding of threshold concepts.[10, 11]

> It has been practitioners who have pointed out the importance of balance between the student's need to discover and the teacher's need to tell . . . In the classroom, it doesn't have to be either-or; it can be a balance of both. Sometimes the content itself makes clear when students should simply be told an answer and when they should be working to discover it on their own.[12]

Threshold concepts may challenge students to change their strongly held ideas of how things work – they are like eureka moments. Once understood, a threshold concept helps students to understand a field of study in a new way.

NEEDS ASSESSMENT: EXPLORING BOTH GAPS AND GOALS

The first step in planning any teaching or learning experience is a needs assessment – an analysis of what learners need or want to know compared with what they already know.[13] In the learner-centered approach, teachers and learners collaborate in defining the outcomes for learning. These are based on an assessment of two potentially divergent sets of learning objectives. On the one hand, there are the gaps in the learner's abilities based on the "official" curriculum – the core requirements for competence; on the other hand are the learner's goals and aspirations – their special interests, perceived weaknesses, and concept of their learning needs for future practice. Effective education requires learners and teachers to find common ground regarding both sets of objectives – to increase the amount of overlap in the two circles in Figure 11.1. While teachers need to respect learners' choices, they should keep in mind that their learners' aspirations might not match what they must learn to achieve competence. Because research suggests that students are often not accurate in their self-assessment[14, 15] and may not be aware of the gaps in their knowledge or skills, teachers might need to guide students to consider different or additional choices. This is especially important in a field of study such as health care where it is vital for learners to achieve competence.[16]

Weimer[12] describes a valuable approach to learner-centered teaching in which she outlines its challenges and values, common reasons for resistance by students and faculty alike, and five key strategies for implementation.

1 The teacher's role changes from authority to guide showing students how to do things, not do it for them. This makes it more likely that their new learning will be connected with what they already know and will make sense to them.
2 The balance of power between teachers and learners must be more equal – decisions about course content, teaching methods, and evaluation should be shared with students but not

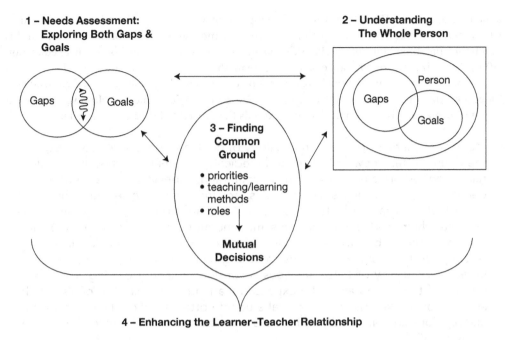

1 – Needs Assessment: Exploring Both Gaps & Goals

Gaps ⇄ Goals

3 – Finding Common Ground

- priorities
- teaching/learning methods
- roles

Mutual Decisions

2 – Understanding The Whole Person

Person

Gaps

Goals

4 – Enhancing the Learner–Teacher Relationship

Figure 11.1 The Learner-Centered Method of Education: Four Interactive Components

transferred wholesale. Research has shown that empowerment of students improves motivation and learning.[17] However, the transfer of power must be made gradually as students learn to make good decisions and assume responsibility for them.

3 Regarding content, less is more![18] Attempts to cover everything they need to know overwhelm students and impede their learning. Effective teachers help learners acquire the fundamental knowledge base they need and, more importantly, guide them to develop their learning strategies to master increasingly complex new material on their own.

4 Create learning environments that encourage students to take more responsibility for their own learning. In a review of autonomy support in medical education,[19] report: "Research suggests that when educators are more supportive of student autonomy, students not only display a more humanistic orientation toward patients but also show greater conceptual understanding and better psychological adjustment".[19] Scheffer et al. found that giving final-year medical students a more autonomous role in patient care was appreciated by patients and the students "were perceived as committed, warm-hearted and competent". They concluded that "an autonomous relationship between student and patient is vital for patient-centeredness".[20]

5 Student assessment should be fair, equitable, and robust, with an emphasis on feedback to support learning. Involving students in determining the methods of assessment and in self- and peer assessment enhances learning and may improve self-assessment. The assessment system should inform learners about their strengths and gaps and guide their ongoing learning plans to assure that they are competent at the time of graduation.

In the past, the transmission perspective on teaching, based on behavioral theories of learning, dominated medical education. Because there is so much to learn and medical error is often blamed primarily (and falsely) on ignorance, medical faculty may feel compelled to use a didactic approach. The recent worldwide adoption of a competency-based model of medical education reinforces our preoccupation with content and standards.[21] Abraham Flexner in his first book, *The American College* (1908),[22] and again in his famous report on medical education (1910),[23] criticized the overreliance on the lecture method. On the other hand, a teacher who is a master of the content and a skilled presenter provides invaluable guidance to medical students, especially when they are being introduced to a new and complex topic.[24-26] However, the quantity of information given in many lectures exceeds the capacity of students to learn it.[27]

> Medical educators often use the analogy of drinking from a firehose to explain the daunting task newly matriculated medical students have chosen to undertake. Frankly, this is not particularly encouraging, especially as the firehose has become larger over the last few decades. Advances in medicine and technology mean that medical students are expected to learn significantly more information than their predecessors in the same amount of time. In addition, they are also expected to be involved in numerous extra-curricular activities, including research and leadership positions to strengthen their residency applications. In fact, lacking any of these activities is considered a shortcoming. There is a paucity of time to do all of the expected learning and look after one's health and personal relationships. "Medical students often sacrifice their own health and relationships with family and friends in the pursuit of their dream to become a physician".[28]

The learner-centered approach shares many features with self-directed learning.[29-31] An early champion of self-directed learning, Malcolm Knowles,[32] defined it this way:

> In its broadest meaning, "self-directed learning" describes a process in which individuals take the initiative, with or without the help of others, in diagnosing their learning needs, formulating learning goals, identifying human and material resources for learning, choosing and implementing appropriate learning strategies, and evaluating learning outcomes.

The Committee on How People Learn II reports on "how difficult it is for people to regulate their own learning in formal educational settings".[33] We are warned to be cautious about overzealous promotion of self-directed learning, a concept based more on rhetoric than evidence. Planning a learning experience involves answering a series of questions – what are the gaps in my knowledge and abilities, what are the priorities for my learning, how is the learning to be accomplished, how and by whom is the learning to be assessed?[34] Learners who are completely self-directed will answer these questions on their own. However, often this task is too daunting, especially for students who are unfamiliar with the content to be learned. "So much work is required to exercise complete control over every aspect of a learning project that it is not practical or worth the effort to try to exercise all that control all the time".[35, 36] For these learners, the questions will need to be answered by the students in consultation with their teachers. There are many reasons to begin by determining students' deepest felt concerns about what matters most in their education. This enhances motivation[37, 38] and personal responsibility for learning. Furthermore, it gives them practice in self-assessment – a critical skill for lifelong learning. However, students may not be aware of all the requirements for competent practice and may have blind spots regarding their own abilities. Addressing these issues is a paramount responsibility of their teachers who must have a clear conception of the knowledge and skills needed for competent practice and the skill to assess students on each of these. In addition, teachers must be able to articulate these learning needs in a manner that is constructive, practical, and makes sense to their learners.

Grow,[39] with an update by Nasri,[40] provides a useful staged model of self-directed learning that matches the teacher's role with the stage of independence of the learner. In stage 1, the learner is "dependent" and needs an authority or coach. Lectures may be appropriate for this stage, especially for new and complex material or when time is limited. The stage 2 learner is "interested" and benefits from guided discussion and goal setting. In stage 3, the learner is "involved" and does well with a facilitator who encourages the student to participate as an equal. The stage 4 learner is "self-directed" and does best with individual work or a self-directed study group. The teacher acts as a consultant.

Teachers will help students understand what is important for practice, not by threatening them with difficult exams, but by providing opportunities to experience the need or desire to know. Students who are motivated to learn choose tasks that will help their learning, work hard at it and persist despite difficulties. Although external rewards can be positive reinforcers for learning, there are many situations where they reduce motivation and performance, e.g., providing an external reward for an activity that was already intrinsically rewarding can reduce intrinsic motivation. Students who are intrinsically motivated learn for the pleasure of learning rather than for higher grades.[41, 42] Positive motivating experiences can take many forms: stories of teachers' own struggles to learn; role-play with simulated patients; seminars with previous students who discuss the evolution of their own understanding of their discipline; discussion with patients about qualities they most admire in physicians. Helping students to reflect on their experiences with patients (what went well and what might have been more effective) encourages them to consider what additional skills they need and how they might improve. Ryan and Deci describe three important conditions learners need to support their intrinsic motivation:

Autonomy concerns a sense of initiative and ownership in one's actions. It is supported by experiences of interest and value and undermined by experiences of being externally controlled, whether by rewards or punishments. *Competence* concerns the feeling of mastery, a sense that one can succeed and grow. The need for competence is best satisfied within well-structured environments that afford optimal challenges, positive feedback, and opportunities for growth. Finally, *relatedness* concerns a sense of belonging and connection. It is facilitated by conveyance of respect and caring. Thwarting of any of these three basic needs is seen as damaging to motivation and wellness.[43]

CASE EXAMPLE

Dr Jacques Boisvert was a first-year family medicine resident in Dr Mary Denzin's community family practice, where he had been observed frequently over the past month during patient encounters. Jacques had consistently demonstrated a conscientious approach to the workup of patients; his case presentations and records were an accurate representation of what he had done; he correctly assessed his need for assistance; and he was not hesitant to seek help appropriately. His patient, Joseph Yong, aged 68, returned for a follow-up regarding his type 2 diabetes and a new problem of right shoulder pain.

Dr Denzin was generally satisfied with Jacques' clinical skills relevant to the assessment and management of diabetes and had observed him care for other patients with poorly controlled diabetes. She was less comfortable with his abilities regarding musculoskeletal problems. In briefing Jacques before seeing the patient, Dr Denzin commented: "I am confident in your skills in dealing with Joseph's diabetes and helping him regain his control of his diabetes. I will leave it to you to tell me if you need any assistance with managing Joseph's diabetes. I remember a few weeks ago you mentioned you would like to learn more about musculoskeletal problems. Would you like me to join you with Joseph when you are ready?" Jacques was encouraged by Dr Denzin's appraisal of his skills in the management of diabetes and relieved that he would be able to learn more about the assessment of shoulder pain.

In a survey of third-year medical students, Hajek and colleagues[44] assessed their common concerns about communicating with patients and compiled a list of 15 issues, ranked in order of importance from the students' perspective, including these top five:

- The patient starts crying or becomes angry with me
- The patient is in pain or emotional distress
- Not understanding the patient
- The patient tells me something important but wants to keep it confidential
- Not knowing the answer to patients' questions.

It is ironic that student manuals frequently offer advice about dress, an issue at the bottom of students' list of concerns, but often do not address more important issues such as "drying up" and not knowing what to ask next. This list by Hajek et al.[44] may assist teachers to be more attentive to students' learning needs.

In a Swedish study by Lumma-Sellenthin, based on group discussions about student-patient interviews

students reported feeling intrusive as they explored the patient's psychosocial situation. They avoided being empathic and felt insecure about coping adequately with emotionally loaded topics. Their difficulties were mainly due to insufficient understanding of the functional relations between psychosocial issues and health conditions.[45]

All students expressed difficulty gaining their patient's trust, assessing their patients' medical histories, and exploring their life situations. Some students felt overwhelmed with irrelevant details. "Requesting information from the patients could elicit moral qualms about appearing too curious and intruding on the patients' privacy, or about 'digging up' emotionally loaded issues that they would not be able to cope with".[45]

In the patient-centered clinical method, it is important for the physician to acknowledge each patient's pre-existing problems so that current issues will be managed in the context of all of the patient's problems. In the same way, teachers need to be cognizant of their students' prior learning experiences. Students are not blank slates. Knowledge of learners' strengths, weaknesses, and special interests accelerates the learning process and increases the potential intensity and complexity of the knowledge, skills, and attitudes that can be mastered. The curriculum can be viewed as a spiral; the same content may be encountered on several occasions, but each time it is assimilated in greater depth. Sometimes such repetition is misunderstood, and students complain that it seems like unnecessary repetition. They need to understand the purpose of revisiting some topics and may need to be challenged by their teachers to dig deeper.

UNDERSTANDING THE LEARNER AS A WHOLE PERSON

In Chapter 10 we elaborated on the developmental issues in becoming a physician; in this chapter we will focus on some of the difficulties students face during their education: stress, burnout, and mental illness. Next, we will address some features of the learning environment that hamper or assist their learning and development: the hidden curriculum and medical student abuse. This framework may be helpful in analyzing the difficulties of a faltering or failing student.

The Learner: Personal Background, Current Situation, and Developmental Issues

Akin to the two important dimensions of understanding patients as whole persons (patients' stage in their life cycle and their context) there are two dimensions for understanding students as whole persons. Teachers need to be aware of the students' background, their life history, personal and cognitive development, and their learning environment.

In the same way that physicians oversimplify their patients' complex problems by focusing on the pathophysiology of disease, so too do teachers oversimplify their students' educational needs by concentrating only on their major learning deficiencies. Teachers may speak of making a "learning diagnosis" in terms of the gaps in students' knowledge, skills, and attitudes compared with the competencies to be achieved. This may be very helpful, as far as it goes, but it may fail to convey an accurate understanding of what the learner, as a person, really needs.[46, 47] Students are different in so many important ways: in previous life experience, courses taken, preferred learning styles, willingness to take risks, self-confidence, and resistance to change.[48] The cultural identity of students has a profound influence on their learning. "Cultural backgrounds of learners are significant because ethnic, racial, linguistic, social, religious or economic differences can cause cultural disconnection leading corruption of motivation to learning".[49] Medical schools worldwide are acknowledging the importance of integrating diversity and inclusion throughout the learning environment, especially recognizing racially minoritized groups.[50] Sir William Osler commented on how individual differences in physicians determine their enjoyment of practice.[51]

In dealing with the many stresses of medical education, pacing is important. When students become overwhelmed by the emotional intensity of a learning experience, they may need a break. Then, restored, they return to the learning environment ready to proceed with the next learning task. For example, helping dying patients come to terms with their mortality is often psychologically draining and students may need emotional respite. This may only happen with the support and permission of their teachers. Noonan describes the value of weekly support sessions for residents.[52]

Eng et al. describe "patient death debriefing sessions" on an inpatient medical oncology rotation – 10-minute debriefing led by the attending physician focusing on internal medicine residents' emotional reactions following each patient's death. "Sessions were guided by a pocketcard tool and did not require faculty training . . . Overall, residents found debriefing sessions helpful, educational, and appreciated attending physician leadership".[53]

CASE EXAMPLE

A few months ago when Dr Sunir Patel had been accepted into the family medicine program as an international medical graduate, he had expressed his deep appreciation and sense of privilege. It had been a long and difficult process to reach this point since immigrating from his war-torn country 5 years earlier. In recent weeks his supervisor, Dr Steinhouse, frequently observed Sunir to be pensive – often lost in thought. Somewhat baffled by his student's change in demeanor, Dr Steinhouse decided to gently explore how her student was managing. Sunir was initially surprised by his supervisor's inquiry and unsure how best to respond. After some consideration he revealed his feelings of confusion. Sunir explained: "The practice of medicine is so different here compared to my country. Back home doctors tell patients that they should do this and that and patients obey. Here we are expected to talk with patients and learn what they want and need – to be patient-centered! This is all so new for me – it is very confusing". Dr Steinhouse probed further: "Are other things different?" Sunir quickly replied: "Oh yes! Back home you would never speak directly to a consultant or a senior resident – you wouldn't even look them in the eye". Sunir sighed, "But here everyone is very friendly and helpful, which is great, but it is so different. Sometimes it is hard to know how to be".

By understanding the challenges Sunir was facing in making the transition from a very hierarchical medical system to one that was both patient- and learner-centered, Dr Steinhouse is guiding her student through this time of adjustment and change.

Even students from the same school and the same class have vastly different abilities and learning needs. It is crucial to identify these so that students are not put into situations where they are too far out of their depth. It is also essential to identify their strengths so that valuable time is not wasted practicing skills already mastered while ignoring areas of deficiency. Students also differ in their stages of personal, cognitive, and professional development, as described in Chapter 10.

The student population has changed dramatically in many medical schools around the world, with the entrance of more women and greater racial and ethnic diversity. The proportion of women entering medical schools has increased dramatically, now exceeding 50% in some countries and 25% in others, reflecting the cultural views of gender roles in the country.[54] However, gender bias remains, resulting in women being underrepresented in leadership positions and slower academic promotion.[55] These changes have the potential to alter the focus and priorities of the curriculum although there is no consensus regarding the impact of these changes.

Many studies have shown differences in communication, working patterns, and patient outcomes between male and female physicians.[56, 57]

Another long-standing inequity in medical education relates to the unfair treatment of racialized populations. The Flexner Report of 1910 led to the closure of all but two Black medical schools.

Flexner based his opinion on the worthiness of candidates to enter medical schools on multiple criteria, including (but not limited to) prior postsecondary education (favoring 2 or more years of college vs. a high school certificate or equivalency test) and standardization of entrance exams for medical schools;

both criteria may have been more prohibitive to Black students based on other discriminatory practices at that time.[58]

In a review of the Flexner report 100 years after its publication, Steinecke and Terrell described the 2-page chapter of the Flexner report titled, "The Medical Education of the Negro", saying that Flexner "promoted the limited education of the African American doctor as a service to 'his own race,' but also for the larger purpose of protecting Whites from the African American population's potential to spread disease".[59]

Kuper and Hodges, in a commentary on the societal context of medical education, suggest:

> An understanding of the impact of inequities on society enables us, at the simplest level, to make them visible to our students. However, we must not assume that patients suffer inequities and physicians do not. Structural inequities exist inevitably at all levels of medical education because it takes place in an inequitable society. Consistent with the critical paradigm, scholars working from this standpoint argue that, in order to address such issues as equitable access to medical education and leadership roles within the discipline, it is necessary to focus on the gender, culture, and racialized hierarchical nature of the profession itself and make efforts to (re)invent a more equitable society.[60]

More recently, educators have recognized the need to integrate LGBTQ-related topics into their curricula.[61] In 2018, the ACGME Board approved a major revision of its Common Program Requirements specifying that residents must demonstrate the following competency: "respect and responsiveness to diverse patient populations, including but not limited to diversity in gender, age, culture, race, religion, disabilities, national origins, socioeconomic status, and sexual orientation".[62]

Another important issue is the effect of stress, substance abuse, and mental illness on the performance of medical students. A survey of 855 medical students representing 49 medical colleges in the United States, "showed that 91.3% and 26.2% of medical students consumed alcohol and used marijuana respectively in the past year, and 33.8% of medical students consumed five or more drinks in one sitting in the past two weeks".[63] In a systematic review and meta-analysis of burnout in medical students, Frajerman et al. found that "one student out of two is suffering from burnout, even before residency".[64] Burnout was studied in this and many other studies using the Maslach Burnout Inventory, which measures three components of burnout: emotional exhaustion, depersonalization, and personal accomplishment.[65] In a study of resident self-reported patient care, burned-out residents were more likely to self-report providing suboptimal patient care at least monthly.[66, 67] In a survey of pediatric resident burnout and attitudes toward patients by Baer et al., residents with burnout, compared to others not reporting burnout, reported they were more likely to provide suboptimal care.[68] In a study of urban family physicians, Lee and colleagues found 42.5% of participants had high stress levels and almost half had high scores for emotional exhaustion and depersonalization.[69]

Starting in 2020, the COVID-19 pandemic introduced an additional stressor for all healthcare workers and resulted in huge changes in medical education. Online platforms replaced classroom and small group instruction, and students were not allowed to participate in clinical care, despite its importance for the development of competence, because of the high risk of infection. A variety of innovative approaches were developed to replace the clerkship experience.[70] In an international systematic review of burnout in physicians during the COVID-19 pandemic, Macaron et al. analyzed 45 observational studies from around the world and concluded:

The COVID-19 pandemic has proven to be an enormous burden on health-care systems across the globe, placing considerable strain on the psychological well-being of all healthcare workers (HCW) involved. The results of this meta-analysis demonstrate that more than half of HCW experienced burn-out at some point during the pandemic. As expected, frontline, compared to second-line HCWs, were found to have higher rates of burnout . . . Lack of personal accomplishment, defined as having a negative outlook on the worth of one's work, was found to be the most affected domain during the COVID-19 pandemic out of the three subscales of the MBI [Maslach Burnout Inventory].[71]

However, on a more encouraging note, Shanafelt[72] describes a number of studies showing how "enhancing meaning in work increases physician satisfaction and reduces burnout." One of these studies, involving an intensive 52-hour curriculum on mindfulness, had large and lasting improvements in burnout, mood disturbance, and attitudes associated with patient-centered care.[73] Cassell describes his personal experience of discovering that getting closer to dying patients reduced the pain associated with their loss.[74]

Despite efforts to reduce the stress experienced by medical students and to provide support services, students continue to suffer from a high prevalence of mental illness. A recent systematic review and meta-analysis estimates the prevalence of depression among medical students to be 27%, which is threefold greater than age-similar norms.[75]

MacLean et al. point out the negative impact of the intense academic demands of medical school and the need to provide formal programs "that promote specific wellness activities focused on the health of students' mind and body, help-seeking behaviors, and the use of healthy coping strategies".[76]

The Saint Louis University School of Medicine introduced changes in the curriculum to reduce stress on students and found that:

significant but efficient changes to course content, contact hours, scheduling, grading, electives, learning communities, and required resilience/mindfulness experiences were associated with significantly lower levels of depression symptoms, anxiety symptoms, and stress, and significantly higher levels of community cohesion, in medical students who participated in the expanded wellness program compared with those who preceded its implementation.[77]

These results suggest that addressing the root causes of stress within the curriculum is more effective than requiring students to come forward to ask for help.

Although teachers should generally not take on the role of therapist with their students, they need to know when their students are struggling with personal issues that might be interfering with their learning, help them to recognize the problem, and direct them to appropriate professional care.

The Context (Opportunities and Constraints of the Learning Environment)

In addition to understanding the cognitive, developmental, and personal struggles of students, a whole-person approach requires the teacher to comprehend the student's learning context.

In addition to the documented curriculum, students and teachers both become aware of the "educational environment" or "climate" of the institution. Is the teaching and learning environment very competitive? Is it authoritarian? Is the atmosphere in classes and field placements relaxed or is it in various ways stressful, perhaps even intimidating? These are all key questions in determining the nature of the learning experience.[78]

The environment of medical education strongly influences what can or will be learned. In the preclinical years of medical school, the course structure, content, and evaluation will steer students' learning. In clinical teaching, case mix, quality of teaching, and practice setting – inpatient, outpatient, primary, secondary, or tertiary – will be the principal influences. Three aspects of the clinical environment will influence the quality of the student's experience – the physical, emotional, and intellectual milieus.

1. *Physical environment:* In ambulatory teaching there should be enough space for students to see patients on their own, without slowing down the whole office, and space for private discussions and feedback between teacher and student. Patient volume and case mix should be adequate to achieve the educational objectives.
2. *Emotional climate:* Students should feel safe. Although there will inevitably be some anxiety inherent in the nature of the work, and students need to feel challenged for optimal learning, students should not be placed in situations where patient safety is jeopardized. Their teachers should be excellent role models of patient-centered care, trained in best practices of clinical teaching, and should include several members of an interprofessional team. Team members should interact effectively and demonstrate respectful communication. Teachers must be approachable, welcome questions from students, and provide frequent feedback to enhance learning. If possible, there should be enough continuity in the relationship between teacher and student to foster mutual respect and trust and opportunities to understand the specific learning needs of each student.
3. *Intellectual climate:* There should be time for reflection and discussion about patient care. Rapid access to learning resources such as the Internet is essential. All members of the team should model intellectual curiosity and ongoing learning from one another. It should be okay to say "I don't know" and use that as a springboard to further learning. General practice in the United Kingdom has pioneered the use of Significant Event Audit as a way for a team to review, analyze, and reflect on an incident that was "significant" to them – usually when something went wrong with patient care. It is an approach to learning from an event through a structured discussion by members of the whole healthcare team who had been involved in the event. Because such discussions can be sensitive and threatening, to use this approach successfully it is important to have strong team dynamics and good leadership.[79]

It is important to remember that medical education is not just about learning a set of knowledge, skills, and attitudes; it is also about changing laypersons into physicians – a profound life-altering transformation, as we described in Chapter 10. The syllabus defines the course of study that students must digest, but it does not describe the intimate personal interactions that bring about this important change. To understand how this occurs we need to examine medical school as a cultural institution.

Why do students concentrate on biomedicine and tend to disregard everything else? Where do they get the message that interviewing, medical humanities, and behavioral science are less important than traditional courses? Even in curricula that espouse a patient-centered mission, students do not take these subjects as seriously as the biological courses. A key to understanding this puzzle is the environment for learning in medical school. One of the key features of the learning environment is the hidden curriculum, which reflects beliefs and values that may not support, and may even be at odds with, the official curriculum. The hidden curriculum is so influential because it is taught by example.[80] It is contagious – students "catch" the lessons of this tacit curriculum through immersion in the system especially through students' relationships with more senior learners and their preceptors. Because it is part of the unspoken culture of medical school, it is not subject to critical reflection but simply taken for granted.[81–83] The same phenomenon is found in all professional schools. Writing from the perspective of nursing, Bevis and Watson describe the hidden curriculum in these terms:

> It is the curriculum in which we are unaware of the messages given by the way we teach, the priorities we set, the type of methods we use, and the way we interact with students. This is the curriculum of subtle socialization, of teaching initiates how to think and feel like nurses. It is the curriculum that covertly communicates priorities, relationships, and values. It colors perceptions, independence, initiative, caring, colleagueship, and the mores and folkways of being a nurse. It is taught by subtle, out-of-awareness things that pervade the whole educational environment: when classes are scheduled, how much time is given a subject in relationship to other subjects, how many test items are assigned a topic or whether or not a term paper is given to the area, who addresses whom in what way, how the teacher responds to students who openly differ in opinion from the teacher, how students are or are not encouraged to work together, and how teachers interact with students. All of these give the value messages to students that shape their learning in this curriculum.[84]

Some of the lessons taught by the hidden curriculum:

- Biology trumps everything else – medicine is essentially applied biology.
- Behavioral issues are just "common sense" – it's not necessary to understand the sciences that explain behavior.
- Patient care comes first, before your needs, health, or illness.
- The humanities are "nice to know" but can be ignored if time is needed to learn important subjects (and time is always needed for more important subjects).
- Demonstrating emotions is an unacceptable sign of weakness and should be avoided in medical practice – it can lead to overinvolvement with patients and interfere with clinical reasoning.
- The more hours a subject has in the curriculum, the more important it is.
- Factual knowledge is more important than attitudes.
- Being able to recite the latest fact is more valued than a deep understanding of concepts.
- Acute care is more important than preventive or chronic care.
- "When you are overwhelmed or at your limit, suck it up and do not ask for help".[85]

Coulehan describes the necessity for role models to counter the negative influences of the hidden curriculum:

> The first requirement for a sea change . . . is to increase dramatically the number of role model physicians at every stage of medical education. By role model

physicians I mean full-time faculty members who exemplify professional virtue in their interactions with patients, staff, and trainees; who have a broad, humanistic perspective; and who are devoted to teaching and willing to forego high income in order to teach. . .. Their presence would dilute and diminish the conflict between tacit and explicit values, especially in the hospital and clinic. The teaching environment would contain fewer hidden messages that say "Detach" while at the same time overt messages are saying "Engage." What trainees need is time and humanism.[86]

One of the most disturbing and intractable problems in medical education is abuse of students and residents. Since the publication of Silver's article[87] on medical student abuse 40 years ago, this "blight on the conscience of the profession" continues.[88] In one study, 72% of medical students reported at least one abusive experience, the most common being yelled at by faculty, residents, and other staff, reported by 54% of students.[89] In a survey of students at 16 nationally representative U.S. medical schools, 42% of seniors reported having experienced harassment, and 84% experienced belittlement during medical school. "Although few students characterised the harassment or belittlement as severe, poor mental health and low career satisfaction were significantly correlated with these experiences".[90]

The University of Colorado School of Medicine (CUSOM) had a higher rate of student mistreatment than the national average. This led to the creation of a student-faculty committee – the Ending Mistreatment Task Force (EMTF) to develop and implement several interventions to address the problem.

Over a five-year period, the EMTF engaged with the student body, clinical clerkship directors, faculty governance leaders, hospital medical staff leaders and the CUSOM administration to develop and implement several interventions that sought to: define mistreatment; respond promptly and confidentially to students' reports of mistreatment and other unprofessional behaviors; address generational misunderstandings; and empower stakeholders (including medical students, faculty leaders, clerkship directors, and administrators). An overriding goal of the EMTF was to reinforce teachers' and learners' shared commitment to a respectful learning environment and high-quality patient care.[91]

Over 6 years, these interventions helped reduce the prevalence of mistreatment reported by students by 36% compared to 4% across all U.S. medical schools.[91]

Olasoji,[92] using a mixed method study of medical students in a Nigerian medical college, found that 80% of students experienced "toxic" practice during bedside teaching encounters with clinical teachers. This included a form of questioning known as "pimping" (asking a series of rapid-fire, often esoteric, questions until the student is unable to answer). When done badly it is a form of teaching by humiliation.[93] 60% of these students reported the incidence but mostly (84.6%) only to fellow students. Many students felt the incident was not important enough to report or felt nothing would be done about it. But 18.8% of students who did not report the incident feared reprisal.[92] Another study analyzed the prevalence of medical student maltreatment by sex, race/ethnicity, and sexual orientation. Based on an analysis of the 2016 and 2017 Association of American Medical College Graduation Questionnaires,

Female, URM [Underrepresented Minorities], Asian, multiracial, and LGB students seem to bear a disproportionate burden of the mistreatment reported in medical schools. It appears that addressing the disparate mistreatment reported will be an important step to promote diversity, equity, and inclusion in medical education.[94]

The following incident, based on a true story, illustrates the type of harassment that remains all too common, despite numerous studies decrying such behavior by teachers. On her first day of clerkship, the medical student arrived on the ward for orientation to her inaugural rotation. While trying to introduce herself, she was initially ignored by the staff physician who was grilling the resident on the team. Finally, he turned in her direction and exclaimed sarcastically, "Oh . . . you're the 'clerkette'!" Turning back to the resident, he commented, "You'll find that clerkettes are all useless".

While the teacher's comment could be interpreted as a failed attempt at humor, most clerks would experience it as humiliating. Clerkette, because it sounds like a feminine term, would make the comment even more hurtful for a female student. Being in a one-down position on a new clinical team, just beginning clerkship, leaves the clerk with several unpleasant emotions – confusion, fear, anger, and perhaps even shame. If the student felt harassed by the teacher's comment, her situation is further complicated by having no recourse because of fear of retribution.

Since the well-publicized Libby Zion case (an 18-year-old patient who died in 1984 from serotonin syndrome misdiagnosed by residents exhausted by 18-hour shifts) there has been a steady attempt to reduce residents' work hours. This case drew widespread attention to the patient safety issues and adverse effects on residents of long shifts without sleep.[95] In the mid-1900s, residents and interns in the United States were on call for 36 hours starting every other night, totaling more than 100 hours per week. In 2011, the Accreditation Council for Graduate Medical Education restricted interns to 16-hour shifts and no more than 80 hours per week.[96] In Europe the restrictions on working hours are even stricter.[97]

A small number of administrations, predominantly in northern Europe, have achieved enviable success in reducing duty hours. Restrictions to 48 hours or less have been confirmed to provide safe care for patients while still achieving satisfactory education and training for staff within an acceptable time frame. These goals seem a long way from fulfilment in the rest of the "developed" world at present.[98]

Studies on the impact of these changes show mixed results. A systematic review of 135 articles on the impact of reduced duty hours (RDH) found that

Recent RDH changes are not consistently associated with improvements in resident well-being, and have negative impacts on patient outcomes and performance on certification examinations. Greater flexibility to accommodate resident training needs is required. Further erosion of training time should be considered with great caution.[99]

A cluster-randomized noninferiority trial of 63 internal medicine residency programs in the United States comparing programs with standard duty hours with programs with more flexible duty hours found that reduced duty hours did not adversely affect 30-day mortality or other measures of patient safety.[100] A separate noninferiority study of sleep and alertness comparing these same programs found no differences in chronic sleep loss or sleepiness.[101] Commenting on these studies, Rosenbaum and Lamas note: "Conspicuously absent in any of these trials is the patient voice. What is the experience of being a hospitalized patient in a world where 'your doctor' is constantly shifting?"[102]

FINDING COMMON GROUND

The central purpose of the patient-centered clinical method is finding common ground – reaching an agreement with patients about the nature of their health problems, the goals of treatment, and a plan describing the roles and responsibilities of patient and clinician. Similarly, the central purpose of the learner-centered method is finding common ground – achieving a common understanding about the priorities for learning, co-planning how these goals will be achieved, and clarifying the roles and responsibilities of the learner and teacher. The other components of each model have inherent benefits; for example, as clinicians or teachers listen intently or share empathic comments, they will deepen their understanding of the other that may even have therapeutic or educational benefit. However, these other components are primarily in the service of reaching a shared decision about what is to be done to improve the patient's sense of wellness or the learner's growth and development as a clinician.

Establishing Priorities

Difficulties arise when there is a conflict between what a student wants to learn and what a teacher wants to teach. When the official curriculum reflects the realities of practice, rather than being a difficult hurdle for students to jump in order to "prove themselves", such conflict is less likely. Also, students may become frustrated when there are so many required competencies that there is no time left to address topics of particular interest or self-assessed need. A learner-centered approach does not hand over the curriculum to the students, but it does respect their intelligence, common sense, and good intentions by involving them in decisions about what to learn, when to learn it, how deeply to focus, and how to evaluate their learning. For example, the value of understanding the family situation of patients may only become relevant to students when they are faced with patients whose family dynamics are central to management.

CASE EXAMPLE

Raymond Zegers, a first-year resident in family medicine, had been an infrequent participant at behavioral science seminars. He argued that "most of this stuff is common sense and I need more time learning about heart failure and COPD [chronic obstructive pulmonary disease]". But then he met Pat! Pat was a 75-year-old crusty woman with metastatic lung cancer who challenged all of her healthcare providers. She seemed to anticipate rejection and was determined to reject them before they rejected her. Raymond could not understand why she insisted on being so difficult. Despite her rough edges, he liked her hard-nosed determination and stoicism. When he was discussing discharge plans with her, he learned that her family had sold all of her belongings and cancelled the lease on her apartment. They had even sold off her clothes and jewelry. Raymond was furious at Pat's family and wondered how they could behave in such a cruel manner. He explored the family dynamics further and discovered that this was not the first time they had treated her this way. He started to understand why Pat kept people at a distance – it would be too dangerous to risk trusting anyone based on a lifetime of betrayal. The seminars on family dynamics started to have more interest for Raymond as he realized how a better understanding of family functioning could help him to provide better care to his patients.

In this case, the learner's struggle to help the patient led to his recognition of a need to learn more about family dynamics. Often, when patients are not doing well, learners blame themselves, even when they have provided appropriate care. As a result, the learner's priorities may be inaccurate. In these situations, the teacher may need to help the learner reflect on why they are feeling guilty and how this is affecting their management of the patient. The learner may need to concentrate on learning more about their feelings than solely about the biomedical topics the learner thinks they missed. The following case illustrates how the teacher helped the resident get past the guilt that was blocking his awareness of the patient's primary needs.

CASE EXAMPLE

Daria Zabian, a second-year family practice resident, after seeing her patient recovering in hospital from a myocardial infarct, wanted to focus her learning on the pharmacological management of cardiac risk factors. The resident had seen this patient in the office about a week before the infarct and wondered if she had missed some subtle warning signs. Daria was determined to provide optimal care for her patient's cardiac problem and failed to recognize the major adjustment the patient was now experiencing. The initial reaction of her supervisor, Dr Leblanc, was to address the importance of understanding the patient's illness experience and the value of good communication in improving adherence and recovery. However, knowing that this might not match the resident's priorities, Dr Leblanc decided to explore the resident's experience with this patient. He discovered that Daria felt somewhat guilty that she had not addressed all of her patient's risk factors before the infarct and was determined to make up for it now. Dr Leblanc asked Daria to tell him more about the office visit – in hindsight, had she in fact missed anything important? Together, they reviewed the medical record. The resident had checked the patient's blood pressure and ordered a serum cholesterol and asked about diet, exercise, and smoking. The patient had mentioned being more tired than usual but had no chest pain or shortness of breath. She was working longer hours than usual, and her elderly mother was requiring more care, but she was planning to take a vacation in the near future. The resident agreed that a vacation would be a good idea and asked the patient to return in 3 months to see how she was doing. Dr Leblanc stated that he agreed with her assessment and plan and complimented Daria on her thorough review.

Dr Leblanc commented: "Even when we have done everything right, we can feel upset when things turn out badly for our patients. Our feelings may lead us to overreact by ordering too many tests or by not tending to the patient's other needs. You are feeling badly for your patient's predicament. I wonder how she is feeling about her current situation?" By supporting Daria, Dr Leblanc modelled the kind of concern he hoped the resident would demonstrate with her patient. This encouraged Daria to recognize that her preoccupation with the biomedical issues was related to vague feelings of guilt and to realize that the patient would benefit from a discussion of her personal reaction to her serious illness.

Teaching and Learning Methods

There are several studies defining the characteristics of excellent clinical teaching that support the use of a learner-centered approach.[103-109] Whether done from the point of view of learners or teachers, or both, these studies agree that clinical teachers should demonstrate the following attributes:

- *Clinical competence, including demonstrating good skills, procedures, and patient care abilities.* They have a humanistic orientation, stressing the social and psychological aspects of patient care. They possess an excellent fund of knowledge and are able to present information in a clear and well-organized fashion. They have mastered the skills of physical examination and are skilled in teaching them. They are prepared to share with students their struggles and success with patients as a model of continuing learning.
- *Enthusiasm for teaching.* They obviously enjoy associating with students and make themselves accessible to them.
- *Supervisory skills.* They are sensitive to patient and student needs simultaneously and involve students actively in patient care and in their own learning. Students particularly value being given increasing patient responsibility as their skills improve.[110] They provide clear and appropriate direction and give frequent constructive feedback. Helpful feedback is the teacher's description of students' effective and ineffective behaviors that shows them how to improve their ineffective behaviors. They emphasize problem-solving by challenging students to discuss their thinking processes and give students an opportunity to practice skills and procedures. They are open to criticism from students, using it to enhance mutual learning.
- *Effective interpersonal skills.* They are sensitive to student concerns, such as feelings of inadequacy, and demonstrate a genuine interest in students through a friendly manner. Whenever possible, they build the self-esteem of students.

In a study of the harmful effects of bias on the teacher-learner relationship, Elks et al. point out that the short-term relationships that characterize much of clinical learning result in inaccurate assessments and leave both teachers and students craving for a deeper connection.

Our students crave relational learning. It is human nature to learn. It is also human nature to learn best from each other. It is human nature to crave direct approval from those who guide us. Medical center faculty, staff, and students are burning out due to a lack of relational experience, which is a human need. Modifying the learning environment to enhance and sustain relationships is key in addressing toxic bias. These are changes that are possible. These are changes that are energizing and vital for us to thrive.[111]

The importance of longer-term rotations for the development of trust and willingness of students to disclose their learning needs and ask for feedback is emphasized in a study by Schut et al. Comments by one of the students highlights their findings:

> Yeah, they know my style, they also know my weaknesses and strengths, I think because it's such a long-term relationship, I feel like it's easier for me to come to them and say I'm struggling with this. . . . It helps to become more vulnerable and I get to be really honest and look for their guidance. Whereas I might not really do that in any of the other settings because I don't want to be judged by the preceptors who don't know me really well, based on one single interaction.[112]

It is important to recognize that our biases against others – often based on gender, ethnic, and religious differences – are implicit or unconscious, and their effects can be devastating. Fortunately implicit bias training and other interventions to mitigate bias are effective including

> bias awareness training, increased exposure to individuals from differing demographic groups, increased participation of individuals from minority groups in key decision-making processes, and the use of structured systematic tools in decision making. These elements are most effective when trainees are active participants in the training process.[113]

In an excellent text on collaborative clinical education, Westberg and Jason describe the qualities of helpful teacher-learner relationships. Particularly effective are collaborative relationships that foster independence:

> Learners are seen as valuable contributors to the teaching-learning partnership and are encouraged to be as actively involved as possible in their learning: generating learning goals, devising strategies for meeting their goals, critiquing and monitoring their progress. Collaborative teachers do not immediately force learners to function as self-directed learners if the learners are not ready for this role. Rather, they start where the learners are and help them become increasingly more independent.[114]

Roles of Teacher and Learner

Clinical teachers have several different roles in their relationships with their students. On the one hand, teachers function as facilitators and role models; they support and encourage students by the force of their own personality. Students incorporate aspects of their teachers into their own developing professional identities and often form close personal relationships with them. On the other hand, teachers are experts, formal authorities, and socializing agents; they are guardians of the traditions of the profession and stand as trustees who decide whether or not each student measures up for admission into the ranks. In this sense, no matter what else they represent in the minds of their students, they are powerful and sometimes intimidating authority figures. Thus, teachers wear many hats and have complex multidimensional relationships with their students.

A survey of medical students beginning year 2, exploring their opinion of the qualities of an ideal role model, found the following key teaching skills: "encourages my learning; is a very good diagnostic clinician; models empathy, respect, compassion; is inspiring; is enthusiastic; has a positive outlook; shows good communication skills".[115]

When teachers switch from a traditional role of telling students everything they need to know to a learner-centered approach where students are required to take more responsibility for their own learning, some students may not be ready. In Chapter 10 we described how students change with experience from a stage of dualism – wanting the one right answer – to one of multiplicity, next a stage of relativism, and finally commitment when they are able to take more control of their learning. It is important that they reach this stage by the time of graduation so that they can continue to learn throughout their years in practice.[116, 117]

The student's role on a healthcare team can be understood using the theory of communities of practice.[118] From this perspective, students' progress through medical school from a position of legitimate peripheral participation, where they are mostly observers on the team, to full participation, where they can make meaningful contributions to patient care.[119]

ENHANCING THE LEARNER–TEACHER RELATIONSHIP

The relational nature of good teaching is captured by Palmer:

> Most important, I learn that my gift as a teacher is the ability to dance with my students, to co-create with them a context in which all of us can teach and learn, and that this gift works as long as I stay open and trusting and hopeful about who my students are.[120]

In a comprehensive review of the role of teacher-learner relationships in medical education, Tiberius et al. conclude: "teacher-learner relationships have an enormous impact on the quality of teaching and learning. By some estimates the teacher-learner relationship explains roughly half of the variance in the effectiveness of teaching".[121] In a list of influences on student achievement, Hattie[122] places teacher–student relationships near the top with an effect size* of 0.72 based on over 900 meta-analyses (an effect size greater than 0.4 is considered worthwhile). Other interventions with a similar effect size include classroom discussion (0.82), teacher clarity (0.75), and feedback (0.75). Good teachers have a desire to help their students learn, which transcends the challenges that teaching creates. Teaching may interfere with clinicians' intimate one-to-one relationships with their patients. It slows them down. It exposes their weaknesses and areas of ignorance. Thus it demands a positive regard and caring for learners even when their behavior may frustrate or upset the teacher. It is essential that clinical teachers "walk the talk" – there must be congruence between the patient-centered clinical method and the process of teaching it. For example, just as patient-centered care must always be provided as part of a healing relationship, so too teaching should be in the context of care for the learner as a developing clinician and not just for their knowledge base. This commitment transcends individual learning problems or specific skills to be learned. It extends into the very being of the learners and challenges them to stretch themselves to their limits. Such learning may require students to experience painful self-discovery or to make difficult personal changes.

CASE EXAMPLE

Brigit Jansen had wanted to be a child psychiatrist since her youth. She had loved caring for young children and had served as an aide at a children's psychiatric facility during her teens. Brigit had also battled with bulimia throughout her late teens and early twenties; hence she was very familiar with the process of psychotherapy. Upon completion of her Bachelor of Education at the age of 22, Brigit decided to apply to medical school. It had been an uphill battle conquering the basic sciences she lacked in her undergraduate education and keeping her bulimia at bay. However, she had succeeded and now was embarking on her child psychiatry residency. Brigit was both excited and anxious. She was eager to work with the younger children but doubted how she might relate to the adolescents, particularly the females who would have an eating disorder like hers. Yet as time went by Brigit became both skilled and assured in her work with adolescents. It was not until her rotation on the inpatient adolescent unit when she was assigned two seriously ill patients with eating disorders that she began to question her ability to work with this patient population. Their issues were too close to her own, and she struggled to keep clear what were their issues and what were her own demons.

Dr Tillman had been her supervisor and mentor since Brigit had joined the residency program. While she had not disclosed her bulimia to him, she realized that it was time to share this information. Her own personal problems were beginning to affect her ability to care for her patients.

What allowed Brigit to expose her feelings about this situation was the trust, respect, and safety that she experienced in the learner–teacher relationship with Dr Tillman. She knew from her past experiences with Dr Tillman that he would not judge her past behavior or question her current situation. He would listen and be there for her. Dr Tillman would invite her "to wonder" what might be causing her present difficulty and how she would overcome this problem. He would respect the boundaries of the learner–teacher relationship. Dr Tillman would not become her therapist but remain her teacher all the while knowing when referral for further professional counseling would be important for Brigit, both personally and professionally.

* Effect size = Average (post-test) – Average (pre-test)/Spread (standard deviation)
Effect size is a standardized approach to measuring the effectiveness of an educational intervention.

Students will often defend against such self-awareness and may find themselves in conflict with their teachers over the need for change. At this stage in the development of their professional identity they often experience ambivalent feelings about their teachers: on the one hand they wish for a dependent relationship where their obligations are spelled out and clearly limited; on the other hand, they resent the imposition of control and long for independent responsibility. Their feelings may vacillate from one extreme to the other depending on the complexity and volume of patient care, fatigue, and feelings of self-efficacy. It is not surprising that intense emotions may develop in the student-teacher relationship replicating similar feelings with other powerful authority figures from the student's past. Working through this transference may enhance the student's self-understanding and prevent similar reactions from occurring in the future. It requires the development of an intimate and trust-based relationship before such intensely personal learning and growth can occur. Continuity in their relationship is the basis for establishing trust and for developing the deep understanding necessary for helping students develop as healers. These decisive personal and contextual issues, so critical in determining what will be learned, and how the teacher can help, cannot be easily communicated from one teacher to another. Robertson describes the importance for teachers to develop the ability to identify and manage unconscious aspects of their relationships with students:

Transference and countertransference are extremely common and have a significant impact on the teacher's relationship with specific learners as well as on the group climate. Most likely, these phenomena are occurring in every course that we teach and are worth our attention. In addition, they are phenomena that by definition are unconscious. We need to go looking for them. As we add our techniques for identifying unconscious associations by ourselves or by the learners to our current repertoire of teacher/learner relationship skills, perhaps we transform our overall capacity to handle the intense emotionality of transference and countertransference and, thereby, to establish effective teacher/learner relationships. If so, we have developed in this area; we have grown.[123]

Supervision of psychotherapists shares many similarities with clinical teaching especially regarding the importance of the relationship between teacher and learner. Alonso summarizes this aspect as follows:

> The development of a clinician from novice to expert is primarily an emotional, maturational process, much like the development of a child from infancy to adulthood . . . It is assumed that a transference relationship will develop between therapist and supervisor and that this transferential field will become a primary vehicle for influencing the student's clinical growth . . . there is a concerted effort to shore up and strengthen the supervisee's healthiest defences, either by reducing the ambiguity or by helping the trainee to tolerate the inevitable confusion of clinical work . . . When difficulty occurs . . . this regression is seen as a healthy and expectable rite of passage . . . In fact, the clinician who never regresses in the course of training is probably avoiding the more difficult levels of learning that occur in the unconscious merger of patient/therapist and may be keeping too great a distance between self and patient.[124]

There are a number of teacher behaviors that contribute to the creation of an impasse with their learners: the need to be admired; the need to rescue; the need to be in control; the need for competition; the need to be loved; the need to work through unresolved prior conflict in the supervisor's own training experience; spillover from stress in the personal or professional life of the supervisor; tension between supervisor and the administration of the institution.[124] This highlights the importance of a healthy and open relationship between teachers and learners characterized by empathy, genuineness, and positive regard.[125] Tiberius describes the central role of relationships in teaching and learning: the relationship between teachers and learners can be viewed as a set of filters, interpretive screens, or expectations that determine the effectiveness of interaction between teacher and student. Effective teachers form relationships that are trustful, open and secure, that involve a minimum of control, are cooperative, and are conducted in a reciprocal, interactive manner. They share control with students and encourage interactions that are determined by mutual agreement. . . . Within such relationships learners are willing to disclose their lack of understanding rather than hide it from their teachers; learners are more attentive, ask more questions, and are more actively engaged. Thus, the better the relationship, the better the interaction; the better the interaction, the better the learning.[126]

CONCLUSION

In this chapter we have described the four components of the learner-centered method of education illustrating the many parallels with the patient-centered clinical method. Key lessons from this chapter are as follows:

- It is important to include learners' ideas and aspirations about what they wish to learn in all educational planning. Incorporating knowledge of learners' strengths, weaknesses, and special interests improves motivation, accelerates the learning process, and increases the potential depth and complexity of the competencies that can be mastered.

- There are two dimensions of understanding the student as a whole person: the student's life history, including personal and cognitive development, and the learning environment. Becoming a physician is a life-altering process, not just the accumulation of competencies. Stress, burnout, and mistreatment can all interfere with learning. The hidden curriculum can have a greater impact on learning than the official curriculum and sometimes it teaches a contrary lesson.
- There are three key elements in finding common ground in the learner-centered approach: (1) establishing priorities, (2) choosing appropriate teaching-learning methods, and (3) determining the roles of both teacher and learner. When teachers and learners collaborate in identifying goals and selecting learning experiences, students are more likely to be successful.
- The way teachers relate to learners will influence the way in which learners interact with patients and is central to their development as effective healers. The relationship between teachers and learners is the dominant influence in creating an effective environment for learning and development.

BEING THERE: CASE ILLUSTRATING BEING LEARNER-CENTERED

Christine Rivet and Judith Belle Brown

It was Monday, a beautiful September morning when Grace, our team nurse, called me at home. She told me that my resident Sam and his wife, Helena, had just had a baby girl. But it didn't make sense – her voice was muted, unreal. "Chris, she's just beautiful. I was just at the hospital with them". Was it the shock that made her voice sound that way? It just didn't match the horror of what she was saying. Did I miss something? Was she really saying that their baby was dead?

"I think you should go over to the hospital". *No, I can't; I can't do it. Don't ask me that. I'm just his supervisor. I don't even know him that well.* He was a first-year resident from a small northern community. New to town. No family here. "You know they don't have any family or close friends here in town. Their parents haven't arrived yet". Sam had been an engineer before going into medicine. A nice guy just a few years younger than me. *What can I do? I certainly can't replace his parents or family.*

I had only met Helena a couple of times at some family medicine outings, and she was very thin, shy, and delicate. She and Sam had been trying to start a family for several years. Finally Helena was pregnant, and everything was going well. Sam was thrilled; even though he was off service he would drop into the family medicine center and describe the progress of her pregnancy. Last week he had told me she was 37 weeks pregnant.

"Chris?"

"What happened? I thought her pregnancy was going so well".

"I don't know. Helena stopped feeling movement, and they did an ultrasound on Friday that showed that the baby had died". *They had known for 2 days?! How could they live through this?*

The hospital was only a 5-minute walk away. When I got up to the maternity floor, I walked down a long hallway to the reception where a nurse was sitting. An unfamiliar setting since I don't do obstetrics. "I'm Dr Rivet. I've been told that Sam and Helena Howell are here and that their baby has died". *I don't belong here. Don't let me go to see them. I shouldn't be allowed. I'm just his supervisor. Not family or close friend. And what can I do to help in such a tragedy?* "Yes, I'll take you. It's just down this hallway". My heart was pounding. What could I say or do? I have three young children. I can't imagine anything more horrible than losing one of my children. *I have no solutions for them – no words of comfort.*

Helena was lying in bed, her face frail and blank. There was a nurse near her and there was Sam standing in the corner. He was holding their baby in his arms wrapped like all newborns in a cocoon of blankets. He came toward me crying. "Would you like to hold her?" *No I couldn't do it. The blankets look like the blankets around all the other new-borns I have ever seen but this baby is dead! I can't hold this baby.* But I nodded yes. And there she was in my arms. As light as a feather. A beautiful baby. Perfect face. Her eyes were closed. She was swaddled in so many blankets that I couldn't feel the cold of her body. *The nurses must do that intentionally.* Her skin must have been cyanotic, but in my memory this baby is pink like all newborns. *I wish I could do something to help you, but I'm overwhelmed by your tragedy.* Then I started to weep as I looked down at their baby.

The expression "just being there" for our patients evokes this tragic event during my early days of being a supervisor. My situation as a supervisor is not unique. All supervisors have been somehow involved in very personal life events of their residents: the sudden death of a parent, severe depression, the breakdown of a marriage. This experience demonstrates the challenges we face when we go beyond the conventional learner-teacher relationship. Yet if we are seeking to teach our students how to extend their relationship with patients beyond the narrow biomedical approach then we must model this behavior.

REFERENCES

1. Flachmann M: Teaching in the twenty-first century. *Teaching Professor.* 1994;8(3):2.
2. Kapp A: *Die andragogic ober bildung im Mannlichen alter. Platons Erziehungslehre, als Padagogik fur die Einzelnen und als Staatspadagogik.* Minden und Leipzig, Germany: Ferdinand Essman, 1833.
3. Henschke JA: *Beginnings of the History and Philosophy of Andragogy 1833–2000.* Knoxville, TN: International Adult and Continuing Education Hall of Fame Repository, TRACE: Tennessee Research and Creative Exchange, University of Tennessee, 2009.
4. Lindeman EC: *The Meaning of Adult Education.* New York: New Republic, 1926. (Reprinted by Windham Press, 2013.)
5. Knowles MS, Holton III EF, Swanson RA, Robinson PA: *The Adult Learner: The Definitive Classic in Adult Education and Human Resource Development,* 9th edition. Abingdon, Oxon: Routledge, 2020.
6. Merriam SB, Bierema LL: *Adult Learning: Linking Theory and Practice.* San Francisco: Jossey-Bass, 2013.
7. Merriam SB, Baumgartner LM: *Learning in Adulthood: A Comprehensive Guide,* 4th edition. Hoboken, NJ: Jossey-Bass, 2020.
8. Kaufman DM: Teaching and learning in medical education: how theory can inform practice. In: Swanwick T, Forrest K, O'Brien BC (Editors): *Understanding Medical Education: Evidence, Theory, and Practice.* Hoboken, NJ: John Wiley & Sons, 2019: 62, 64.
9. Dennick R: Constructivism: reflections on twenty five years teaching the constructivist approach in medical education. *International Journal of Medical Education.* 2016;7:200–205.

10. Liljedahl M, Palmgren PJ, McGrath C: Threshold concepts in health professions education research: a scoping review. *Advances in Health Sciences Education.* 2022;27:1457–1475.
11. Jones H, Hammond L: Threshold concepts in medical education: a scoping review. *Medical Education.* 2022;56:983–993.
12. Weimer M: *Learner-Centered Teaching – Five Key Changes to Practice*, 2nd edition. San Francisco: Jossey-Bass, 2013: 22.
13. Thomas PA, Kern DE, Hughes MT, Tackett SA, Chen BY: *Curriculum Development for Medical Education. A Six-Step Approach*, 4th edition. Baltimore: Johns Hopkins University Press, 2022.
14. Lu F-I, Takahashi SG, Kerr C: Myth or reality: self-assessment is central to effective curriculum in anatomical pathology graduate medical education. *Academic Pathology.* 2021;8. https://doi.org/10.1177/23742895211013528.
15. Andrade, HL: A critical review of research on student self-assessment. *Frontiers in Education.* 2019;4(87). https://doi.org/10.3389/feduc.2019.00087.
16. Lucey CR, Thibault GE, ten Cate O: Competency-based, time-variable education in the health professions: crossroads. *Academic Medicine.* 2018;93(3):S1–S5.
17. Chaghari M, Saffari M, Ebadi A, Ameryoun A: Empowering education: a new model for in-service training of nursing staff. *Journal of Advances in Medical Education and Professionalism.* 2017;5(1):26–32.
18. Lessing JN, Pierce RG, Dhaliwal G: Teaching more about less: preparing clinicians for practice. *American Journal of Medicine.* 2022;135(6):673–675.
19. Williams GC, Deci EL: The importance of supporting autonomy in medical education. *Annals of Internal Medicine.* 1998;129(4):303–308.
20. Scheffer C, Valk-Draad MP, Tauschel D, et al.: Students with an autonomous role in hospital care – patients perceptions. *Medical Teacher.* September 2018;40(9):944–952. https://doi.org/10.1080/0142159X.2017.1418504.
21. Caverzagie KJ, Nousiainen MT, Ferguson PC, et al.: Overarching challenges to the implementation of competency-based medical education. *Medical Teacher.* 2017;39(6):588–593.
22. Flexner A: *The American College: A Criticism*. New York, NY: Century, 1908. (Reprinted by Arno Press; *New York Times*, 1969).
23. Flexner A: *Medical Education in the United States and Canada. Bulletin No. 4.* New York, NY: Carnegie; Foundation for the Advancement of Teaching, 1910.
24. Pratt DD, Associates. *Five Perspectives on Teaching in Adult and Higher Education.* Malabar, FL: Krieger Publishing, 1998.
25. Matheson C: The educational value and effectiveness of lectures. *Clinical Teacher.* 2008;5:218–221.
26. Lowe RC, Borkan SC: Effective medical lecturing: practice becomes theory – a narrative review. *Medical Science Educator.* 2021;31:935–943.
27. Young JQ, van Merrienboer J, Durning S, ten Cate O: Cognitive load theory: implications for medical education: AMEE guide no. 86. *Medical Teacher.* 2014;36:371–384.
28. Morcos G, Awan OA: Burnout in medical school: a medical student's perspective. *Academic Radiology.* June 2023;30(6):1223–1225. https://doi.org/10.1016/j.acra.2022.11.023.
29. Murad MH, Coto-Yglesias F, Varkey P, et al.: The effectiveness of self-directed learning in health professions: a systematic review. *Medical Education.* 2020;44(11):1057–1068.
30. Loeng S: Self-directed learning: a core concept in adult education. *Education Research International.* 2020;2020:1–12

31. Ricotta DN, Richards JB, Atkins KM, et al.: Self-directed learning in medical education: training for a lifetime of discovery. *Teaching and Learning in Medicine – An International Journal.* 2021;34(5):530–540.

32. Knowles MS: *Self-Directed Learning – A Guide for Learners and Teachers.* Chicago: Follett Publishing, 1975: 18.

33. National Academies of Sciences, Engineering, and Medicine: *How People Learn II: Learners, Contexts, and Cultures.* Washington, DC: National Academies Press, 2018: 73. https://doi.org/10.17226/24783.

34. Doyle T: *Learner-Centered Teaching: Putting the Research on Learning into Practice.* Sterling, VA: Stylus Publishing, 2011.

35. Cheren M: Helping learners achieve greater self-direction. In: Smith RM (Editor): *Helping Adults Learn How to Learn.* San Francisco, CA: Jossey-Bass, 1983: 27.

36. Buch AC, Rathod H, Naik MD: Scope and challenges of self-directed learning in undergraduate medical education: a systematic review. *Journal of Medical Education.* 2021;20(1):e114077.

37. Svinicki MD: New directions in learning and motivation. *New Directions for Teaching and Learning.* 1999;80:5–27.

38. Svinicki MD, McKeachie W: *McKeachie's Teaching Tips,* 14th edition. Belmont, CA: Wadsworth, 2013.

39. Grow G: Teaching learners to be self-directed. *Adult Education Quarterly.* 1991;41:125–149.

40. Nasri NM: Self-directed learning through the eyes of teacher educators. *Kasetsart Journal of Social Sciences.* 2019;40:164–171.

41. Pink D: *Drive: The Surprising Truth about What Motivates Us.* New York, NY: Riverhead Books, 2011.

42. Hidi S: Revisiting the role of rewards in motivation and learning: implications of neuroscientific research. *Educational Psychology Review.* 2016;28:61–93. https://doi.org/10.1007/s10648-015-9307-5.

43. Ryan RM, Deci EL: Intrinsic and extrinsic motivation from a self-determination theory perspective: Definitions, theory, practices, and future direction. *Contemporary Educational Psychology.* 2010;61:1. https://doi.org/10.1016/j.cedpsych.2020.101860.

44. Hajek P, Najberg E, Cushing A: Medical students' concerns about communicating with patients. *Medical Education.* 2000;34(8):656–658.

45. Lumma-Sellenthin A: Talking with patients and peers: medical students' difficulties with learning communication skills. *Medical Teacher.* 2009;31:528–534.

46. Lacasse M, Théorêt J, Skalenda P, et al.: Challenging learning situations in medical education: innovative and structured tools for assessment, educational diagnosis, and intervention. Part 1: history and data gathering. *Canadian Family Physician.* 2012;58(4):481–484.

47. Rath VL, Mazotti L, Wilkes MS: A framework to understand the needs of the medical students of the future. *Medical Teacher.* 2020;42(8):922–928.

48. Curry L: Individual differences in cognitive style, learning style and instructional preference in medical education. In: Norman GR, van der Vleuten CPM, Newbie DI (Editors): *Handbook of Research in Medical Education.* Dordrecht: Kluwer Academic, 2002.

49. Altugan AS: The relationship between cultural identity and learning. *Procedia – Social and Behavioral Sciences.* 2015;186:1159–1162.

50. Forrest D, George S, Stewart S, et al.: Cultural diversity and inclusion in UK medical schools. *Clinical Teacher.* 2022;19:213–220.

51. Osler W: *Aequanimitas with Other Addresses to Medical Students, Nurses and Practitioners of Medicine,* 3rd edition. London: Blakiston Division; McGraw-Hill Book Company, 1932: 423.

52. Noonan WD: Must an internship be miserable? The pharos of alpha omega alpha-honor medical society. *Alpha Omega Alpha*. 1 January 1998;58(3):19–23, 180.

53. Eng J, Schulman E, Jhanwar SM, et al.: Patient death debriefing sessions to support residents' emotional reactions to patient deaths. *Journal of Graduate Medical Education*. 2015;7(3):430–436.

54. Ramakrishnan A, Sambuco D, Jagsi R: Women's participation in the medical profession: insights from experiences in Japan, Scandinavia, Russia, and Eastern Europe. *Journal of Women's Health*. 2014;11:927–934.

55. Newman C, Templeton K, Chin EL: Inequity and women physicians: time to change millennia of societal beliefs. *Permanente Journal*. 2020;24:20.024. https://doi.org/10.7812/TPP/20.024.

56. Mast MS, Kadji KK: How female and male physicians' communication is perceived differently. *Patient Education and Counseling*. 2018;101:1697–1701.

57. Hedden L, Barer ML, Cardiff K, et al.: The implications of the feminization of the primary care physician workforce on service supply: a systematic review. *Human Resources for Health*. 2014;12:32. www.human-resources-health.com/content/12/1/32.

58. Daher Y, Austin ET, Munter BT, et al.: The history of medical education: a commentary on race. *Journal of Osteopathic Medicine*. 2021;121(2):163–170.

59. Steinecke A, Terrell C: Progress for whose future? The impact of the Flexner "report on medical education for racial and ethnic minority physicians in the United States". *Academic Medicine*. 2010;85:236–245.

60. Kuper A, Hodges B: Medical education in its societal context. In: Dornan T, Mann K, Scherpbier A, Spencer J (Editors): *Medical Education Theory and Practice*. Oxford: Churchill Livingstone Elsevier, 2011: 39–48.

61. Pregnall AM, Churchwell AL, Ehrenfeld JM: A call for LGBTQ content in graduate medical program requirements. *Academic Medicine*. 2021;96(6):828–835.

62. Accreditation Council for Graduate Medical Education. *ACGME Common Program Requirements (Residency) Effective July 1 2022*. Retrieved 28 February 2023: 21. www.acgme.org/globalassets/PFAssets/ProgramRequirements/CPRResidency_2022v2.pdf.

63. Ayala EE, Roseman D, Winseman JS, Mason HRC: Prevalence, perceptions, and consequences of substance use in medical students. *Medical Education Online*. 2017;22. https://doi.org/10.1080/10872981.2017.1392824.

64. Frajerman A, Morvan Y, Krebs M-O, et al.: Burnout in medical students before residency: a systematic review and meta-analysis. *European Psychiatry*. 2019;55:36–42.

65. Williamson K, Lank PM, Cheema N, et al.: Comparing the Maslach burnout inventory to other well-being instruments in emergency medicine residents. *Journal of Graduate Medical Education*. 2018:532–536.

66. Shanafelt TD, Bradley KA, Wipf JE, et al.: Burnout and self-reported patient care in an internal medicine residency program. *Annals of Internal Medicine*. 2002;136(5):358–367.

67. Dyrbye LN, Massie Jr FS, Eacker A, et al.: Relationship between burnout and professional conduct and attitudes among US medical students. *JAMA*. 2010;304(11):1173–1180.

68. Baer TE, Feraco AM, Tuysuzoglu Sagalowsky S, Williams D, Litman HJ, Vinci RJ: Pediatric resident burnout and attitudes toward patients. *Pediatrics*. 1 March 2017;139(3).

69. Lee FJ, Stewart M, Brown JB: Stress, burnout, and strategies for reducing them. *Canadian Family Physician*. 2008;54(2):234–235.

70. Frenk J, Chen LC, Chandran L, et al.: Challenges and opportunities for educating health professionals after the COVID-19 pandemic. *Lancet*. 2022;400:1539–1556.

71. Macaron MM, Segun-Omosehin OA, Matar RH, et al.: A systematic review and meta analysis on burnout in physicians during the COVID-19 pandemic: a hidden health-care crisis. *Frontiers in Psychiatry*. 2023;13:1071397, 11. https://doi.org/10.3389/fpsyt.2022.1071397.

72. Shanafelt TD: Enhancing meaning in work: a prescription for preventing physician burn-out and promoting patient-centered care. *JAMA*. 2009;302(12):1338–1340.

73. Krasner MS, Epstein RM, Beckman H, et al.: Association of an educational program in mindful communication with burnout, empathy, and attitudes among primary care phy-sicians. *JAMA*. 2009;302(12):1284–1293.

74. Cassell EJ: *The Nature of Healing: The Modern Practice of Medicine*. New York, NY: Oxford University Press, 2013.

75. Drybye L, Sciolla F, Dekhtyar M: Medical school strategies to address student well-being: a national survey. *Academic Medicine*. 2019;94(6):861–868.

76. MacLean L, Booza J, Balon R: The impact of medical school on student mental health. *Academic Psychiatry*. 2016;40:89–91.

77. Slavin SJ, Schindler DL, Chibnall JT: Medical student mental health 3.0: improving student wellness through curricular changes. *Academic Medicine*. 2014;89(4):573–577.

78. Roff S, McAleer S: What is educational climate? *Medical Teacher*. 2001;23(4):333–334.

79. Bowie P, McNaughton E, Bruce D, et al.: Enhancing the effectiveness of significant event analysis: exploring personal impact and applying systems thinking in primary care. *Journal of Continuing Education in the Health Professions*. 2016;36(3):195–205.

80. Bandura A: *Social Foundations of Thought and Action: A Social Cognitive Theory*. Englewood Cliffs, NJ: Prentice Hall, 1986.

81. Hafferty FW: Beyond curriculum reform: confronting medicine's hidden curriculum. *Academic Medicine*. 1998;73(4):403–407.

82. Inui TS: *A Flag in the Wind: Educating for Professionalism in Medicine*. Washington, DC: Association of American Medical Colleges, 2003.

83. Lawrence C, Mhlaba T, Stewart KA, et al.: The hidden curricula of medical education: a scoping review. *Academic Medicine*. 2018;93(4):648–656.

84. Bevis O, Watson J: *Towards a Caring Curriculum: A New Pedagogy for Nursing*. Sudbury, MA: Jones & Bartlett, 2000: 75–76.

85. Pearl R: *Uncaring: How the Culture of Medicine Kills Doctors and Patients*. New York, NY: Hachette Book Group, 2021: 77.

86. Coulehan J: You say self-interest, I say altruism. In: Wear D, Aultman JM (Editors): *Professionalism in Medicine: Critical Perspectives*. New York, NY: Springer, 2006: 116.

87. Silver HK: Medical students and medical school. *JAMA*. 1982;247:309–310.

88. Rees CE, Monrouxe LV: "A morning since eight of just pure grill": a multischool qualita-tive study of student abuse. *Academic Medicine*. November 2011;86(11):1374–1382. https://doi.org/10.1097/ACM.0b013e3182303c4c.

89. Kumar P, Basu D: Substance abuse by medical students and doctors. *Journal of the Indian Medical Association*. 2000;98(8):447–452.

90. Frank E, Carrera JS, Stratton T, et al.: Experiences of belittlement and harassment and their correlates among medical students in the United States: longitudinal survey. *BMJ*. 2006;333(7570):682.

91. Lind KT, Osborne CM, Badesch B, et al.: Ending student mistreatment: early successes and continuing challenges. *Medical Education Online*. 2019;25:1690846, 1, 2. https://doi.org/10.1080/10872981.2019.1690846.

92. Olasoji HO: Broadening conceptions of medical student mistreatment during clinical teaching: message from a study of "toxic" phenomenon during bedside teaching. *Advances in Medical Education and Practice*. 2018;9:483–494.

93. Chen DR, Priest KC: Pimping: a tradition of gendered disempowerment. *BMC Medical Education*. 2019;19:345.

94. Hill KA, Samuels EA, Gross CP, et al.: Assessment of the prevalence of medical school mistreatment by sex, race/ethnicity, and sexual orientation. *JAMA Internal Medicine*. 2020;180(5):663–665.

95. Woodrow SI, Segouin C, Armbruster J, et al.: Duty hour reforms in the United States, France, and Canada: is it time to refocus our attention on education. *Academic Medicine*. 2006;81(12):1045–1051.

96. Rosenbaum L, Lamas D: Residents' duty hours: toward an empirical narrative. *New England Journal of Medicine*. 2012;367(21):2044–2049.

97. Moonesinghe SR, Lowery J, Shahi N, et al.: Impact of reduction in working hours for doctors in training on postgraduate medical education and patients' outcomes: systematic review. *BMJ*. 2011;342:d1580.

98. Temple J: Resident duty hours around the globe: where are we now? *BMC Medical Education*. 2014;14(Suppl 1):S8. www.biomedcentral.com/1472-6920/14/S1/S8.

99. Ahmed N, Devitt KS, Keshet I, et al.: A systematic review of the effects of resident duty hour restrictions in surgery – impact on resident wellness, training, and patient outcomes. *Annals of Surgery*. 2014;259:1041–1053.

100. Silber JH, Bellini LM, Shea JA, et al.: Patient safety outcomes under flexible and standard resident duty hour rules. *New England Journal of Medicine*. 2019;380(10):905–914.

101. Basner M, Aasch DA, Shea JA, et al.: Sleep and alertness in a duty-hour flexibility trial in internal medicine. *New England Journal of Medicine*. 2019;380(10):915–923.

102. Rosenbaum L, Lamas D: Eyes wide open – examining the data on duty-hour reform. *New England Journal of Medicine*. 2019;380(10):969–970.

103. Kilminster S, Cottrell D, Grant J, et al.: AMEE guide no. 27: effective educational and clinical supervision. *Medical Teacher*. 2007;29(1):2–19.

104. Yeates PJA, Stewart J, Barton JR: What can we expect of clinical teachers? Establishing consensus on applicable skills, attitudes and practices. *Medical Education*. 2008;42(2):134–142.

105. Sutkin G, Wagner E, Harris I, et al.: What makes a good clinical teacher in medicine? A review of the literature. *Academic Medicine*. 2008;83(5):452–466.

106. Skeff KM, Stratos GA: *Methods for Teaching Medicine*. Philadelphia, PA: American College of Physicians, 2010.

107. Reilly JB, Bennett N, Fosnocht K, et al.: Redesigning rounds: towards a more purposeful approach to inpatient teaching and learning. *Academic Medicine*. 2015;90(4):450–453.

108. Silkens MEWM, Chahine S, Lombarts KMJMH, Arah OA: From good to excellent: improving clinical departments' learning climate in residency training. *Medical Teacher*. 2018;40(3):237–243.

109. Fantaye AW, Kitto S, Hendry P, et al.: Attributes of excellent clinician teachers and barriers to recognizing and rewarding clinician teachers' performances and achievements: a narrative review. *Canadian Medical Education Journal*. 2022;13(2):57–72.

110. Alguire PC, DeWitt DE, Pinsky LE, et al.: *Teaching in Your Office: A Guide to Instructing Medical Students and Residents*, 2nd edition. Philadelphia, PA: ACP Press, 2008.

111. Elks ML, Johnson K, Anachebe NF: Morehouse school of medicine case study: teacher-learner relationships free of bias and discrimination. *Academic Medicine*. 2020;95(Suppl 12):S88–S92.

112. Schut S, van Tartwijk J, Driessen E, van der Vleuten C, Heeneman S: Understanding the influence of teacher–learner relationships on learners' assessment perception. *Advances in Health Sciences Education*. May 2020;25:441–456.

113. Plews-Ogan ML, Bell TD, Townsend G, et al.: Acting wisely: eliminating negative bias in medical education – part 2: how can we do better? *Academic Medicine*. 2020;95(12):S16–S22.

114. Westberg J, Jason H: *Collaborative Clinical Education: The Foundation of Effective Health Care*. New York, NY: Springer, 1993: 92, 93.

115. Burgess A, Oates K, Goulston K: Role modelling in medical education: the importance of teaching skills. *The Clinical Teacher*. 2016;13:134–137.

116. Bhandari B: Cultivating self-directed learning skills in the budding doctors: an attempt to transform an "Indian medical graduate" into a "lifelong learner". *South-East Asian Journal of Medical Education*. 2021;15(1):65–67.

117. Witt EE, Onorato SE, Schwartzstein RM: Medical students and the drive for a single right answer. *ATS Scholar*. 2022;3(1):27–37.

118. Wenger E: *Communities of Practice – Learning, Meaning, and Identity*. Cambridge: Cambridge University Press, 1998.

119. Gonzalo JD, Thompson BM, Haidet P, et al.: A constructive reframing of student roles and systems learning in medical education using a communities of practice lens. *Academic Medicine*. 2017;92(12):1687–1694.

120. Palmer PJ: *The Courage to Teach: Exploring the Inner Landscape of a Teacher's Life*. 10th anniversary edition. San Francisco, CA: Jossey-Bass, 2007: 74, 75.

121. Tiberius RG, Sinai J, Flak EA: The role of teacher-learner relationships in medical education. In: Norman GR, van der Vleuten CPM, Newble DI (Editors): *International Handbook of Research in Medical Education*. Dordrecht: Kluwer Academic Publishers, 2002: 463.

122. Hattie J: *Visible Learning for Teachers: Maximizing Impact on Learning*. New York, NY: Routledge, 2012: 251.

123. Robertson DL: Emotion and professors' developmental perspectives on their teaching. In: Wehlburg CM (Editor): *In-Chief: New Directions for Teaching and Learning, No. 153*. Wiley Periodicals, Spring 2018: 15. https://doi.org/10.1002/tl.20276.

124. Alonso A: *The Quiet Profession: Supervisors of Psychotherapy*. Toronto, Canada: Collier Macmillan, 1985: 47, 48.

125. Rogers C: *Client-Centered Therapy: Its Current Practice Implications and Theory*. Cambridge, MA: Riverside Press, 1951.

126. Tiberius RG: The why of teacher/student relationships. *Teaching Excellence: Toward the Best in the Academy*. 1993;5(8):1–5.

Challenges in Learning and Teaching the Patient-Centered Clinical Method

W WAYNE WESTON AND JUDITH BELLE BROWN

In the previous chapter describing the learner-centered method of education, we outlined a framework for teachers applying this approach to teaching. In this chapter we present some of the common challenges faced by those who strive to learn, teach, and practice the patient-centered clinical method.

Teaching and learning the patient-centered clinical method is demanding for many reasons. First, we will describe issues related to the nature of clinical practice and patient–practitioner communication; second, we will elaborate on challenges specific to being a teacher of the patient-centered clinical method.

THE UNRECOGNIZED COMPLEXITY OF PATIENT–PRACTITIONER COMMUNICATION

Students and clinicians have been talking all their lives; it feels natural and seems easy. Consequently, some students think they do not need any instruction on communication. And once they have learned the basics, most students, especially postgraduate students, feel that further instruction on communication is a waste of time. They have failed to realize the complexity of patient–practitioner communication.

> Communication is a little like sex. It is a normal function and most of us think we are good at it and some are, but many aren't. Superior clinical communication is a learned skill. Speaking with patients, families, and colleagues calls for a studied blend of selective curiosity, quiet intensity, and the ability to attend to what is *not* being said.[1]

Nimmon and Regehr, in a year-long study of "the place of social networks in people's efforts to make meaning about their own health,"[2] point out that physicians are only one part of a patient's network of resources, including family members, friends, workplace or school associates, and

DOI: 10.1201/9781003394679-16

acquaintances used to make sense of their health problems and decide on their preferred health behaviors. It is far more complex than the prevailing notion that people simply consult physicians to gain an understanding of their health concerns and the best way to manage them. It is important for physicians to discuss with patients what they have learned about their problems from others, including "Dr. Google," especially when it is at variance with what the physician has advised. Clinicians who react defensively or angrily risk losing the patient's confidence and cooperation.

Koopman and colleagues describe the importance for clinicians to acknowledge the work patients do to prepare for a doctor's visit. Patients with chronic conditions have usually looked up health information on the Internet including disease-specific foundations, chat rooms, and blogs.

> Patients often come to health interactions armed with stories from "others" to share at health encounters. In our study, the proactive information-seeking behaviour that patients engaged in often helped them to make sense of their symptoms or learn about interventions for their condition, which shaped their interactions with health practitioners. While the information patients gain from social media does not necessarily trump health practitioners' recommendations, the knowledge accrued may be an avenue to equalise the relationship between patients and health practitioners, thereby empowering patients for health interactions.[3]

Communication skills are usually taught in the first 2 years of medical school, often as part of a clinical skills course, where students also learn history taking and physical examination skills. In recent years, communication courses include practice with simulated patients and, by the time they reach clerkship, most students have acquired basic skills for engaging with real patients. However, the clinical setting is more complex and unpredictable than the well-organized and structured communication lab; not only must students concentrate on applying good communication techniques such as open-ended inquiry, active listening, and empathy, but also they must gather a comprehensive medical history, conduct an accurate physical examination, consider the differential diagnosis, and, together with the patient, develop a tentative plan of management. And real patients are sick – often very sick! Their illnesses may make it hard for them to provide clear answers to the student's many questions and may diminish their capacity to engage in a dialogue about treatment choices. It is not surprising that the lessons learned in the communication lab do not transfer easily to the clinical setting.

Experts in teaching communication skills[4-6] point out that there are three broad categories of communication skills (content, process, and perceptual skills) that students must learn to integrate when they interact with patients.

- Content skills are *"what health care professionals communicate"* – they include taking a history, conducting the functional inquiry, and performing the physical examination. They also include exploration of the patient's illness experience and finding common ground.
- Process skills are *"how they do it"* – how they build their relationship with the patient and how they provide structure to the interview. This includes the way they ask questions (whether open-ended or closed) as well as non-verbal communication, and how they pick up on patient cues. Finally, it addresses the strategies they use to attend to the flow of the interview and make the organization of the interview overt.

- Perceptual skills are *"what they are thinking and feeling"* – the intrapersonal aspects of the interaction. They include clinical reasoning skills, thoughts, and feelings for and about the patient and also include student's values, beliefs, and biases related to the patient, and awareness of distractions.

In Ofri's sensitive analysis of the role of emotions in the care of patients, she states:

Understanding the positive and negative influence of emotions in the doctor–patient interaction is a crucial element in maximizing the quality of medical care. Every patient deserves the best possible care that doctors can offer. Learning to recognize and manage the emotional subtexts is a critical tool on both sides of the exam table.[7]

Sommer et al. conducted a validation study of a teaching skills assessment tool based on the patient-centered method and learner-centered approach inspired by the Calgary-Cambridge model and found it has high reliability and can be used as a tool to assist clinical teachers to improve their skills in teaching communication skills.

In this study, we developed a teaching skills descriptive observation tool for peer review. Through the research methods and processes used, we empha-sised the similarities between the patient-centered approach using the interview structure according to the Calgary-Cambridge model and the learner-centered approach, as we believed that the recognition of these similarities would facili-tate the transfer of competencies from the clinician's level to the teacher's role, thereby helping the clinical teachers to more easily master the expected teach-ing competencies.[8]

According to cognitive load theory, performance degrades when the learner is overloaded.[9] Cognitive load theory assumes that working memory is limited – humans can attend to only a limited number of concepts at once.[10] An expert has learned to "chunk" concepts together to free up space in working memory, but the novice is still struggling to know what goes together. For example, a novice has a hard enough time simply attending to all the elements of the functional inquiry until, with repeated practice, they can perform without referring to a checklist. Each element of the three broad categories of communication skills is gradually mastered, separate from the others, with repetition. However, in the fast-paced and messy setting of clinical prac-tice, even an experienced clinician can become overwhelmed by the multiple factors that must be considered simultaneously. Imagine an office visit in which the patient says to her physi-cian: "I'm really concerned about this chest pain I've been having." And then she places her fist against her chest and the clinician notices a tear in her eye. At the same time, he hears a knock on the office door. How does the physician decide whether to first address the chest pain: "What does it feel like, how long does it last, what makes it better or worse? Are you having pain right now?" Or perhaps it would be better to explore her mood: "You seem upset; can you tell me about it?" And what about the distracting knock on the door? How can the physician handle that without losing this special moment in the interview? To top it off, he realizes he is already 20 minutes behind in his schedule, and he promised to attend his son's football game after school. The cognitive load can be overwhelming.

Communication training focuses on one component at a time and provides opportunities to practice and receive feedback. Thus, students are able to learn the skills for taking a medical history and the process of interviewing. In some programs they will explore their personal reactions to patients and to being clinicians. Smith et al.[11] explored the importance of developing learners' awareness of interfering emotions and beliefs. For example, believing that emotions are harmful and should be avoided in medical interviews, or feeling that all interruptions are rude, that clinicians should remain in control of the interview at all times, or believing that clinicians should carefully keep their distance from patients. These beliefs could prevent clinicians from exploring difficult or painful issues, make it harder for patients to express their opinions, and result in a cold interaction between clinician and patient that is inimical to patient-centered care. Training in emotional intelligence (EI) has been shown to be

> favorably associated with physician and physician trainee wellness, decreasing burnout, improved physician-patient relationships, and perhaps better patient outcomes, the integration of EI into medical school curricula continues to be inadequate. Key barriers to wider implementation of EI include insufficient awareness, lack of time and/or financial resources, and paucity of qualified faculty.[12]

Strategies to enhance physician self-awareness include mindfulness training.[13, 14] Other approaches include classroom discussions of emotionally challenging clinical situations, regular or even impromptu support group discussions, Balint groups, family-of-origin group discussions, literature in medicine discussion groups, personal awareness groups, and behavioral science/interpersonal skills curricula.[15] Halpern[16] describes how physicians can learn to empathize with patients even when they are in conflict by "an ongoing practice of engaged curiosity. Activities that can help in this process include meditation, sharing stories with colleagues, writing about doctoring, reading books, and watching films conveying emotional complexity." Often the personal qualities, described here earlier under perceptual skills, are taught in courses on professionalism. Clinical reasoning, if it is taught at all, is usually addressed in a separate course or left to the clerkship or residency. Rarely is there time for, or attention given to, integration of all three sets of skills. As a result, students adopt a survival strategy to avoid being overwhelmed by the complexity of the patient–physician encounter; they focus on conducting a good history and establishing a credible diagnosis and appropriate management plan. It is during their clinical training where students and residents need more guidance in learning to integrate the three categories of communication skills. It is unfortunate that, when they need it most, so little has been offered to students after the first 2 years of medical school. Rosenbaum describes students' decline in communication skills during medical education and lists the key contributing factors:

> 1) lack of formal communication skills training during clinical clerkships; 2) informal workplace teaching failing to explicitly address learner clinical communication skills; 3) emphasizing content over process in relation to clinician-patient interactions; 4) the relationship between ideal communication models and the realities of clinical practice; and 5) clinical teachers' lack of knowledge and skills to effectively teach about communication in the clinical workplace.[17]

Recognizing the complexity and importance of communication between patients and physicians in the critical care setting, the Cumming School of Medicine in Calgary, Alberta, developed a longitudinal integrated curriculum for fellows in critical care medicine based on Kern's 6-step model[18] for curriculum development. A needs assessment, based on a literature review and survey of members of the critical care team informed the curriculum structure. Five 4-hour classroom sessions were developed consisting of 45-minute interactive presentations followed by 3-hours of small group simulation practice. The SPIKES (setting, perception, invitation, knowledge, empathy, summarize, and strategize)[19] protocol was used as the framework for all five sessions. Scenarios for the simulations were based on challenging clinical events that the fellows had encountered. Actors familiar with medical education courses were prepared with a description of the scenario and guidance on how to respond to cues, but scripts were not provided. Instead, they were instructed to "respond to nuances of interpersonal interaction in the moment."[20] Evaluation included feedback from peers and trained facilitators in the classroom setting and feedback in the clinical setting from ICU patients' family members and clinicians.[20]

Van Weel-Baumgarten and colleagues, in Nijmegen, the Netherlands, developed a program to integrate communication and consultation skills. Unlike many schools, the undergraduate curriculum in Nijmegen delays teaching communication skills until near the end of the preclinical years and continues training throughout the three clinical years. The educational rationale was

1. To introduce communication skills not as a separate skill but integrated with medical content
2. To provide training just before each clerkship starts, so students can immediately practice what they have learned during training ("just in time learning")
3. To reinforce and further develop communication skills throughout their clinical training.[21]

Each clinical block in the curriculum included 1–4 weeks of preparation for the types of patients the students were likely to observe and participate in caring for on that rotation and ended with a 1-week classroom-based session where students reflected on issues raised during that block. Students had opportunities to practice communication and consultation skills with simulated patients focused on the clinical conditions relevant to each discipline-based block. In the surgical block, students learned their suturing skills on a simulated "bleeding" head wound in a wig the simulated patient was wearing while they practiced their skills of reassuring an anxious patient and explaining what they were doing. Ninety-eight percent of students agreed, "It is important that communication is taught integrated with medical content."[21]

Schopper et al. conducted a study focused on senior medical students' insights related to their experiences of observation and feedback for teaching communication skills during the clinical years.

> The majority of students reported rarely being observed interviewing, and they reported receiving feedback even less frequently. Students valued having communication skills observed and became more comfortable with observation the more it occurred. Student-identified challenges included supervisor time constraints and grading based on observation. Most feedback focused on information gathering and was commonly delayed until well after the observed encounter.[22]

Typical of comments by the students is,

> I also don't feel like I'm watched nearly enough in my interactions with patients. You know, because otherwise I could go through a 4-week rotation and never have anybody watch me, and never know if I'm, like, asking the right questions . . . or if it would be better to ask them a different way.[22]

Wouda and van de Wiel[23] express doubt that "expertise in professional communication can be fully attained during medical training." There are many reasons for this, including lack of curriculum time devoted to communication and the complexity of the skills to be learned. They refer to the seminal work on the development of expertise by Ericsson[24, 25] and suggest that it is only after years of practice that physicians can master the full spectrum of communication skills. In deliberate practice, unlike the way most people practice, students must avoid rote learning or settling into a comfortable routine, and they must set themselves new goals that raise the bar on their abilities. They must force themselves to reflect on their performance and continually strive for improvement. The learning conditions for deliberate practice are

(a) clear and comprehensive objectives about which skills have to be learned and how to teach them in simulated consultations, (b) stimulating learning tasks of short duration with opportunities for immediate feedback, reflection and corrections, (c) ample opportunities for repetition and gradual refinements of performance, (d) possibilities for individual students to rehearse their existing skills frequently in different sorts of consultations and to acquire new skills in challenging consultations of an increasing complexity, and (e) transfer of the learned skills into real life consultations/clinical practice.[23]

However, if students fail to recognize the importance of learning more about communication skills, they are unlikely to exert the effort needed.

Additional challenges were created by the COVID-19 pandemic leading to a medical education revolution, which some felt was overdue.[26] In order to limit spread of the virus, many medical schools limited medical student participation in ward rounds and switched classroom courses to online learning. Lectures were recorded for synchronous or asynchronous delivery. Platforms such as Zoom or Facetime were used for synchronous small group teaching. Because these changes have been effective, they may well be continued in a hybrid pre-clerkship curriculum along with more traditional teaching methods. The biggest challenge has been finding ways to assure clinical competence without excessive risk of infection. Sukumar et al. describe a novel virtual rounds curriculum for medical students' internal medicine clerkship including following virtually the course of at least one patient each week, listening to hospital rounds, and delivering an oral presentation. The goals were to become familiar with ward rounds and to develop skills in delivering oral presentations including articulating clinical reasoning.[27]

Zuo and Juvé describe how faculty development needs to change to assist teachers in managing the huge changes occurring in medical education resulting from the COVID-19 pandemic:

The COVID-19 pandemic created an urgent need for staff development. New skills were required to perform the necessary tasks of restructuring lectures from in-person to online, staying up to date on frequently changing health care guidelines and continuing activities important for career advancement. However, COVID-19 has created many challenges for staff development, including the inability to meet in-person, travel restrictions to conferences, over-whelming clinical demands on already overextended faculty members and the increased need to focus on personal health and safety. Although current challenges were immediately met with solutions borne out of an emergency, questions remain on how to identify and sustain best practices and further evolve staff development beyond the immediate crisis.[28]

THE NATURE OF CLINICAL PRACTICE

Clinical practice often seems arduous enough when limited to the diagnosis and treatment of disease; suggesting to clinicians that they must also consider patients' perspectives on their health and illness experience, as well as the social context in which patients live their lives, may seem overwhelming. This is especially true for young clinicians who are struggling to learn their craft. Several characteristics of practice pose difficulties for learning. Hippocrates commented on this 2000 years ago in his aphorism: "Life is short and the Art long; the occasion fleeting; experience fallacious, and judgment difficult."[29] The long hours, lack of sleep, and the personally draining nature of patient care often leave students and practitioners exhausted and emotionally spent. Physicians, in this state, may have little energy to invest in learning to be patient-centered. In the long run, we argue, patient-centered care is more rewarding for both doctors and patients. However, when doctors are harried, they are tempted to focus narrowly on the patient's presenting complaint alone and to end the visit quickly by ignoring any other concerns the patient may have thereby contributing to the problem of patient nondisclosure of concerns. It is important for physicians to realize that patients frequently (over 60%) withhold medically relevant information from their physicians because of not wanting to be judged or hear how harmful their behavior is.[30] In a similar, more worrisome study, over 40% of patients withheld information from clinicians about imminent threats (depression, suicidality, abuse, or sexual assault) most commonly because of feeling embarrassed or not wanting to be judged or lectured.[31]

Giroldi et al. note that patients express at least one worry in 90% of consultations but usually express their worries implicitly by presenting cues. In order to learn how GPs recognize these cues, they used stimulated recall interviews with GPs, using their own video-recorded consultations, to explore how they recognized their patients' cues. They concluded:

> Identifying patients' worries by adequately picking up and exploring patient cues is crucial for effective reassurance. GPs recognise worry by detecting a variety of specific non-verbal, verbal, and behavioural cues and cues based on foreknowledge. GPs' reflections have given insight into the variety and nature of patient cues and have highlighted that cues occur throughout the whole consultation. The accuracy of the interpretation that doctors attribute to the cue should always be verified with the patient.[32]

Although there are undeniable time pressures in practice, sometimes clinicians are caught up in "busy work" to avoid the emotional demands of practice. Without a commitment to continuing personal growth and self-awareness, practitioners may not confront the reasons for their avoidance. The following case serves as an example.

CASE EXAMPLE

Michael Wong, a first-year internal medicine resident, described his discomfort with the recent death of his patient. He found the experience painful because in spending time with the patient he had developed a relationship. Unlike the deaths of other patients who had remained strangers, this patient's death touched him deeply. Michael almost wished he had not become attached and was ambivalent about allowing himself to become vulnerable again. This experience was a turning point in his education; the opportunity to discuss his feelings with his peers and teachers helped him to accept his pain as a necessary part of his learning and growth. Michael realized that protecting himself from further painful experiences, by avoiding getting to know his patients, would rob him of one of the most valued aspects of practice. He also recognized that his relationship with the patient was the most helpful element of his care.

DISCOMFORT WITH FINDING COMMON GROUND

In Chapter 6, we examined the role of finding common ground as the lynchpin of the patient-centered clinical method. Here, we explore the challenges teachers encounter in guiding their students to master the skills they need to find common ground with their patients. Many clinical teachers find teaching about finding common ground particularly challenging. The case study of Piotr in Chapter 6 is a powerful reminder to respect and support patients who choose decisions based on what most matters to them even when clinicians might make different choices.

It may be particularly difficult for young physicians, still struggling to develop their self-confidence as professionals, to share power with their patients. The following example illustrates some of the challenges in finding common ground, in this instance, due to a need to explore the patient's understanding of his symptoms first.

CASE EXAMPLE

Melvin Langer, aged 42, presented to Rebecca Bridge, a second-year family medicine resident, convinced that he had been misdiagnosed. At his last appointment at the clinic 2 weeks previously, he complained of symptoms similar to what he experienced with Graves' disease 10 years ago. He was adamant that this was a recurrence of his hyperthyroidism. However, he had been treated with radioactive iodine at the time of his diagnosis of Graves' disease, and his most recent thyroid-stimulating hormone blood test was consistent with hypothyroidism. Based on this, Dr Bridge had diagnosed hypothyroidism and gave him a prescription for an increased dose of levothyroxine. On this follow-up visit, Dr Bridge was surprised by Mr Langer's agitation. He was normally a very pleasant and humorous individual, but today he appeared angry and frustrated. When she inquired how he was doing on the increased thyroid medication, he retorted, "Not well at all! I'm feeling the same as I did when I had Graves' disease. I am convinced I have too much thyroid, not too little, so I did not take the new pills." Dr Bridge felt herself getting annoyed and defensive. She felt she had provided correct advice based on a careful assessment of his medical condition and thought to herself, "My treatment was appropriate; I don't know how I can handle his anger and noncompliance." Feeling at a loss, she consulted her preceptor. Recognizing her frustration with this patient, the preceptor helped her understand that the most important issue was the patient's conviction that the diagnosis was wrong. Until that was addressed, trying to change Mr Langer's mind about management would be futile. Resuming her interview with Mr Langer, Dr Bridge acknowledged that she had not fully explored his understanding of his symptoms. As she listened carefully to his explanation, Mr Langer became remarkably calmer. As they explored the conflict between his lab results and his symptoms, Mr Langer mentioned that he was taking diet pills that he ordered on the Internet. Dr Bridge wondered if the symptom of feeling "revved up" might be related to an unknown ingredient in the diet pills. Together they developed a plan for management over the next week. Because Mr Langer was reluctant to take an increased dose of his levothyroxine, Dr Bridge agreed that he would continue the lower dose of thyroid medication and would repeat his thyroid-stimulating hormone blood test in a week. As well, Mr Langer would discontinue his diet pills. Having now established a trusting relationship they were able to agree on a management plan.

THE IMPORTANCE OF SELF-AWARENESS AND GUIDED SELF-ASSESSMENT

McWhinney challenges medicine to become a self-reflective discipline:

> We can only attend to a patient's feelings and emotions if we know our own, but self-knowledge is neglected in medical education, perhaps because the path to this knowledge is so long and hard. Egoistic emotions often come disguised as virtues and we all have a great capacity for self-deception. But there are pathways to this knowledge and medical education could find a place for them. Could medicine become a self-reflective discipline? The idea may seem preposterous. Yet I think it must, if we are to be healers as well as competent technologists. . . . The fault line runs through the affect-denying clinical method which dominates the modern medical school. Not until this is reformed will emotions and relationships have the place in medicine they deserve. Finally, to become self-reflective, medicine will have to go through a huge cultural change. In these changes, general practice is already some distance along the way. The importance of being different is that we can lead the way.[33]

Medical education involves confronting powerful emotions.[34] In a gripping account of his experience in the anatomy lab, as a first-year medical student, Crichton describes his experience of how sawing a skull in half taught him to turn off his emotions at times which would otherwise overwhelm him.

> Somewhere inside me, there was a kind of click, a shutting off, a refusal to acknowledge, in ordinary human terms, what I was doing. After that click, I was all right. . . . The best doctors find a middle position where they are neither overwhelmed by their feelings nor estranged from them. This is the most difficult position of all, and the precise balance – neither too detached nor too caring – is something few learn.[35]

Commenting on Crichton's account, Neighbour describes the importance of physicians being able to turn off their emotions when necessary, which he called "Crichton's switch." "Difficult it may be, but finding a way to that centre ground between the extremes of emotional involvement and indifference is surely one of the core tasks for an emerging professional."[36]

Clinicians who explore patients' cues to personal problems quickly find themselves discussing intensely intimate issues. When confronted with having a serious illness, patients often wonder about its meaning for them and their families. For example, it may raise fundamental questions such as "Why me?" or "What will happen to my children if I die?" Other patients may present with symptoms that reflect their concerns about their relationships or employment. These situations may trigger questions and feelings in practitioners' minds related to their own current relationships or to unresolved issues from their families of origin. As a result, young clinicians with little life experience may be overwhelmed by their feelings and thus distance themselves for self-protection. Additionally, they may form relationships with some patients that unconsciously replicate troubled relationships from their past; without insight the practitioner is likely to become entangled in the same difficulties.

Because the patient-provider relationship is so intensely personal, such difficulties are inevitable at times. Students and young clinicians need opportunities to develop self-awareness. These issues must be addressed with sensitivity by the teacher, taking into consideration the student's level of comfort in discussing their feelings. Often this can be done in a small group, such as a Balint group,[37, 38] so that all students learn from one another's insights; but sometimes this may be too threatening or overwhelming. Opportunities for one-to-one discussion also need to be available. Another approach to self-awareness is the use of narrative, as described in Chapter 10. Self-awareness is an important aspect of what Epstein describes as mindful practice. He outlines five forms of self-awareness:

> Intrapersonal self-awareness helps the physician be conscious of his or her strengths, limitations, and sources of professional satisfaction. . . . Interpersonal self-awareness . . . allows physicians to see themselves as they are seen by others and helps to establish satisfactory interpersonal relationships with colleagues, patients, and students. . . . Self-awareness of learning needs allows physicians to recognize areas of unconscious incompetence and to develop a means to achieving their learning goals. Ethical self-awareness is the moment-to-moment cognizance of values that are shaping medical encounters. Technical self-awareness is necessary for self-correction during procedures such as the physical examination, surgery, computer operations, and communication.[39]

He goes on to discuss the implications for teachers: "The teacher's task is to invoke a state of mindfulness in the learner, and, thus, the teacher can only act as a guide, not a transmitter of knowledge."[39] Kern and colleagues describe the importance of powerful experiences, which evoke strong feelings, as a stimulus for personal growth particularly if they are accompanied by introspection, a helping relationship, or both.

> Powerful experiences occur commonly in medicine but may lack optimal conditions for personal growth. To promote practitioner personal growth, medical settings may wish to explore methods to promote introspection, helping relationships, and the acknowledgement of powerful experiences when they occur.[40]

The ability to assess one's abilities and learning needs is important during medical education and essential after graduation for the maintenance of competence. However, several studies[41-45] indicate "humans are poor at producing self-generated summative assessments of their own performance or ability."[46] However, a few studies indicate that students are able to correctly assess their abilities compared with supervisor assessments. For example, Torres and Cochran found that students were able to accurately identify their strengths and weaknesses in a midclerkship self-evaluation compared with supervisor evaluations.[47] One reason for the discrepancy in results of studies of self-assessment is lack of consensus regarding a definition of self-assessment.[48] Eva and Regehr emphasize, "personal unguided reflections on practice simply do not provide the information sufficient to guide performance improvements adequately."[46] In a summary of articles on self-assessment, Sargeant comments, "Like the old fable 'The Blind Man and the Elephant' we each have a sense of what self-assessment looks like from where we are standing, from our own unique context." She goes on to stress the importance of seeking feedback and explicit information from external sources and using that information to guide continuing learning. Equally important for self-assessment are several internal factors such as reflection, mindfulness, openness and curiosity.[49]

Several strategies can be utilized to enhance self-assessment skills. Watching a video of their interviewing improved the accuracy of students' assessment of their interviewing performance. Reviewing a video with faculty increased the accuracy of surgical residents' self-assessment of their surgical skills. The opportunity for benchmarking – reviewing the performance of other students for comparison with their own performance – improved self-assessment for high-performing students but not for poor-performing students.[50, 51] Scaffidi et al. studied the impact of video review on the self-assessment ability of novice endoscopists. They concluded:

> Accurate self-assessment requires appropriate external standards for measuring one's performance and the ability to judge the extent to which one's own performance meets those standards. Providing novices with a video of their own performance as well as a benchmark performance likely enhances self-assessment accuracy as it provides trainees with high-quality data which they can use to interpret their own performance and compare it to an explicit standard.[52]

Final-year medical students' self-assessment of their suturing ability in a simulated environment showed moderate correlation with expert assessor scores. There was no improvement in their self-assessment after reviewing a video recording of their performance. However, after viewing a video recording of an ideal performance – the "benchmark performance" – their self-assessed scores showed strong correlation with expert scores of their performance ($r = 0.83$; $p < 0.0001$).[53] Poirier et al. describe an interprofessional error disclosure simulation training program for dental, nursing, and pharmacy students. Use of video recordings made a significant difference in student self-assessment for communication and process categories of error disclosure and appeared to enhance learning about the skills needed for interprofessional error disclosure.[54]

Sargeant et al. describe how learners and physicians informed their self-assessments in clinical settings by utilizing data from both internal and external sources. A "gut feeling" that one is not doing well in a particular area might stimulate seeking out opportunities to learn more about that topic. However, without external feedback, many learners will not recognize their deficiencies. Because feedback from trusted, credible supervisors was notable for its absence, learners sought feedback from peers, often through informal discussions related to how they handled similar situations. The authors of this qualitative study noted the "tensions between wanting to know how one is doing and fear of learning one is not doing as well as one should."[55] One value of portfolios is that they make it more likely that a learner will reflect on a patient event that did not go well rather than ignoring it to avoid the discomfort of recognizing ones error.[56, 57] Using a smartphone app plus group coaching sessions promoted residents' reflections in the workplace.[58] Another important study by Mann et al.[59] explores how tensions between people might hamper self-assessment – for example, worrying about damaging a relationship with a colleague or student by providing honest feedback.

Some researchers draw a distinction between summative self-assessment ("guess your grade") and self-monitoring – "moment-by-moment awareness of performance during a task."[60] Schön[61] referred to this as "reflection in action." For example, experienced surgeons slow down and pay more attention to parts of a surgical procedure that are unusual or more complicated. Epstein and colleagues suggest that "self-monitoring is characterized by an ability to attend, moment-to-moment, to our own actions; curiosity to examine the effects of those actions; and willingness to use those observations to improve behavior and patterns of thinking in the future." They suggest that these skills can be enhanced by practicing mindfulness techniques to cultivate an "observing self"[62] that helps to resist the tendency of going on automatic pilot. One way of improving the ability to stay focused and attentive to the patient is practicing paying attention to one's breathing while clearing the mind of everything else and, when the mind wanders, bringing attention back to the breathing over and over again. Clinical teachers can help students develop their curiosity, another important feature of mindfulness, by encouraging them to ask themselves reflective questions such as

- If there were data that I ignored, what might they be?
- What am I assuming that might not be true?
- Did I avoid premature closure?
- Is there another way in which I can formulate this patient's story and/or my response?
- What are important aspects of the present situation that differ from previous situations?
- How might prior experiences be affecting my response to this situation?
- What would a trusted peer say about how I am managing or feeling about this situation?[62]

Eva and Regehr[46] suggest that students be taught the habit of "self-directed assessment seeking." Students should learn how to gather evidence about their knowledge and performance from a variety of sources (personal reflection and reading, peer assessment, review questions, objective structured clinical examinations, and feedback from patients and supervisors) and use this multisource feedback to inform their self-assessments, which can then be used to guide their ongoing learning. Weak students tend to discount feedback that is too much at variance with their self-assessments and may benefit from counseling from a peer or mentor to place the feedback in context – guidance on how to use the feedback to improve performance rather than as an assessment of their worth as clinicians.[63] Students at all levels might benefit from practice sessions in which they learn, with role-play, how to ask their supervisors to observe them and provide feedback. This strategy would likely be more effective than exhorting faculty to provide more feedback.

The following example describes a teaching intervention that promoted self-awareness.

CASE EXAMPLE

In a teaching practice, Sarah Pinchot, a first-year family medicine resident, stepped out of an interview to consult with her supervisor. This was the second time she had seen the patient for tension-type headaches. Tony Sanatani, a 45-year-old executive, was not improving, and he initiated this visit in order to be referred for a CT scan. The resident was frustrated and angry with what she described as an "abuse of the system." Her attempt to persuade Mr Sanatani that the test was unnecessary terminated in a heated disagreement. Dr Pinchot felt her medical knowledge had been rejected and her professional credibility undermined. She needed to win this argument!

While the resident was describing her frustration and the standoff with her patient, the supervisor recognized Dr Pinchot's vulnerability and need for support. But, from previous knowledge of Mr Sanatani, the supervisor understood his request probably stemmed from the death of his uncle from a brain tumor 6 months ago. The teacher's task was to help the resident ventilate her feelings and then to help her explore why she had fallen into a win-lose relationship with the patient. Dr Pinchot needed to understand how both she and her patient had contributed to this impasse. Then she had to find a way to convert the struggle into a win-win outcome. The resident recognized that her recurrent conflict with authority figures led her to experience Mr Sanatani's request for reassurance as a demand for an unnecessary test and a challenge of her medical competence. Instead of exploring his fears, she reacted by defending herself. Dr Pinchot dismissed the patient's request as unwarranted and the fight was on. After realizing what had happened, Dr Pinchot was able to return to the patient, acknowledge that they had reached an impasse and ask if they could begin again. This culminated in an exploration of the patient's concerns and fears about the headaches. Following a careful neurological examination and discussion about why a brain tumor was highly unlikely, the patient was prepared to consider other causes for his headaches.

Later, Dr Pinchot sat down with her supervisor to discuss options for exploring her problem with authority figures. The supervisor's recognition of Dr Pinchot's vulnerability had prevented him from criticizing her error and engaging in a parallel struggle, which would have replicated the student's difficulties with authority. Instead, his nonjudgmental stance encouraged the development of her self-awareness.

For the most part, as physicians grow in their personal and clinical wisdom, they become more comfortable with the uncertainties of medicine and the complexities of their patients' problems; but ongoing self-reflection is essential to promote a deepening understanding of the patient–physician relationship. In an inspiring paper, gastroenterologist McLeod reflects on his struggle to achieve self-awareness:

I worked to keep my emotions and intuitions from influencing medical decisions because they were subjective and not measurable. I became adept at hiding the feelings of vulnerability and helplessness that I felt when my patients died, and those of anger and frustration with "hateful" patients. . . . As a result I became increasingly isolated from my own emotions and needs; I shared less with my colleagues at work. I evolved a workaholic lifestyle with the subconscious expectation that others would figure out my needs and satisfy them because I was "doing so much." I did not take the risk of identifying and asking for what I needed. I hid behind a mask of pseudocompetence and efficiency. I let power, money, and position take the place of empowerment, love, and meaning. But because they were substitutes for my primary needs, they were never enough.[64]

OVEREMPHASIS ON THE CONVENTIONAL MEDICAL MODEL

There are several features of medical education and professional socialization that may interfere with learning an effective clinical approach to the familiar problems presented by patients. Medical training indoctrinates students to see patients' problems as derangements of the "body-machine" and to be concerned about missing some rare but deadly disease. As a result, most students and many physicians attempt to find a disease to explain each of their patients' complaints. This may result in over-investigation, unnecessary referral, and over-prescribing. Also, patients' personal concerns may receive little attention because physicians are concentrating all of their thought and energy on ferreting out pathology. This is not surprising since, until recently, the majority of medical students' clinical experience was in large tertiary care hospitals where they were exposed to very seriously ill patients. While more education has shifted to community sites, the aging population and associated multimorbidity reinforces the focus on the conventional medical model. Although worldwide reductions in duty hours varied considerably among countries[65] and was associated with meaningful improvements in physician safety and health in some studies, many clinicians are still often overworked and may have little time to do anything but tend to the grave physical needs of their patients.[66]

It is understandable that young physicians will use the framework they are most familiar with – the conventional medical model. Even experienced physicians, when stressed or overwhelmed by the problems of a patient, will often revert to a simplistic focus on conventional medical diagnosis even if they have learned and have used a more sophisticated and comprehensive patient-centered approach.

One of our students, in describing her struggle to use the patient-centered clinical method, expressed her fears that she would be mandated to relinquish the conventional medical model altogether:

> I want to remember that stuff (textbook information), you know! Not only did I work hard to learn it and to remember it for a short while, and it has helped me to fend off attendings in the past, but even without the quizzing, it is a form of security, a teddy bear of sorts. Beyond that, sometimes it's a source of pride, of excitement, of fun, of conversation with colleagues, a worldly treasure. Yeah, I know it's a treasure moths will soon destroy (to coin a phrase), but meanwhile I am trying to live in a world that demands these things!

The conventional medical model has a long history of success and is highly respected in our culture, but it allows physicians to remain comfortably distant from patients and their problems. Also, if doctors do their best (biomedically speaking) and their patients do not improve, the physicians need feel no blame. If the patient did not "comply" with the doctor's "orders" then the lack of improvement is inappropriately blamed on the patient. Students and physicians need to learn a more appropriate clinical method, one that incorporates the power of the conventional medical model, but which is not constrained by its narrow focus on disease. Such a clinical method cannot be learned all at once. Students may need to learn each component of the patient-centered clinical method separately, and they will also require opportunities to practice integrating their clinical skills into a unified whole.

CONCENTRATION ON HISTORY TAKING RATHER THAN LISTENING TO THE PATIENT

Students in first-year medical school have little difficulty learning how to inquire about patients' ideas and expectations concerning their illnesses, but as they progress through medical school, they become consumed by the task of making the right diagnosis, and their interviews become less patient-centered.[67-69] This may be a consequence of the emphasis on taking a thorough history of each disease and completing a comprehensive functional enquiry. Much less attention is given to open-ended exploration of the patient's feelings and ideas. Commenting on an observational study of "inductive foraging" in 132 consultations in family practice,[70] Launer was struck with how these physicians started their history taking with open-ended queries unlike the more structured history taking approach taught in medical school. He wonders,

> Could we teach medical students to work in this way from the outset of their training? . . . Abandoning the notion of taking a history and replacing it with the idea of listening to the story could be a vital step in creating more humane and equitable interactions in medicine.[71]

Without practice, most young doctors feel uncomfortable enquiring about patients' personal lives. Often there is concern that patients will become emotional and perhaps cry or show anger; they worry that they will open up a "can of worms" that they will not be able to handle. Physicians' training tends to make them cautious about trying new approaches with patients where they feel uncertain about the outcome; they are also reluctant to try unfamiliar techniques if they feel uncomfortable or awkward. The commonest excuse given to avoid asking about patients' personal concerns is lack of time. However, it is not efficient use of time to search for a disease that is not present or to ignore a major source of patients' distress such as their fear or concern about the possible cause and implications of their symptoms.

Alternately, when physicians are learning the patient-centered clinical method, they mistakenly equate it with a "psychosocial functional enquiry." The following example typifies this common misunderstanding.

> When a patient presented with concerns about her severe sore throat and about how long she was going to be off school the resident interrupted her story with: "Wait, I need to get to know more about your personal situation. Where did you grow up? What was your childhood like? Was there much conflict in your family?" These questions would be very useful in the appropriate context, but in this case they seemed unconnected from the patient's practical concerns about receiving effective treatment and getting back to school as soon as possible. The physician needed to be sensitive to any cues about how this patient's home and school situation were related to her illness but was not being patient-centered by imposing a psychosocial inquiry.

TEACHER INEXPERIENCE

Teachers often go through stages in their development. They start out motivated by fear – fear that they do not know enough about the content and will be found out. Brookfield describes how novice teachers sometimes feel like imposters:

> Impostership means that many of us go through our teaching lives fearing that at some unspecified point in the future we will undergo a humiliating public unveiling. We wear an external mask of control, but beneath it we know that really we are frail figures, struggling not to appear totally incompetent to those around us.[72]

With experience, teachers move to the next stage – they are more confident now and want to show how much they know. Tompkins describes this stage:

> I had finally realized that what I was actually concerned with and focused on most of the time were three things: a) to show the students how smart I was, b) to show them how knowledgeable I was, and c) to show them how well-prepared I was . . . I had been putting on a performance whose true goal was not to help the students learn but to perform before them in such a way that they would have a good opinion of me.[73]

In the third stage, teachers are comfortable with their knowledge and skills and can focus on the learners and their needs instead of on themselves.

It takes considerable experience, first as a doctor and then as a clinical teacher, before a physician is able to integrate second-hand information from students about patients in order to make good decisions. To make the task even more complex, teachers are trying to assess not only the patient's problems but also the student's learning needs. To achieve this, teachers must consider many different factors at the same time. First, there are several questions about students: Did they establish a comfortable relationship with the patient that allowed them to mention everything on their mind? Did the student pick up on all the important cues the patient gave? Did the student mention to the teacher all their concerns about the patient, or did the student avoid those topics that might have disclosed their own ignorance? What are the student's blind spots? Unless the teacher has prior knowledge of the students or has witnessed their conduct in actual interviews with patients, it may be difficult to answer many of these questions. It is important to establish a climate of acceptance, where students are not criticized for admitting ignorance. Students need to know that the teacher is depending on the information they gather to make important management decisions; hence they must state where they are confused or uncertain so that the teacher will explore or double-check these areas.

Second, there are questions to be considered about the patients: What more information does the physician need to make a reasonable diagnosis? Why did the patient present now? What are the patient's feelings, ideas, and expectations about the problem and how are they affecting their life? Here, too, prior knowledge is invaluable. However, unless teachers have seen the patient-student interactions, they must depend on obtaining second-hand information from students. Here is where a patient-centered case report, described in Chapter 13, is an invaluable tool for both the learner and the teacher.

Finally, inexperienced teachers may be concerned about their reputation among their students and may feel a need to prove themselves by demonstrating their excellence as clinicians. The dilemma for physicians who are teaching a patient-centered approach is that the value system of the medical school may be at odds with this approach. As a result, excellence may be defined in terms of one's technical prowess and diagnostic acumen and may give little credit to one's ability to relate to patients.

In clinical teaching, the discussion may focus on the latest treatment for the patient's problem, leaving no time for exploring the patient's illness experience. For young students, desperate for unambiguous answers in the chaotic and messy domain of clinical practice, knowing the latest treatments for various diseases is highly valued. Because they have not yet learned how to deal with uncertainty, students may reward teachers who can provide black-and-white answers and discount teachers who urge them to address not only the patient's diseases but also the patient's health and illness experiences in the context of their life setting. Thus, students' needs for certainty and simplicity, coupled with the teacher's need for acceptance by peers, can have a powerful adverse influence on novice teachers.

COMPETING DEMANDS ON TEACHERS

Full-time faculty are pulled in many different directions at once. The destructive myth of faculty members as triple threats – expected to be exemplary clinicians, outstanding researchers, and superb teachers – casts faculty into impossible situations of role overload. Pololi et al. surveyed a randomized sample of full-time faculty from 26 representative US medical schools, 21% had seriously considered leaving academic medicine.

> Significant predictors of intention to leave included feeling vulnerable and unconnected to colleagues, moral distress, perceptions of the culture being at times unethical, and feelings of being adversely changed by the culture. Low self-efficacy and sense of engagement and a lack of alignment of faculty members' personal values with perceived institutional values also predicted intention to leave.[74]

A survey of job satisfaction among members of one department of family medicine found that job satisfaction was associated with lower levels of emotional exhaustion through their work and a feeling of effectiveness in achievement within their job. In addition, they found that being born in Canada was associated with twice the likelihood of job satisfaction compared to foreign-born academics (similar to results in a US study[75]). Job satisfaction was three times more likely among faculty rating the quality of mentoring they received as being very good or excellent and two times more likely among those who rated teamwork between physicians and staff and among other physicians as being very good or excellent.[76]

Faculty members are increasingly finding themselves stretched thin and forced to set priorities. Too often it is time for teaching that is cut back, since there are fewer institutional rewards for these activities than for research or clinical care.[77] Teaching the patient-centered approach may be time-consuming considering that teachers would want to observe student-patient interactions, provide constructive feedback, and adequately explore students' personal issues that may be evoked by the discussion. Community preceptors are also expected to be exemplary role models and remain available to care for their patients. They often provide learning opportunities for undergraduate and postgraduate students and many serve on professional organizations that depend on their involvement. As a result, they too experience role strain.

To avoid replicating their teachers' lifestyle and to prevent burnout, students may impose inappropriate limitations on the responsibilities they will assume. One outcome of the establishment of rigid boundaries between their personal and professional lives is lost opportunities for learning and growth. Examples of such behavior in primary care include working in settings where the hours of work are limited, interactions are superficial, and complex problems are referred; limiting hours of practice or range of services provided (e.g., refusal to provide home visits, hospital visits, intrapartum care, or palliative care). Specialists may reduce their responsibilities by shortening their office hours or by limiting their scope of practice.

While more effective time management will ease some of the competing demands on teachers, the answer is not that simple. Each teacher must discover how to balance patients' needs, students' needs, personal and family needs, and their own professional needs. Thus it is important for teachers to strike a balance for themselves to be effective role models for their students. However, there is a limit on what individual teachers can do to remedy their working conditions;

schools of medicine must also make changes. There needs to be a better match between what faculty members are asked to do and academic promotion guidelines. In particular, teaching needs to be as recognized and rewarded by promotion as research. Irby and O'Sullivan describe the remarkable scholarly progress over the past 30 years to define the preparation needed for educator roles, faculty development programs to prepare teachers, and criteria for rewarding the scholarship of teaching. Acknowledging that research is still more highly valued and rewarded than teaching, they describe a holistic approach to correct this inequality:

> Education scholars have advanced our understanding of the unique knowledge of educators and have provided guidance on its development. Expanded definitions of scholarship, clarity on educator roles and criteria for evaluating excellence in these roles offer the tools necessary to achieve the vision articulated in the Edinburgh declaration.[78] Yet, strong advocacy is needed to translate these insights into practice so that educators are rewarded and retained at similar rates to researchers. This will continue to be a challenging task because of the powerful influences of culture, history and social structures of universities and teaching hospitals that continue to privilege researchers over teachers. Educational leaders will need to be persistent in advocating for changes in policies and procedures that develop and reward teaching excellence and educational scholarship.[79]

TEACHER OVERPROTECTIVENESS

Including students in patient care changes the patient–doctor relationship and creates several challenges for teachers. Clinical teaching makes the doctor's job more complicated – the teacher, in this context, is responsible not only for the quality of patient care but also for the quality of the student's learning experience. Sometimes the two responsibilities seem to be at odds. Physician discomfort in these situations may interfere with student learning. Doctors may be more hesitant to allow students to practice on their patients than the patients are themselves.[80, 81] For example, physicians may falsely assume that their patients would not want to discuss their feelings about their illness with a student. This may be a reflection more of the physician's discomfort than the patient's uneasiness. Most patients are willing to allow medical students to participate in their care, provided the students are appropriately supervised and not trying to do something for which they are ill-prepared and that patients have granted informed consent.[82-84] Towle et al. describe the increasing involvement of patients in the education of health and social care professionals and how it benefits patients and professionals:

> The literature provides evidence that learning from patients plays a role in the development of clinical reasoning, communication skills, professional attitudes, empathic understanding and an individualized approach to the patient; it also motivates students by providing relevance and context. . . . Benefits to patients involved in education include satisfaction in giving back to the community, having an influence on the education of future professionals, and increased self-esteem and empowerment.[85]

It is essential that teachers do not undermine the student's position with patients. Whenever possible, teachers should function as consultants to the student and emphasize their agreement with their approach. However, if the student has made an error, the facts need to be addressed honestly. One approach is for the teacher and student to excuse themselves from the examining room to allow for frank discussion. When they both return, the student discusses with the patient the error and the new plans for treatment. With postgraduate students in an ambulatory setting, the patient may have already gone home before the error is noted. In this situation, it is essential that the patient be contacted to correct the mistake as quickly as possible. Not everyone will be comfortable with such candor in this age of litigation, even though openness reduces medicolegal risks. Such honesty reassures patients that the monitoring system works and that a teaching practice offers the advantage of at least two opinions on their problems. In addition, this provides an important opportunity for residents to learn the skills of honest disclosure of error, an important aspect of patient-centered care and one that is often poorly taught.[86, 87]

TEACHERS AS ROLE MODELS

The most important teaching method used by clinical teachers is role modeling. Daniel Tosteson, former dean of Harvard Medical School, emphasized this central responsibility of teachers: "We must acknowledge . . . that the most important, indeed the only, thing we have to offer our students is ourselves. Everything else they can read in a book."[88] Whether or not they are aware of it, medical school teachers act as models of the profession for students and house staff – either as good examples to emulate or bad examples to avoid.[89] Teachers must recognize that they are being role models at all times, not just when they are teaching but also in social situations (e.g., making a derogatory comment about a patient in an elevator). Whatever is taught in the preclinical years of medical school is either accepted or rejected by students depending on whether they see "real doctors" doing it. For example, exhortations to "listen to the patient" will be scoffed if most clinicians routinely conduct disease-centered interviews and cut-off patients' attempts to express their concerns.

In a qualitative study at the School of Medicine at Tehran University of Medical Sciences using semi-structured interviews of three categories of people who dealt with known role models (medical students, graduates with previous exposure to known role models, and faculty members who worked as colleagues with known role models). Analysis of the interviews found five characteristics of outstanding role models in medical education: excellent character, effective coach and mentor, inspiring medical leader, expert clinical teacher, and professional physician.[90] A few examples highlight the special qualities of these physicians:

> *"All the people who were associated with Prof. X remembered his calmness, humility, and dignity. He believed that if we want to succeed in life, we should set aside our pride. By avoiding our instincts, we will be ready to rise up, learn, and evolve."*
>
> *"In addition to teaching medical sciences, he taught us to practice medicine. What he taught us was about life and ethics. By providing examples, he tried to teach us how to practice medicine."*
>
> *"He knew how to attract the students' attention and win their hearts. Many professors have a high level of knowledge, but their words have no power. Prof . . . was a great example in this respect."*
>
> *"A role model should put himself/herself in patients' shoes and understand their concern."*[90]

In order to develop and nurture excellent teachers, the institution must reward those who spend time with students and residents as well as time in workshops and faculty development activities honing their own skills. Cruess and colleagues describe the profound influence of the culture of the medical school and the hidden curriculum on role modeling. For example, an institutional culture that promotes overwork, leaving insufficient time for harried clinical teachers to promote the type of reflective practice needed to demonstrate best practices among students, is detrimental to effective role modeling. Similarly, a culture that tolerates inadequate clinical care or poor interpersonal relationships inhibits positive modeling, as do administrative decisions that fail to show appreciation and support, both financial and non-financial, of those who are trying to be exemplary.[91] Many faculty decry the problems created by the medical culture and give up on ever changing it, but DiCorcia and Learman describe how the steps taken at the Indiana University School of Medicine (IUSM) to change the culture of the medical school to foster the development of professionalism resulted in a marked improvement in medical student graduates' overall satisfaction with their medical education.

The key elements of the culture change at IUSM included affirmation of core organizational values, implementation of appreciative and relational strategies as part of a relationship-centred care initiative (RCCI), revisions in admissions criteria, and alignment of compensation incentives with important qualitative aspects of faculty performance.[92]

In a seminal study of clinical teachers in three medical schools in Quebec, Beaudoin and colleagues surveyed all senior clerks and second-year residents about their perceptions of the qualities of their teachers. Almost half of the clerks and one-third of the residents perceived that most of their teachers did not display humanistic characteristics in their role as caregivers and teachers (e.g., valuing contact with patients as an important part of patient care, concern about the overall well-being of patients and not just their presenting complaints, spending time educating patients about their health problems); 75% of clerks agreed that their teachers seemed unconcerned about how their patients adapted psychologically to their illnesses; 78% felt their teachers did not try to understand students' difficulties; and 77% felt their teachers did not try to support students who were having difficulties. Residents were somewhat less critical suggesting that perhaps they were being socialized to accept these deficiencies in patient care and teaching. The authors speculate: "Perhaps their perceptions show how difficult it becomes to attain high standards of humanistic care when health care personnel must deal with increasing strains, constraints and uncertainties. Under these circumstances, perhaps there are limits to one's caring."[93]

Wright and Carrese[94] conducted in-depth interviews with 29 highly regarded role models at two large teaching hospitals and analyzed the interview transcripts for major themes. Strong clinical skills were considered essential but insufficient for effective role modeling. Consistency of good behavior was indispensable and truly distinguished role models stepped up their performance in difficult and demanding situations. They sought out opportunities to model particular skills and to teach aspects of medicine that tend to be neglected such as professionalism. Personal qualities were mentioned by all of the role models, particularly interpersonal skills, positive outlook, and commitment to excellence and growth. Teaching skills were also mentioned by all, especially establishing rapport with learners, developing specific teaching philosophies and methods, and being committed to the growth of learners.

A number of barriers to role modeling were mentioned – being impatient and overly opinionated, being quiet, and being overextended.

Students can have mixed experiences in learning the patient-centered clinical method as opportunities for learning from their role models may vary. In focus group interviews with clinical clerks at Western University, students described their observations of their role models and the conflict they experienced in the transition from theory to practice. As one student said, "I think we have been trained well but putting it into practice is another story."

The following comments highlight students' awareness that the patient-centered clinical method is applicable to all physicians and not just family doctors.

> I think that any specialist can be just as patient-centered as the family doctor. It's just how you approach it.

Furthermore, a paucity of role models in the specialities was a concern.

> We don't have the role models in the specialities to reinforce it. I think that time is just an excuse. In an extra minute you can do so much more. Being patient-centered affects everything from helping you with your diagnosis to helping with your treatment plan and management.

As one student observed

> It's hard to be optimistic about the way we're going to practice patient-centered medicine when we have no role models.

The following comment illustrates the negative effect a role model can have on students when they are attempting to apply patient-centered concepts to clinical practice:

> If you're laughed at by physicians for using this, and they say, "Don't bother with those questions," you stop doing it. Your residents will be directing a lot of your learning along the next two years and when they say, "You don't want to piss off your Attending. He hates those patient-centered questions." So you're not going to ask patients, "What are your ideas about your illness?"

When role modeling was effective, it provided a powerful and memorable learning experience.

> One orthopaedic surgeon I had for clinical methods, I still remember this, I was FIFEing the patient and I found out that the patient had diabetes and was worried about their upcoming surgery, and possible complications. When I told the surgeon that, he didn't laugh at me; he didn't think it was ridiculous. He then went in to see the patient and said, "So do you have any concerns about the upcoming surgery?" And they talked about it. It only took a few minutes.

Learning from role models is both a conscious and unconscious process.[95] At an unconscious level, learners will "catch" the values, attitudes, and behaviors of their teachers by observing their actions and the consequences of their actions.[96] They may be pleasantly surprised (or perhaps horrified) when others comment on how much they have become like their teachers. The literature on apprenticeship describes how a novice learns complex skills and concepts from a master.[97] Often these skills are so complex that they cannot be put into words. Reber[98] describes this as implicit learning – "the acquisition of knowledge that takes place largely independently of conscious attempts to learn and largely in the absence of explicit knowledge about what was acquired." Students can learn the particulars of good patient–physician communication (e.g., using open-ended questions or reflective listening) in a formal setting with simulated patients. Their teachers can give them descriptions and examples of how to use these skills in talking with patients and provide specific, focused feedback on how they are doing. However, putting these skills together with all the other skills needed for an effective dialogue with a real patient is a much more complex task. This is where role modeling is most effective. Their teachers may be able to demonstrate the skills even though they are at a loss for words to describe exactly how to do it.[99, 100] Polanyi likened this to how we are able to recognize the faces of acquaintances without being able to describe how we identify them. Such tacit skills "can be communicated only by example not by precept."[101]

However, even though it is difficult, and sometimes impossible, to articulate some of the skills students and residents must learn, it is important to make an effort to describe them as best we can. Mohammadi et al. point out the importance of role models explicitly demonstrating their actions and explaining to students what they are performing and why.[102] This will deepen their learning and reduce the risk of misinterpreting their observations of their teachers – for example, observing how their teacher calmed an angry, anxious patient and established common ground might look like magic until they have a chance to discuss this encounter with their teacher and, together, identify the specific strategies used. By elaborating on their observations, they are more likely to apply these skills when confronted with a similar situation. Egnew and Wilson conducted focus groups and long interviews with students and faculty to explore the characteristics of exemplary role models. One key finding was the opinion that effective role models needed "role modelling consciousness." "Role models who made the implicit explicit by articulating the relational qualities they were attempting to portray and the interpersonal struggles they experienced were highly valued by our respondents."[103]

CONCLUSION

In this chapter we have described some of the challenges experienced by both teachers and learners as they endeavor to learn, teach, and practice the patient-centered clinical method. These challenges include personal, professional, and systemic aspects. Each one affects the others. Thus solutions are not simple and must include tackling the educational challenges in concert. It is particularly important to acknowledge the unrecognized complexity of patient-practitioner communication, the continuing influence of the conventional medical model, and discomfort with finding common ground. Teachers are pulled in many different directions and inadequately recognized for their powerful influence as role models for the socialization of students in the health professions. Learning to be patient-centered cannot happen in isolation but must be respected and reinforced at all levels of professional education.

REFERENCES

1. Taylor RB: *Medical Wisdom and Doctoring: The Art of 21st Century Practice*. New York, NY: Springer, 2010: 53.
2. Nimmon L, Regehr G: The complexity of patients' health communication social networks: a broadening of physician communication. *Teaching and Learning in Medicine*. 2018;30(4):352–366.
3. Koopman WJ, LaDonna KA, Kinsella EA, Venance SL, Watling CJ: Getting airtime: exploring how patients shaped the stories they tell health practitioners. *Medical Education*. 2021;00:1–10. https://doi.org/10.1111/medu.14561.
4. Kurtz S, Silverman J, Benson J, et al.: Marrying content and process in clinical method teaching: enhancing the Calgary-Cambridge guides. *Academic Medicine*. 2003;78(8):802–809.

5. Kurtz S, Silverman J, Draper J: *Teaching and Learning Communication Skills in Medicine*, 2nd edition. Oxford: Radcliffe Publishing, 2005.

6. Silverman J, Kurtz S, Draper J: *Skills for Communicating with Patients*, 3rd edition. Boca Raton, FL: CRC Press, 2013.

7. Ofri D: *What Doctors Feel: How Emotions Affect the Practice of Medicine*. Boston: Beacon Press, 2013: 5.

8. Sommer J, Lanier C, Perron NJ, et al.: A teaching skills assessment tool inspired by the Calgary-Cambridge model and the patient-centered approach. *Patient Education and Counseling*. 2016;99:600–609.

9. Young JQ, Van Merrienboer J, Durning S, ten Cate O: Cognitive load theory: implications for medical education: AMEE guide no. 86. *Medical Teacher*. 2014;36:371–384.

10. Miller GA: The magical number seven, plus or minus two: some limits on our capacity for processing information. *Psychological Review*. 1956;63(2):81–97.

11. Smith RC, Dorsey AM, Lyles JS, et al.: Teaching self-awareness enhances learning about patient-centered interviewing. *Academic Medicine*. 1999;74(11):1242–1248.

12. Uchino R, Yanagawa F, Weigand B, et al.: Focus on emotional intelligence in medical education: from problem awareness to system-based solutions. *International Journal of Academic Medicine*. 2015;1:9–20.

13. Epstein RM: *Attending: Medicine, Mindfulness, and Humanity*. New York: Scribner, 2017.

14. Horton J: *We Are All Perfectly Fine: A Memoir of Love, Medicine and Healing*. Toronto: Harper Perennial, 2021.

15. Benbassat J, Baumal R: Enhancing self-awareness in medical students: an overview of teaching approaches. *Academic Medicine*. 2005;80:156–161.

16. Halpern H, Morrison S: Narrative-based supervision. In: Owen D, Shohet R (Editors): *Clinical Supervision in the Medical Profession: Structured Reflective Practice*. New York, NY: Open University Press, 2012.

17. Rosenbaum ME: Dis-integration of communication in healthcare education: workplace learning challenges and opportunities. *Patient Education and Counseling*. 2017;100:2054–2061.

18. Thomas PA, Kern DE, Hughes MT, et al. (Editors): *Curriculum Development for Medical Education: A Six-Step Approach*, 4th edition. Baltimore: Johns Hopkins University Press, 2022.

19. Buckman, R: Breaking bad news: the S-P-I-K-E-S strategy. *Community Oncology*. 2005;2:138–142.

20. Roze des Ordons A, Doig CJ, Couillard P, Lord J: From communication skills to skilful communication: a longitudinal integrated curriculum for critical care fellows. *Academic Medicine*. 2017;92(4):501–505.

21. Van Weel-Baumgarten E, Bolhuis S, Rosenbaum M, et al.: Bridging the gap: how is integrating communication skills with medical content throughout the curriculum valued by students? *Patient Education and Counseling*. 2013;90(2):177–183.

22. Schopper H, Rosenbaum M, Axelson R: "I wish someone watched me interview": medical student insight into observation and feedback as a method for teaching communication skills during the clinical years. *BMC Medical Education*. 2016;16:286, 1, 3. https://doi.org/10.1186/s12909–016–0813-z.

23. Wouda JC, van de Wiel HBM: The communication competency of medical students, residents and consultants. *Patient Education and Counseling*. 2012;86(1):57–62.

24. McGaghie WC, Barsuk JH, Wayne DB: Mastery learning with deliberate practice in medical education. *Academic Medicine*. 2015;90(11):AM Last Page.

25. Ericsson E, Pool ZR: *Peak: Secrets from the New Science of Expertise*. London: Bodley Head, 2016.
26. Torda A: How COVID-19 has pushed us into a medical education revolution. *International Medical Journal*. 2020;50:1150–1153.
27. Sukumar S, Zakaria A, Lai CJ, et al.: Designing and implementing a novel virtual rounds curriculum for medical students' internal medicine clerkship. *MedEdPORTAL*. 2021;17:11106.
28. Zuo L, Juvé AM: Transitioning to a new era: future directions for staff development during COVID-19. *Medical Education*. 2020:55:104–107.
29. Adams F: *The Genuine Works of Hippocrates*. Birmingham, AL: Classics of Medicine Library, 1985: 697.
30. Levy AG, Scherer AM, Zikmund-Fisher BJ, et al.: Prevalence of and factors associated with patient nondisclosure of medically relevant information to clinicians. *JAMA Network Open*. 2018;1(7):e185293.
31. Levy AG, Scherer AM, Zikmund-Fisher BJ, et al.: Assessment of patient nondisclosures to clinicians of experiencing imminent threats. *JAMA Network Open*. 2019;2(8):e199277.
32. Giroldi E, Timmerman A, Veldhuijzen W, et al.: How doctors recognize that their patients are worried: a qualitative study of patient cues. *Patient Education and Counseling*. 2020;103:220–225.
33. McWhinney IR: The William Pickles lecture 1996: the importance of being different. *British Journal of General Practice*. 1996;46(408):433–436.
34. Helmich E, Diachun L, Joseph R, et al.: "Oh my God, I can't handle this!": trainees emotional responses to complex situations. *Medical Education*. 2018;52(2):206–215.
35. Crichton M: *Travels*. New York: Vintage, 2014: 10.
36. Neighbour R: *The Inner Physician*. London: Royal College of General Practitioners, 2016: 221.
37. Balint M: *The Doctor, His Patient and the Illness*, 3rd edition. Philadelphia, PA: Churchill Livingstone, 2000.
38. Player M, Freeddy JR, Diaz V, et al.: The role of Balint group training in the professional and personal development of family medicine residents. *International Journal of Psychiatry in Medicine*. 2018;53(1–2):24–38.
39. Epstein RM: Mindful practice. *JAMA*. 1999;282(9):833–839.
40. Kern DE, Wright SM, Carrese JA, et al.: Personal growth in medical faculty: a qualitative study. *Western Journal of Medicine*. 2001;175(2):92–98.
41. Fleming M, Vautour D, McMullen M, et al.: Examining the accuracy of residents' self-assessments and faculty assessment of behaviors in anesthesiology. *Canadian Medical Education Journal*. 2021;12(4):17–26.
42. Lu F-I, Takahashi SG, Kerr C: Myth or reality: self-assessment is central to effective curriculum in anatomical pathology graduate medical education. *Academic Pathology*. 2021;8:1–6.
43. Melrose S: Balancing reflection and validity in health profession students' self-assessment. *International Journal of Learning, Teaching and Educational Research*. 2017;16(8):65–76.
44. Eva KW, Cunnington JPW, Reiter HI, et al.: How can I know what I don't know? Poor self-assessment in a well-defined domain. *Advances in Health Sciences Education*. 2004;9(3):211–224.
45. Davis DA, Mazmanian PE, Fordis M, et al.: Accuracy of physician self-assessment compared with observed measures of competence: a systematic review. *JAMA*. 2006;296(9):1094–1102.

46. Eva KW, Regehr G: "I'll never play professional football" and other fallacies of self-assessment. *Journal of Continuing Education in the Health Professions.* 2008;28(1):14–19.

47. Torres MB, Cochran A: Accuracy and content of medical student midclerkship self-evaluations. *American Journal of Surgery.* 2016;211:1153–1157.

48. Andrade H: A critical review of research on student self-assessment. *Frontiers in Education.* 2019;4(87):1–13.

49. Sargeant J: Toward a common understanding of self-assessment. *Journal of Continuing Education in the Health Professions.* 2008;(1):1–4.

50. Martin D, Regehr G, Hodges B, et al.: Using videotape benchmarks to improve the self-assessment ability of family practice residents. *Academic Medicine.* 1998;73(11):1201–1206.

51. Hodges B, Regehr G, Martin D: Difficulties in recognizing one's own incompetence: novice physicians who are unskilled and unaware of it. *Academic Medicine.* 2001;76(Suppl 10):S87–S89.

52. Scaffidi MA, Walsh CM, Khan R, et al.: Influence of video-based feedback on self-assessment accuracy of endoscopic skills: a randomized controlled trial. *Endoscopy International Open.* 2019;7:E678–E684.

53. Hawkins SC, Osborne A, Schofield SJ, et al.: Improving the accuracy of self-assessment of practical clinical skills using video feedback: the importance of including benchmarks. *Medical Teacher.* 2012;34(4):279–284.

54. Poirier TI, Pailden J, Jhala R, et al.: Student self-assessment and faculty assessment of performance in an interprofessional error disclosure simulation training program. *American Journal of Pharmaceutical Education.* 2017;8(3):Article 57.

55. Sargeant J, Armson H, Chesluk B, et al.: The processes and dimensions of informed self-assessment: a conceptual model. *Academic Medicine.* 2010;85(7):1212–1220.

56. Van Tartwijk J, Driessen EW: Portfolios for assessment and learning: AMEE guide no. 45. *Medical Teacher.* 2009;31(9):790–801.

57. Heeneman S, Driessen EW: The use of a portfolio in postgraduate medical education – reflect, assess and account, one for each or all in one? *GMS Journal for Medical Education.* 2017;34(5):1–12.

58. Könings K, van Berlo J, Koopmans R, et al.: Using a smartphone app and coaching group sessions to promote residents' reflection in the workplace. *Academic Medicine.* 2016;91(3):365–370.

59. Mann K, van der Vleuten C, Eva K, et al.: Tensions in informed self-assessment: how the desire for feedback and reticence to collect and use it can conflict. *Academic Medicine.* 2011;86(9):1120–1127.

60. McConnell MM, Regehr G, Wood TJ, et al.: Self-monitoring and its relationship to medical knowledge. *Advances in Health Sciences Education.* 2012;17:311–323.

61. Schön DA: *Educating the Reflective Practitioner.* San Francisco, CA: Jossey-Bass, 1987.

62. Epstein RM, Siegel DJ, Silberman J: Self-monitoring in clinical practice: a challenge for medical educators. *Journal of Continuing Education in the Health Professions.* 2008;28(1):5–13.

63. Eva KW, Regehr G, Gruppen LD: Blinded by "insight": self-assessment and its role in performance improvement. In: Hodges BD, Lingard L (Editors): *The Question of Competence: Reconsidering Medical Education in the Twenty-First Century.* Ithaca, NY: Cornell University Press, 2012.

64. McLeod ME: Doctor-patient relationship: perspectives, needs, and communication. *Official Journal of the American College of Gastroenterology: ACG.* 1 May 1998;93(5):676–680.

65. Temple J: Resident duty hours around the globe: where are we now? *BMC Medical Education.* 2014;14(Suppl 1):S8, 2.

66. Weaver MD, Landrigan CP, Sullivan JP, et al.: The association between resident physician work hour regulations and physician safety and health. *American Journal of Medicine.* 2020;133(7):e343–e354.

67. Wilcox MV, Orlando MS, Rand CS, et al.: Medical students' perceptions of patient-centeredness of the learning environment. *Perspectives in Medical Education.* 2017;4:44–50.

68. Rasasingam D, Kerry G, Gokani S, et al.: Being a patient: a medical students' perspective. *Advances in Medical Education and Practice.* 2017;8:163–165.

69. Ishikawa H, Son D, Eto M, et al.: Changes in patient-centered attitude and confidence in communicating with patients: a longitudinal study of resident physicians. *BMC Medical Education.* 2018;18:20.

70. Michiels-Corsten M, Weyland AM, Gold J, et al.: Inductive foraging: patients taking the lead in diagnosis, a mixed-methods study. *Journal of Family Practice.* 2022;39(3):479–485.

71. Launer J: Is taking a history outmoded? Why doctors should listen to stories instead. *Postgraduate Medical Journal.* 2022;98:236.

72. Brookfield S: *The Skillful Teacher: On Technique, Trust, and Responsiveness in the Classroom,* 2nd edition. San Francisco, CA: Jossey-Bass, 2006: 80.

73. Tompkins J: Pedagogy of the distressed. *College English.* 1990;52(6):653–660.

74. Pololi LH, Krupat E, Civian JT, et al.: Why are a quarter of faculty considering leaving academic medicine? A study of their perceptions of institutional culture and intentions to leave at 26 representative U.S. medical schools. *Academic Medicine.* 2012;87(7):859–869.

75. Corley EA, Sabharwal M: Foreign-born academic scientists and engineers: producing more and getting less than their US-born peers? *Research in Higher Education.* December 2007;48:909–940.

76. Krueger P, White D, Meaney C, et al.: Predictors of job satisfaction among academic family medicine faculty. *Canadian Family Physician.* 2017;63:e177–e185.

77. Fantaye AW, Kitto S, Hendry P, et al.: Attributes of excellent clinician teachers and barriers to recognizing and rewarding clinician teachers' performances and achievements: a narrative review. *Canadian Medical Education Journal.* 2022;13(2):57–72.

78. World Federation for Medical Education: Medical education the Edinburgh declaration. *Medical Education.* 1988;22(5):481–482.

79. Irby DM, O'Sullivan PS: Developing and rewarding teachers as educators and scholars: remarkable progress and daunting challenges. *Medical Education.* 2018;52:58–67.

80. Muller-Juge V, Pereira AC, Rieder A, et al.: A medical student in private practice for a 1-month clerkship: a qualitative exploration of the challenges for primary care clinical teachers. *Advances in Medical Education and Practice.* 2018;9:17–26.

81. Weston WW: The teacher-student-patient relationship in family practice: common dilemmas. *Canadian Family Physician.* 1989;35:139–143.

82. Mwaka AD, Taremwa S, Adoch W, et al.: Patients' attitudes towards involvement of medical students in their care at university teaching hospitals of three public universities in Uganda: a cross sectional study. *BMC Medical Education.* 2022;22:519.

83. Iqbal MZ, Bukhamsin EY, Alghareeb FY, et al.: Participation of medical students in patient care: how do patients perceive it? *Journal of Family Medicine and Primary Care.* 2020;9:3644–3651.

84. Rockey NG, Ramos GP, Romanski S, et al.: Patient participation in medical student teaching: a survey of hospital patients. *BMC Medical Education*. 2020;20:142. https://doi.org/10.1186/s12909-020-02052-1.

85. Towle A, Farrell C, Gaines ME, et al.: The patient's voice in health and social care professional education. *International Journal of Health Governance: The Vancouver Statement*. 2016;21(1):18–25.

86. Swinfen D, Labuschagne M, Joubert G: Disclosing medical errors: how do we prepare our students? *BMC Medical Education*. 2023;23:191.

87. Kim CW, Myung SJ, Eo EK, Chang Y: Improving disclosure of medical error through educational program as a first step toward patient safety. *BMC Medical Education*. 2017;17:52.

88. Tosteson DC: Learning in medicine. *New England Journal of Medicine*. 1979;301(13):690–694.

89. Wear D, Zarconi J, Dhillon N: Teaching fearlessness: a manifesto. *Education for Health (Abingdon)*. 2011;24(3):668–675.

90. Ahmady S, Kohan N, Namazi H, et al.: Outstanding qualities of a successful role model in medical education: students and professors' points of view. *Annals of Medicine and Surgery*. 2022;82:104652.

91. Cruess SR, Cruess RL, Steinert Y: Role modelling making the most of a powerful teaching strategy. *BMJ*. 2008;336(7646):718–721.

92. DiCorci MJ, Learman LA: Changing the educational environment to better support professionalism and professional identity formation. In: Cruess RL, Cruess SR, Steinert Y (Editors): *Teaching Medical Professionalism*, 2nd edition. Cambridge: Cambridge University Press, 2016: 261–274.

93. Beaudoin C, Maheux B, Côté L, et al.: Clinical teachers as humanistic caregivers and educators: perceptions of senior clerks and second-year residents. *CMAJ*. 1998;159(7):765–769.

94. Wright SM, Carrese JA: Excellence in role modelling: insight and perspectives from the pros. *CMAJ*. 2002;167(6):638–643.

95. Steinert Y: Educational theory and strategies for teaching and learning professionalism. In: Cruess RL, Cruess SR, Steinert Y (Editors): *Teaching Medical Professionalism*. Cambridge: Cambridge University Press, 2009.

96. Bandura A: *Social Foundations of Thought and Action: A Social Cognitive Theory*. Englewood Cliffs, NJ: Prentice Hall, 1986.

97. Rassie K: The apprenticeship model of clinical medical education: time for structural change. *New Zealand Medical Journal*. 2017;130(1461):66–72.

98. Reber AS: *Implicit Learning and Tacit Knowledge: An Essay on the Cognitive Unconscious*. Oxford: Oxford University Press, 1993: 5.

99. Tucker M, Balmer DF, Gowda D: Impact of explicit, implicit, and extra curricula on students' learning of the history and physical examination. *MedEdPublish*. 2017;6:136. (Last updated 2021)

100. Brown PC, Roediger III HL, McDaniel MA: *Make it Stick – The Science of Successful Learning*. Cambridge, MA: Belknap Press of Harvard University Press, 2014: 56–60.

101. Polanyi M: *Knowing and Being: Essays by Michael Polanyi*. London: Routledge & Kegan Paul, 1969: 54.

102. Mohammadi E, Shahsavari H, Mirzazadeh A, et al.: Improving role modeling in clinical teachers: a narrative literature review. *Journal of Advances in Medical Education & Professionalism*. 2020;8(1):1–9.

103. Egnew TR, Wilson HF: Role modelling the doctor-patient relationship in the clinical curriculum. *Family Medicine*. 2011;43(2):99–105.

13

The Case Presentation as a Teaching Tool for Patient-Centered Care

THOMAS R FREEMAN

INTRODUCTION

In their simplest form, cases represent an individual patient's problem or situation, an attempted solution and the outcome, typically from the perspective of the physician. Their organization may vary but reflect the culture from which they derive. They have been the fundamental way that physicians have thought about and communicated their work from antiquity to the present day. They are virtually ubiquitous in the practice of medicine and family physicians have difficulty discussing medical issues without referring to individual cases.[1] Case reports dominated the medical literature of the 19th century, essentially constituting medical knowledge and represented the main method of knowledge translation. With the rise of scientific medicine in the late 19th and early 20th century, the focus shifted from diagnosis of the patient to diagnosis of the disease, and the differential diagnosis became the primary clinical method. By the mid-20th century, the influence of evidence-based medicine had relegated case reports to the lowest level in the hierarchy of knowledge, and they began to disappear from the pages of medical journals and textbooks. Nevertheless, they continued to be used in bedside teaching and rounds.

A resurgence of interest in case reports and presentations began to occur around 2007 brought about by recognition of their importance in education, their potential for generating new hypotheses, shedding light on rare conditions not amenable to large scale or randomized control studies, and identification of adverse drug effects.[2-4] This stimulated interest in standardizing case reports for ease of aggregation for research or development of case series beginning with the CAse REport (CARE) guidelines[5] and modifications for different disciplines including surgery, (Surgical CAse REport or SCARE),[6] chiropracty, homeopathy, and therapeutic massage.[7-9] As of 2015, there were more than 160 peer-reviewed journals representing a wide variety of medical specialties, devoted to publishing case reports.[2] Arguments have been made for inclusion of case reports as part of systematic reviews,[10] and protocols for evaluating the suitability of reports for inclusion in such reviews have been published.[11]

In education, case reports have long been recognized as fundamental in developing physician practice and transmitting practical knowledge.[12] Sir William Osler outlined in his natural method of teaching the subject of medicine as follows: "In the natural method of teaching,

DOI: 10.1201/9781003394679-17

the student begins with the patient, continues with the patient, and ends his studies with the patient, using books, and lectures as tools, as a means to an end".[13] All clinical success is measured as an N of 1.[14] Case reports are recognized as useful in teaching basic observation, clinical reasoning,[15] ethics, hypothesis generation, and pattern recognition[16] and outperform lectures in improving clinicians' cognitive knowledge and recall.[17] The case method remains a "signature pedagogy of medicine" and "the center of medical education and, indeed, the center of all medical communication about patients".[18]

It is important to distinguish between case presentations, case reports, and case records. Case records are principally the written working tool of practice intended to make a record of pertinent patient information, investigations, and therapy to ensure continuity of care and to communicate with other members of a healthcare team. Case reports are short, usually verbal descriptions of patient details related to the immediate encounter and are commonly used in teaching venues such as hospitals, clinics, and offices. Case presentations are longer, formal expositions of a patient or patients, from initial presentation, through to diagnosis, therapeutic initiatives and outcomes as well as references to the relevant medical literature. This chapter focuses on case presentations and case reports.

Although the use of the word "case" itself has been challenged as impersonal or even dehumanizing,[19] it remains the way clinicians refer to their work and will be the term used in this chapter.

THE CONVENTIONAL CASE PRESENTATION

Though himself a prolific publisher of cases, Sir William Osler's enormously influential work, *The Principles and Practice of Medicine*, published in 1892, focused on diseases, their etiology, symptomatology, diagnosis, and treatment. Cases only appeared occasionally as illustrative charts or in the footnotes. Perhaps recognizing that patients don't present to the physician with a diagnosis, Richard Cabot published his multi-volume compendium of 385 cases to demonstrate the clinical method of the differential diagnosis.[20] These cases typically began with a narrative paragraph describing the patient and their initial presentation, including a brief history of the onset of symptoms and the patient's living circumstances and occupation. This was followed by a longer history and description of physical and laboratory findings, ending with the outcome of treatment and final diagnosis. The opening paragraph of a typical case presentation by Richard Cabot[20] reads as follows:

> A married woman of forty-two consulted me March 17, 1904, for long-standing headaches which had been present, off and on, during the last five years, since an attack of "grip", followed by deafness and ringing in the left ear. The patient lives in a very malarious suburb of Boston, but has never had the disease as far as she knows.

Cabot goes on to demonstrate how the diagnosis of methemoglobinemia was made and the case concludes with a follow-up 3 years later.

By the latter half of the 20th century case presentations had assumed a relatively standard format that eschewed narration and focused more on the disease than on the patient. Such formats begin with a brief description of the patient's presenting complaint, followed by history of present illness, past medical history, family history, social history, patient profile, and examination findings. These items are augmented by results of investigation such as laboratory work, imaging, pathology reports, a problem list, and management plan. This form of case presentation accurately reflects the conventional clinical method, one based on the biomedical model.[21] Medicine had shifted from consideration of individual cases to diseases and diagnosis became the chief work of medicine. The evidence-based medicine movement continued the shift away from consideration of individual cases to large, randomized trials.

The written medical record was greatly improved by the method described by Weed,[22] and his Problem-Oriented Medical Record has been widely accepted. This method made problems, rather than diseases, the organizing principle of the record and separated subjective and objective elements. This form of written record has had a great influence on the format of oral case presentations as well.

The biopsychosocial model proposed by Engel[23] was an attempt to apply systems theory to clinical problems. This model, along with the recognition that psychological and social factors play a role in illness events, has led to the inclusion of these topics in many case presentations.

The electronic health record introduced new dimensions into record keeping introducing a "third person" into the examining room competing with the patient for attention[24] as well as raising concerns of its effects on clinician cognition and clinical reasoning[25, 26] as well as communication.[27]

CRITICISMS OF THE CONVENTIONAL CASE PRESENTATION AND REPORT

The conventional case history or report as described has been criticized for being heavily dependent on scientific language, which, although seemingly precise, leaves much of reality aside.[28] Abstract scientific language excludes the human, lived experience (lifeworld) of patients and obscures the fact that where illnesses are unique, disease labels are classificatory terms only.[29] This problem is as true of chronic illness as it is of acute illness.[30] By minimizing the importance of the patient's story and subjective experience, the conventional case history separates biological processes from the person (depersonalization) and minimizes the physician's role in producing findings or observations.[31-34] This form of presentation is primarily doctor- and disease-centered. "The message is clear, disease counts; the human experience of illness does not".[31] The expectations of general internal medicine consultants regarding the content of oral case presentations continue to neglect this issue.[35-37]

From a phenomenological perspective, the clinical encounter can be viewed as a hermeneutical exercise involving the interpretation of multiple "texts". These consist of the "experiential text" of illness as lived by the patient, the "narrative text" arising from history taking, the "physical text" of the patient's body as objectively examined and the "instrumental text" constructed by diagnostic technologies. Such a hermeneutic model poses a number of questions, the most important being: "How can the ill person, both as text and co-interpreter, be restored to centrality in the clinical encounter?"[38]

ADDRESSING THE CRITICISMS OF THE CONVENTIONAL CASE PRESENTATION

The recognized shortcomings of the conventional case presentation have taken on greater importance with the recognition of how the language used in medical education contributes to the "hidden curriculum" (mentioned in Chapter 11 of this book). The way that medical students are taught to talk about patients also teaches them how to think about them and how to define their relationship.[39] Anspach[40] points out that the presentation of case histories is an important part of the medical training of students, interns, and residents. Usually presented before an audience of peers and senior medical people, these presentations are important for both their content and as part of the socialization process. They are a powerful way of teaching and reinforcing a particular worldview. Such exercises are important in the development of professional identity.[41] They are a method for communicating standards of practice[42] and can serve to teach management of uncertainty in clinical judgement[43] as well as ethical values.[44] Learning to balance the use of evidence with the particulars of a case serves to foster in the learner the development of practical knowledge.

Hawkins[45] advocates the method of the clinical biography of AR Luria, in which the scientific and humanistic are complementary, each representing different attitudes to the human experience. She points out that case history and biography are similar, in that they involve a lot of interpretation and are to be understood in the "context" of the narrative.

In the conventional case presentation, the patient's perspective is, to some extent, represented under the heading "subjective". The symptoms described therein have been described as an important source of medical knowledge[46] and need to receive more emphasis. This is more widely recognized in the hermeneutic approach to medicine.[47]

Efforts to change the focus of case histories to include more accurate descriptions of patients as persons range from the elegant literary work of Luria[45] and Sacks[48] to the innovative and pragmatic teaching methods of Donnelly,[49] Charon,[50, 51] and Cassell.[52]

Donnelly[33, 49] suggests that the human aspects of medicine can be addressed by teaching stories (which pay attention to what has happened in the interior world) instead of chronicles (which stick simply to a recitation of events). He asked house staff to include in the history one or two sentences about what the patient's understanding of the illness was and how it affects their life, in an effort to help the physician empathize more accurately.

Charon[50, 51] states that the physician's effectiveness increases with empathy and the physician teaches the "empathic stance" by asking medical students to write stories about their patients. These stories are considered as adjuncts to the hospital chart and do not replace the traditional case write-ups. Charon has suggested that the students are molded into the kind of doctor their teachers want by becoming the kind of writer their teachers want.[53] Reflective exercises over the course of medical training have been found to support students in developing capacity for expressing complex interior, interpersonal, perceptual experiences.[54] Launer[55] has extended the narrative approach to the supervisor/supervisee relationship when the latter is describing a patient or client that presents a challenge. This may facilitate the presentation of the case as well as model how this can be done with the patient. "By showing a capacity for holding onto uncertainty and avoiding inappropriate foreclosure, supervisors can model the same capacity for others".[55]

Cassell advises medical trainees that writing succinct summaries of patients is a skill that must be developed:

Include a brief personality description. Follow with a description in succinct terms of the patient's background, education and employment, current family (married or single, children) or other significant relationship. Following that there should be a brief description of the patient's physical appearance. Start with the patient's appearance prior to undressing. If there are distinguishing features of speech or presentation of self they should be mentioned. Then focus on the unclothed appearance-body habitus, general development, musculature, and prominent distinguishing features such as major birthmarks, scars, or deformities. The whole description is usually not more than a paragraph.[52]

Narrative medicine has developed a literature in its own right[51, 54-60] and has helped inform our understanding of how we seek meaning in the events of our lives. Evaluation of the impact of narrative medicine workshops for faculty[61] and narrative medicine programmes[62, 63] have found evidence of a positive impact on attitudes, knowledge, and skills, but it remains unclear whether these changes are felt by patients or positively impact care. For the most part, however, the narrative format lacks the structure desirable in transmitting important knowledge quickly in clinical settings. There remains the need for a bridge between the thin description of the conventional case presentation and the thick description of the narrative approach, especially in the teaching of students and house staff. Basic changes must occur in the way that medicine is taught. Integrated narrative and evidence-based case reports have been advocated and published such as combining narrative in the standard case report and placing the history of present illness at the end.[64, 65] The CARE guidelines for written case reports call for the patient to share their perspective "whenever possible".[5] It is hoped that by including the patient perspective there will be a shift in the understanding of disease "away from narrow biological processes to more holistic, socioculturally grounded understandings of wellness and deviations from it".[66] The *Canadian Medical Association Journal* (CMAJ) has introduced a section called "360 Cases" that consist of a brief case summary followed by personal reflections from up to four individuals involved in the case, one of whom must be the patient or caregiver or family member.[67] The intent is to highlight interpersonal and systemic aspects of care that are typically missing from case reports.[5]

The absence of clear instructions on how case presentations should be done may result in acquisition of unintended professional values and delayed development of effective communication skills. "Teaching and learning of oral presentation skills may be improved by emphasizing that context determines content and by making explicit the tacit rules of presentation".[68]

The patient-centered clinical method is strengthened by a method of case presentation that reflects the same values.

DESCRIPTION OF THE PATIENT-CENTERED CASE PRESENTATION

The following is a description of a full case presentation method to be carried out at special end-of-rotation teaching sessions or Grand Rounds.

In a sharp departure from the conventional case report, which focuses on the organic pathology of the patient, the patient-centered case presentation (PCCP) gives primacy to the patient and the total experience of the illness and associated pathology. Unlike the conventional method, in which "the objective truths of medicine are recorded in the 'language of abstraction'" and are not "related to the existence of the individual patient",[69] the PCCP regards objective truth as of less interest when it is not related to the individual.

The PCCP focuses on an "acquaintance with particulars".[70] It begins with a description of the particulars of the case under study and then proceeds to a discussion of the general – that is, other cases or studies that may share similar features. There may be a discussion of a single case or several cases that seem to express a common theme.

The PCCP, by going from the particular to the general and from the subjective to objective and back again, performs a cycle that ultimately informs the presenter with a greater understanding of the patient.

Table 13.1 compares the conventional case presentation and the PCCP and highlights how the items of information of the conventional approach are incorporated into the PCCP.

1. *The Patient's Chief Concern or Request.* When possible, a brief narrative in the patient's voice begins this section of the presentation. This is followed by a statement of the symptomatology as well as the illness behavior[71] that brought the patient to the encounter. It should address the patient's actual reason for coming. Room needs to be made for the caregiver's voice in circumstances where a patient is in need of assistance from a family member or other individual.[72]

2. *The Patient's Health and Illness Experience.* A description of the experience of the illness should include some quotations from the patient that particularly illustrate the subjective quality of the illness. For example, when discussing an individual for whom pain is a predominant feature, it would be appropriate to include the pain descriptors that the patient used in communicating the discomfort. Knowing the metaphors that patients use to describe their illness gives the clinician greater insight, understanding, and empathy. The language for the metaphoric landscape is "not found in traditional textbooks of medicine,

Table 13.1 Comparison of Conventional and Patient-Centered Case Presentation

Conventional Case Presentation	Patient-Centered Case Presentation
Chief complaint	Patient's chief concern or request
History of present illness	Patient's health and illness experience; Quotes from the patient; Meaning of health and aspirations; Feelings, ideas, effects on function, expectations
Past medical history, Medications, Allergies, Observations	Disease • History of present illness • Past medical history • Review of systems • Physical exam • Laboratory etc.
Family history	Person • Patient profile • Individual life cycle phase
Patient profile	Context Proximal (e.g.) • Family history • Genogram Distal (e.g.) • Culture • Ecosocial
Review of systems	Patient–doctor relationship (The clinical encounter) The Dyad itself • Transference/Countertransference issues • Finding common ground • Problems • Goals • Roles

Table 13.1 *(Continued)* Comparison of Conventional and Patient-Centered Case Presentation

Conventional Case Presentation	Patient-Centered Case Presentation
Physical exam	Assessment (Problem list)
Laboratory database	General discussion
	Illness experience – literature (pathographies, poetry)
	Medical literature
	Clinical epidemiology
	Pathophysiology; other case reports; medical anthropology.
Problem list	Proposed management plan
General assessment	
Proposed plan	

but in articulate memoirs of illness, insightful fiction, poetry, drama, and the examined experience of our own illnesses and those of our family and friends".[49] As in the patient-centered clinical method, the patient's feelings, ideas, effects on function, and expectations are presented here, including the significance of the symptoms to the patient. A statement of the patient's meaning of health and how the patient's illness affects their ability to achieve a state consistent with their particular aspirations in this regard is appropriate (corresponding to the Health and Illness Experience portions of Figure 1.1 in Chapter 1).

3. *Observations.* The observation portion of the presentation involves the Disease, Person, and Context dimensions shown in the diagram (Figure 1.1 in Chapter 1). This section is subdivided into observations about the disease, including the standard elements of the medical history (history of present illness, past medical history, genetic information if available and appropriate, review of systems, physical examination findings, and relevant laboratory work), issues related to the person (patient profile, life cycle phase), and context (e.g., family, employment, culture community. See Chapter 5).

4. *The Patient–Clinician Relationship (The Clinical Encounter).* This involves a discussion of not only the technical management issues (e.g., drug and nondrug therapies) but also a discussion of how the patient–clinician dyad can be developed into a healing relationship.[52] Issues of self-awareness, feelings about the patient, and struggles to make effective connections are appropriate, as are any issues related to finding common ground between the doctor and the patient. See Chapter 6 for a detailed description of finding common ground and Chapter 7 for more on enhancing the relationship.

5. *Assessment (Problem List).* This section summarizes the issues that need further assessment or intervention in any of the five areas of health, disease, illness, person, or context.

6. *General Discussion.* Having discussed the particulars of the case, the presentation then turns to the general issues raised by the case. The issues selected for discussion are chosen by the presenter from elements of the case which they found most interesting, puzzling or disturbing. In this way, the case helps to instruct the presenter. General issues can be subdivided into those that relate to the experience of the illness and those issues related to pathophysiology, epidemiology, psychology, sociology, and medical anthropology.

First-person accounts of the experience of illnesses have become common. Literature and poetry provide many examples of individuals who have written in a lucid and illuminating way of their personal experience of an illness.[73-82] In addition, the movie industry has focused on this area and occasionally a short video can very effectively communicate the trials of a particular sickness.[83] It will be necessary for faculty to accumulate a usable bibliography of such material, as it, not only in journals but also in newspapers, magazines, books, and illness blogs are common on the Internet,[84] and work has been undertaken on content analysis of cancer blogs.[85] Indeed, this type of writing has recently undergone a resurgence, and an acquaintance with it will provide the presenter with improved insights into the patient's experience of the illness.

This section of the PCCP includes a discussion of any relevant medical literature pertaining to the case. It should incorporate the current understanding of any pathology or clinical epidemiology (i.e., prevalence, natural history, the sensitivity and specificity and predictive value of any tests, effects of intervention).

This section also demonstrates knowledge of the published scientific literature concerning the disturbed psychological and social functions that have been observed in other individuals with similar problems.

Comparison of the case to any published cases of a similar nature will help to draw attention to what is unique and what is shared in those facing similar problems.

7. *Proposed Therapeutic Approach.* This is an opportunity to use the information gleaned from the discussion of the general issues and to integrate this knowledge into a therapeutic approach.

CASE EXAMPLE

Thomas R Freeman

Janna M: "He was my main support . . . he did everything".

Chief Concern: "I don't want to get up again. He was my main support; he did everything". Janna has been wheeled into the office by her adult son, Mike.

Health and Illness Experience: Mike relates that his mother, who is 72, has refused to get up since her husband Tiva, his father, died suddenly 3 weeks ago. As far as anyone knew Tiva had been a healthy 76-year-old retired construction worker when he collapsed while working in the yard. Janna, like everyone else, was shocked, in despair, and didn't move from a chair in the bedroom for several days. She needed assistance to get to the bathroom stating that her feet felt "like lead". She took to her bed: "I don't want to get up again. He was my main support. He did everything". Now she needs assistance to get into and out of bed and has been incontinent of urine. She has lost interest in everything including her crocheting and spends most of her time staring out the window and weeping.

A discussion with her son provided further detail. His parents were married for almost 50 years and, as his mother said, Tiva was very much the patriarch of the family, while Janna controlled the household. Janna and Tiva were married in their 20s and immigrated to Canada in their early 30s. They have lived in their own home for the past 20 years and had two children: the son, Mike, and a daughter, Louise. Louise came home from overseas to help look after her mother. Mike also said that Janna's health had been "slipping" for the last couple of years as she found walking to be difficult, which they attributed to her arthritic hips. She had become less active in their church and local social club. He and his sister had been wondering about the onset of dementia.

Observations: Janna's past medical history includes mild hypertension and type 2 diabetes as well as osteoarthritis of the hips. There have been periods of anxiety related to marital problems, but no known physical trauma. She had an appendectomy in her late 20s and delivered her two children without complications. She underwent a hysterectomy for fibroids in her mid-40s. *Medications:* Metformin 500 mg twice a day; enalapril 10 mg once a day; naproxen 250 BID if needed for hip pain.

She remained in her wheelchair to begin the physical examination. Leaning on her right elbow with her hand supporting her chin, her answers were slow, and she stared at the wall. She exhibited a depressed affect. She was able to move her arms reluctantly. There was mild rigidity of the upper limbs, but no cogwheeling. BP 135/90; HR 86/min and regular. HS normal. Chest clear but poor inspiratory effort. Cranial nerves intact. With her son's assistance, we moved her to an examining table to complete the examination. Examination of the cranial nerves was normal. Deep tendon reflexes, with the exception of absent ankle reflexes were normal. Strength was diminished in all limbs but particularly the legs. The plantar reflex was equivocal bilaterally. In the standing position she was unsteady and unwilling to take a step unaided.

A brief test of cognitive function (Montreal Cognitive Assessment, MoCA©) scored 18, in the mild cognitive impairment range.

An office urine test was normal with no evidence of infection. Blood tests were carried out including complete blood count, renal function, liver function; thyroid and B12 were all within normal limits. The HbA1$_c$ was 7.2. A CT scan of the brain revealed moderately dilated ventricles bilaterally.

Patient–clinician relationship: Over the 8 years that she had been a patient in the practice, her visits were primarily for monitoring diabetes and hypertension and helping to manage her hip pain. She was usually easy to connect with and conveyed a calm demeanor. Her presentation this day was a marked contrast and the alarm raised by the apparent suddenness of her immobility was accentuated by her son who was trying to cope with the recent death of his father. The atmosphere in the examining room was strained with anxiety and grief. The rapidity of her physical decline was alarming.

ASSESSMENT

1. Rapid decline in mobility
2. Urinary incontinence
3. Moderately dilated ventricles of the brain
4. Depressed affect
5. Grief
6. Mild cognitive decline
7. Diabetes type 2 – controlled
8. Hypertension – controlled
9. Osteoarthritis of hips

DISCUSSION

The close association of rapid onset of immobility and her husband's death, upon whom she was very dependent, combined with mild cognitive impairment initially raised the issue of whether it represented a form of functional cognitive disorder.[86, 87] Cognitive symptoms can also occur with functional movement disorders and, in the past, such presentations were named conversion pseudodementia but were exceedingly rare.[88] This condition was characterized by cognitive impairment, regression, and physical dependency. While Janna's presentation was dramatic and closely timed to her husband's death, the predominant symptomatology was difficulty standing and walking and the cognitive impairment was mild, so a diagnosis of functional cognitive disorder was set aside.

Janna presented with a depressed affect, but in the context of the grief reaction to her husbands' sudden death, whether she was clinically depressed would only become apparent with further follow up. The relationship of depression to dementia in the elderly is well known, but whether it is a risk factor, a prodromal symptom, or unrelated remains unclear.[89]

The symptom cluster of gait disturbance, urinary incontinence, and dementia (Hakim's triad) all of which Janna presented, is a hallmark of idiopathic normal pressure hydrocephalus (iNPH). The gait in iNPH is described as "magnetic" as if the feet are glued to the floor. Both urinary and fecal incontinence are possible. In the early stages it may be confused with Parkinson's or Alzheimer's disease. Psychiatric symptoms including aggressive behavior, psychosis, and obsessive-compulsive disorder are common and may respond to antidepressants or antipsychotics.[90] The prevalence of iNPH among the elderly is estimated to be between 0.41% and 2.4% and may represent up to 6% of all dementias.[91] In a 10-year follow-up study of a population of elderly (more than 70 years of age) in Japan, the incidence was 1.2/1000 person years, and there appeared to be subclinical or preclinical states before the condition became symptomatic.[92] Relief of the hydrocephalus by means of large volume cerebrospinal fluid (CSF) extraction through lumbar puncture (LP) is followed by a dramatic improvement in mobility and cessation of incontinence. Insertion of a ventricle-peritoneal (VP) shunt sustains these advantages but is not without physical and psychosocial problems including shunt revisions.[93] In a 10-year follow up of 127 patients with VP shunts quality of life improved for 79% over the first 5 years post-shunt but declined gradually in thereafter.[94]

First-person accounts of iNPH can be found on the Internet and are helpful for providing insight into the subjective experience of the condition before and after VP shunt.[95] What is noteworthy in many of these accounts is the length of time and varied symptomatology that arise before the classic triad becomes apparent. Difficulty concentrating, reduced problem-solving skills, being easily distracted, difficulty focusing eyes, irritability, and drowsiness are commonly mentioned. The wide range of symptoms and the slow progression likely contributes to the prolonged time to diagnosis.

THERAPEUTIC PLAN

A referral was made to neurology and a subsequent MRI of the brain confirmed moderately dilated ventricles bilaterally and no evidence of other lesions. An LP found a normal opening pressure. A large volume drainage of CSF resulted in a marked improvement in Janna's ability to stand and walk. This was followed 3 weeks later by surgery to put in place a VP shunt.

Follow-up was arranged for counseling related to grief and possible depressive disorder with the team social worker. A fuller evaluation of cognitive function was arranged to take place several months after insertion of VP shunt.

KEY TAKEAWAYS

Idiopathic normal pressure hydrocephalus in the elderly is not uncommon. There may be vague and varied symptomatology prior to the presentation of the classic triad and the observations of family members are important in providing collateral information crucial to the diagnosis. If iNPH is confirmed on LP, a VP shunt is effective in alleviating many of the symptoms.

SHORT FORM OF THE PATIENT-CENTERED CASE REPORT

In day-to-day clinical work in the office or ward, it is necessary to use a shortened form of case presentation while continuing to emphasize the values of patient-centered medicine. In these settings learners should be instructed to begin with the patient's name and then describe the patient's chief concern or request; the patient's health and illness experience; a brief summary of proximal context such as family and occupation. This is followed by the relevant physical findings and any laboratory/imaging results and suggested plan. When learners lapse into a truncated and impersonal case description (e.g., "I have a 54-year-old woman with pain and weakness in her shoulders and hips"), they must be gently but firmly instructed in "re-humanizing" their report by beginning with the patient's name, followed by the elements of the shortened PCCP.

ADVANTAGES OF THE PATIENT-CENTERED CASE PRESENTATION

Case presentations are viewed as "highly conventionalized linguistic rituals" that serve to socialize physicians in training to a particular worldview.[40] Usually cases in medical education are chosen to highlight general principles and what are understood to be the underlying mechanisms of disease and illness. Actual practice, however, engages with a complex network of biological, psychological, pathological, and social forces that are missing from the traditional version of case presentations and reports. The PCCP, by placing the patient at the center of the presentation, reinforces the centrality of the person rather than the disease, including these elements in the process of clinical reasoning. In this way, it can serve to instill a more humane form of medicine and reinforce the basic values inherent in the patient-centered clinical method. It does this without sacrificing the more conventional type of information found in the conventional case presentation.

A PCCP is strong pedagogical mode of education for students transitioning from the prepositional knowledge emphasized in early medical education to knowledge-in-practice, requiring "learners to embrace a situation in all its holistic complexity".[96]

In increasing numbers of medical schools there has been a shift away from passive learning (i.e., lectures) to a less structured format in which learners take greater responsibility for setting learning goals. This is more effective at developing "lifelong learners". Nevertheless, it is not an unusual experience, after starting into practice, to feel somewhat at a loss as to how to continue to be well informed. The rapid expansion of medical knowledge makes it impossible for any individual to always be completely up-to-date. Therefore, it is necessary that the practicing physician have a method for continuing medical education that takes into account one's individual learning needs. Most experienced physicians acknowledge that their most demanding teachers are ultimately their patients. The PCCP, when a part of medical education, develops a useful framework for later use by practicing physicians when considering their challenging cases. It recognizes the role of the patient in teaching us what we most need to know.

The usual reasons stated for making a written case report are (a) a unique case, (b) a case of unexpected association, and (c) a case of unexpected events.[97] The philosophy of the PCCP is that *every* case is unique and may, indeed, often, involve the unexpected. The only necessary motivation for undertaking a PCCP is a desire to come to a deeper understanding of the patient.

CONCLUSION

The patient-centered case presentation is a method of presenting cases in medicine that is consistent with new clinical methods. It recognizes that case presentations are an important part of the socialization of physicians in training as well as other health care professionals. Inclusion of the human aspects of illness serves to reinforce an attitude of "patient-centeredness".

REFERENCES

1. McWhinney IR, Freeman TR: *McWhinney's Textbook of Family Medicine.* Oxford; New York: Oxford University Press, 2016: 21.
2. Akers KG: New journals for publishing medical case reports. *Journal of the Medical Library Association: JMLA.* April 2016;104(2):146.
3. Zabielska M: Reporting on individual experience: a proposal of a patient-centered model for the medical case report. *Communication and Medicine.* 2019;16(3):292–303.
4. Cook S, Burton M, Glasziou P: Efficacy and safety of the "mother's kiss" technique: a systematic review of case reports and case series. *CMAJ.* November 2012;184(17):E904–E912. https://doi.org/10.1503/cmaj.111864.
5. Gagnier JJ, Kienle G, Altman DG, et al.: The CARE guidelines: consensus-based clinical case reporting guideline development. *Journal of Medical Case Reports.* 2013;7:223. https://doi.org/10.1186/1752-1947-7-223.
6. Agha RA, Fowler AJ, Saeta A, Barai I, Rajmohan S, Orgill DP, Afifi R, Al-Ahmadi R, Albrecht J, Alsawadi A, Aronson J: The SCARE statement: consensus-based surgical case report guidelines. *International Journal of Surgery.* 1 October 2016;34:180–186.
7. Budgell B: Guidelines to the writing of case studies. *Journal of the Canadian Chiropractic Association.* December 2008;52(4):199.
8. Van Haselen RA: Homeopathic clinical case reports: development of a supplement (HOM-CASE) to the CARE clinical case reporting guideline. *Complementary Therapies in Medicine.* 1 April 2016;25:78–85.
9. Munk N, Boulanger K: Adaptation of the CARE guidelines for therapeutic massage and bodywork publications: efforts to improve the impact of case reports. *International Journal of Therapeutic Massage & Bodywork.* September 2014;7(3):32.
10. Sampayo-Codera M, Miguel-Huguet R, Malfeltone A, Perez-Garcia JM, Llombert-Cussac A, Cortes J, Pardo A, Perez-Lopez J: The values of case reports in: systematic reviews form rare diseases: the example of enzyme replacement therapy (ERT) in patients with mucopolysaccharidosis type II. *International Journal of Environmental Research and Public Health.* 2020;17(18):6590.
11. Nambiema A, Sembajwe G, Lam J, Woodruff T, Mandrioli D, Chartres N, Fadel M, Le Guillou A, Valter R, Deguigne M, Legeay M, Bruneau C, LeRoux G, Descatha A: A protocol for the use of case reports/studies and case series in systematic reviews for clinical toxicology. *Frontiers in Medicine* 2021;8:708380.
12. Cannon WB: The case method of teaching systematic medicine. *Boston Medical and Surgical Journal.* 1990;142:31–36.
13. Osler W: The natural method of teaching the subject of medicine. *Journal of the American Medical Association.* 15 June 1901;36(24):1673–1679.
14. Koch CA, Fülöp T: Case reports: old-timers and evergreens. *Journal of Medical Case Reports.* 2018;12:355. https://doi.org/10.1186/s13256-018-1889-3.

15. Bannister SL, Hanson JL, Maloney CG, Raszka Jr WV: Using the student case presentation to enhance diagnostic reasoning. *Pediatrics.* August 2011;128(2):211–213.
16. Packer CD, Katz RB, Iacopetti CL, et al.: A case suspended in time: the educational values of case reports. *Academic Medicine.* 2017;92:152–156.
17. Greenberg LW, Jewett LS: The impact of two teaching techniques on physicians' knowledge and performance. *Journal of Medical Education.* 1985;60:390–395.
18. Hunter KM: *Doctors' Stories – The Narrative Structure of Medical Knowledge.* Princeton, NJ: Princeton University Press, 1991: 247.
19. Murakawa M: A multitude of voices and worlds: towards a new model of the medical case report. *Token: A Journal of English Linguistics.* 2013;2.
20. Cabot RC: *Differential Diagnosis: Presented Through an Analysis of 385 Cases*, volume 1, 3rd edition. Philadelphia; London: W. B. Saunders Company, 1917: 39.
21. How to Present a Patient: A Step-To-Step Guide. www.studentdoctor.net/2018/06/28/oral-case-presentation/.
22. Weed LL: *Medical Records, Medical Education and Patient Care.* Chicago, IL: Year Book Medical Publishers, 1969.
23. Engel GL: The need for a new medical model: a challenge for biomedicine. *Science.* 1977;196(4286):129–136.
24. Lown BA, Rodriguez D: Lost in translation/How EHRs structure communication, relationships and meaning. *Academic Medicine.* 2012;7(4):392–394.
25. Wisner K, Lyndon A, Chesla CA: The electronic health record's impact on nurses' cognitive work: an integrative review. *International Journal of Nursing Studies.* June 2019;94:74–84. https://doi.org/10.1016/j.ijnurstu.2019.03.003.
26. Nijor S, Rallis G, Lad N, Gokcen E: Patient safety issues from information overload in electronic medical records. *Journal of Patient Safety.* 1 September 2022;18(6):e999–e1003. https://doi.org/10.1097/PTS.0000000000001002.
27. Shachak A, Reis S: The impact of electronic medical records on patient-doctor communication during consultation: a narrative literature review. *Journal of Evaluation in Clinical Practice.* August 2009;15(4):641–649.
28. Schwartz MA, Wiggins O: Science, humanism and the nature of medical practice: a phenomenological view. *Perspectives in Biology and Medicine.* 1985;28(3):331–361.
29. McCullough LB: The abstract character and transforming power of medical language. *Soundings.* 1989;72(1):111–125.
30. Gerhardt U: Qualitative research on chronic illness: the issue and the story. *Social Science and Medicine.* 1990;30(11):1149–1159.
31. Donnelly WJ: Medical language as symptom: doctor talk in teaching hospitals. *Perspectives in Biology and Medicine.* 1986;30(1):81–94.
32. Donnelly WJ: The language of medical case histories. *Annals of Internal Medicine.* 1997;127(11):1045–1048.
33. Donnelly WJ: Patient-centered medical care requires a patient-centered medical record. *Academic Medicine.* 2005;80(1):33–38.
34. Khan M: The perspective of medical communication on the biomedical model of practice and patient centeredness: a review of the language of medical case presentations genre. *International Journal of Linguistics, Literature and Translation.* 2019;2(3):71–80.
35. Green EH, Durning AJ, DeCherrie L, et al.: Expectations for oral case presentations for clinical clerks: opinions of internal medicine clerkship directors. *Journal of General Internal Medicine.* 2009;24(3):370–373.

36. Green EH, DeCherrie L, Fagan MJ, Sharpe BA, Hershman W: The oral case presentation: what internal medicine clinician-teachers expect from clinical clerks. *Teaching and Learning in Medicine*. January 2011;23(1):58–61. https://doi.org/10.1080/10401334.2011.536894.

37. Williams DE, Surakanti S: Developing oral case presentation skills: peer and self-evaluations as instructional tools. *Ochsner Journal*. 20 March 2016;16(1):65–69.

38. Leder D: Clinical interpretation: the hermeneutics of medicine. *Theoretical Medicine*. 1990;11(1):9–24.

39. Lingard L, Haber RJ: Teaching and learning communication in medicine: a rhetorical approach. *Academic Medicine*. 1 May 1999;74(5):507–510.

40. Anspach RR: Notes on the sociology of medical discourse: the language of case presentation. *Journal of Health and Social Behavior*. 1998;29(4):357–375.

41. Jarvis-Selinger S, Halwani Y, Joughin K, Pratt D, Scott T, Snell L: *Supporting the Development of Residents as Teachers: Current Practices and Emerging Trends*. Members of the FMEC PG Consortium, 2011.

42. Spafford MM, Lingard L, Schryer CF, Hrynchak PK: Tensions in the field: teaching standards of practice in optometry case presentations. *Optometry and Vision Science*. 1 October 2004;81(10):800–806.

43. Holmes SM, Ponte M: En-case-ing the patient: disciplining uncertainty in medical student patient presentations. *Culture, Medicine, and Psychiatry*. June 2011;35:163–182.

44. Charon R, Montello M (Editors): *Stories Matter: The Role of Narrative in Medical Ethics*. New York, NY: Routledge, 2002.

45. Hawkins AH: AR Luria and the art of clinical biography. *Literature and Medicine*. 1986;5(1):1–5.

46. Malterud K: Symptoms as a source of medical knowledge: understanding medically unexplained disorders in women. *Family Medicine*. 1 October 2000;32(9):603–611.

47. Wardrope A, Reuber M: The hermeneutics of symptoms. *Medicine, Health Care and Philosophy*. 2022;25:395–412. https://doi.org/10.1007/s11019-022-10086-z.

48. Sacks O: Clinical tales. *Literature and Medicine*. 1986;5:16–23. https://doi.org/10.1353/lm.2011.0299.

49. Donnelly WJ: Righting the medical record: transforming chronicle into story. *Soundings*. 1 April 1989:127–136.

50. Charon R: To render the lives of patients. *Literature and Medicine*. 1986;5:58–74. https://doi.org/10.1353/lm.2011.0295.

51. Charon R: Narrative and medicine. *New England Journal of Medicine*. 26 February 2004;350(9):862–864. https://doi.org/10.1056/NEJMp038249.

52. Cassell EJ: *The Nature of Healing: The Modern Practice of Medicine*. New York, NY: Oxford University Press, 2013: 81, 248.

53. Charon R: Doctor-patient/reader-writer: learning to find the text. *Soundings*. 1989;72(1):137–152.

54. Miller E, Balmer D, Hermann MN, Graham MG, Charon R: Sounding narrative medicine: studying students' professional identity development at Columbia University College of physicians and surgeons. *Academic Medicine*. February 2014;89(2):335.

55. Launer J: *Narrative-Based Practice in Health and Social Care: Conversations Inviting Change*, 2nd edition. London; New York: Routledge; Taylor & Francis, 2018.

56. Charon R, DasGupta S, Hermann N: *The Principles and Practice of Narrative Medicine*. New York, NY: Oxford University Press, 2017.

57. DasGupta C, Irvine H, Colon M, Spiegel S: *The Principles and Practice of Narrative Medicine*. New York: Oxford University Press, 2017.

58. Greenhalgh T, Hurwitz B: *Narrative Based Medicine: Dialogue and Discourse in Clinical Practice*. London: BMJ Books, 1998.

59. Greenhalgh T: Narrative based medicine: narrative based medicine in an evidence based world. *BMJ*. 1999;318(7179):323–325.

60. Launer J: *Narrative-Based Primary Care: A Practical Guide*. Oxford: Radcliffe Medical Press, 2002.

61. Liben S, Chin K, Boudreau JD, Boillat M, Steinert Y: Assessing a faculty development workshop in narrative medicine. *Medical Teacher*. 1 December 2012;34(12):e813–e819.

62. Remein CD, Childs E, Pasco JC, et al.: Content and outcomes of narrative medicine programmes: a systematic review of the literature through 2019. *BMJ Open*. 2020;10:e031568. https://doi.org/10.1136/bmjopen-2019-031568.

63. Milota MM, van Thiel GJMW, van Delden JJ: Narrative medicine as a medical education tool: a systematic review. *Medical Teacher*. 2019;41(7):802–810.

64. Reis S, Hermoni D, Livingstone P, Borkan J: Integrated narrative and evidence based case report: case report of paroxysmal atrial fibrillation and anticoagulation. *BMJ*. 11 November 2002;325(7371):1018.

65. Bayoumi AM, Kopplin PA: The storied case history. *CMAJ*. 2004;171(6):569–570.

66. Ankeny R: Chapter 6 in knowing and acting in medicine. In: Robyn Bluhm (Editor): *The Role of Patient Perspectives in Clinical Case Reporting*. London; New York: Rowman & Littlefield, 2017.

67. Saigle V, Miller J, Dumez V, Patrick K: Embedding patient voices in CMAJ. *CMAJ*. 12 July 2021;193(27):E1046–E1047.

68. Haber RJ, Lingard L: Learning oral presentation skills: a rhetorical analysis with pedagogical and professional implications. *Journal of General Internal Medicine*. 2001;16(5):309–314.

69. Wulff HR, Andur S, Rosenberg R: *Philosophy of Medicine: An Introduction*. Oxford: Blackwell Scientific Publications, 1986: 132.

70. McWhinney IR: An acquaintance with particulars . . . *Family Medicine*. 1989;21(4):296–298.

71. McWhinney IR: Beyond diagnosis: an approach to the integration of behavioural science and clinical medicine. *New England Journal of Medicine*. 1972;287(8):384–387.

72. McCabe M, You E, Tatangelo G: Hearing their voice: a systematic review of dementia family caregivers' needs. *Gerontologist*. 1 October 2016;56(5):e70–e88.

73. Styron W: *Darkness Visible*. New York, NY: Random House, 1990.

74. Mukand J: *Vital Lines: Contemporary Fiction about Medicine*. New York, NY: St. Matin's Press, 1990.

75. Cousins N: *Anatomy of an Illness as Perceived by the Patient*. New York, NY: WW Norton, 1979.

76. Broyard A: *Intoxicated by My Illness: And Other Writings on Life and Death*. New York, NY: Clarkson Potter Publishers, 1992.

77. Frank A: *At the Will of the Body: Reflections on Illness*. Boston, MA: Houghton, Mifflin, 1991.

78. Heshusius L: *Inside Chronic Pain – An Intimate and Critical Account*. Ithaca, NY: Cornell University Press, 2009.

79. Carel H: *Illness: The Cry of the Flesh*. Stocksfield, UK: Acumen Publishing, 2008.

80. Stein M: *The Lonely Patient: How We Experience Illness*. New York, NY: HarperCollins, 2007.

81. Atkins CGK: *My Imaginary Illness: A Journey into Uncertainty and Prejudice in Medical Diagnosis*. Ithica, NY: Cornell University Press, 2010.

82. Hadas R: *Strange Relation – A Memoir of Marriage, Dementia and Poetry*. Philadelphia, PA: Paul Dry Books, 2011.

83. Alexander M, Lenahan P, Pavlov A (Editors): *Cinemeducation: Using Film and Other Visual Media in Graduate and Medical Education*, volume 2. London: Radcliffe Publishing, 2012.

84. https://blog.feedspot.com/chronic_illness_blogs/.

85. Kim S: Content analysis of cancer blog posts. *Journal of the Medical Library Association*. 2009;97(4):260–266.

86. McWhirter L, Ritchie C, Stone J, Carson A: Functional cognitive disorders: a systematic review. *Lancet Psychiatry*. 1 February 2020;7(2):191–207.

87. Cabreira V, McWhirter L, Carson A: Functional cognitive disorder: diagnosis, treatment, and differentiation from secondary causes of cognitive difficulties. *Neurologic Clinics*, 15 March 2023.

88. Peritogiannis V, Zafiris S, Pappas D, Mavreas V: Conversion pseudodementia in the elderly: a review of the literature with case presentation. *Psychogeriatrics*. March 2008;8(1):24–31.

89. Wiels W, Baeken C, Engelborghs S: Depressive symptoms in the elderly – an early symptom of dementia? A systematic review. *Frontiers in Pharmacology*. 7 February 2020;11:34.

90. Micchia K, Formica C, De Salvo S, Muscarà N, Bramanti P, Caminiti F, Marino S, Corallo F: Normal pressure hydrocephalus: neurophysiological and neuropsychological aspects: a narrative review. *Medicine*. 3 March 2022;101(9).

91. Conn HO: Normal pressure hydrocephalus (NPH): more about NPH by a physician who is the patient. *Clinical Medicine (London)*. April 2011;11(2):162–165. https://doi.org/10.7861/clinmedicine.11-2-162.

92. Iseki C, Takahashi Y, Wada M, Kawanami T, Adachi M, Kato T: Incidence of idiopathic normal pressure hydrocephalus (iNPH): a 10-year follow-up study of a rural community in Japan. *Journal of the Neurological Sciences*. 15 April 2014;339(1–2):108–112.

93. Mitchell KA, Zelko I, Shay T, Horen S, Williams A, Luciano M, Huang J, Brem H, Gordon CR: The impact of hydrocephalus shunt devices on quality of life. *Journal of Craniofacial Surgery*. 1 July 2021;32(5):1746–1750.

94. Grasso G, Torregrossa F: The impact of cerebrospinal fluid shunting on quality of life in idiopathic normal pressure hydrocephalus: a long-term analysis. *Neurosurgical Focus*. 1 April 2023;54(4):E7.

95. www.hydroassoc.org/voices-from-our-community-milton-newman-shares-his-story-of-nph/.

96. Fraser SW, Greenhalgh T: Coping with complexity: educating for capability. *BMJ*. 2001;323:799. https://doi.org/10.1136/bmj.323.7316.799.

97. Morris BAP: Case reports: boon or bane? In: Norton PG et al. (Editors): *Primary Care Research: Traditional and Innovative Approaches*. Newbury Park, CA: Sage Publications, 1991.

PART FIVE

Research on Patient-Centered Care

INTRODUCTION

MOIRA STEWART

The four chapters in this part of the book present reviews of research literature and descriptions of relevant measures. The role of Chapters 14 and 15 is to help clinicians and teachers learn about the value of the patient-centered clinical method. Chapter 14 explores the nature and experience of patient-centered care through qualitative and mixed methods studies. Chapter 15 reviews recent trials of patient-centered innovations and their impact on both clinician wellness (and burnout) and patient self-reported outcomes. Chapter 16 presents the measure of patient perception of patient-centeredness. Chapter 17 displays the observation measure of patient-centered consultations. These two measures have been requested over 200 times from 25 countries and have been translated into eight languages.

DOI: 10.1201/9781003394679-18

14

Using Qualitative Methodologies and Mixed Methods Approaches to Illuminate Patient-Centered Care

JUDITH BELLE BROWN AND BRIDGET L RYAN

In this chapter, we examine evidence gleaned from select studies using a qualitative or a mixed methods approach, which demonstrate the universality of the patient-centered clinical method as well as illuminate one or more of the interactive components of the patient-centered clinical method.

Qualitative research explores the nature and experience of being human, eliciting in-depth descriptions or holistic interpretations to enhance understanding. In qualitative inquiry, the researcher and research participant together strive to capture the motives, meanings, and expectations of participants to construct the interpretation of their subjective experience. By describing a participant's unique experience, qualitative research helps attain a deeper and richer understanding of patients' challenges and helps clinicians be more sensitive and compassionate in their delivery of patient-centered care. Qualitative research can elucidate our understanding of phenomena for which we have limited knowledge and can give voice to the silenced, empowering them to share their stories. Qualitative research can help unravel complex and conflicting perspectives on a problem or situation. Qualitative inquiry can stimulate a quantitative research question or alternatively provide explanation of quantitative results. Methodological approaches using qualitative inquiry include ethnography, grounded theory, and phenomenology.[1, 2] Rich accounts of patient stories can be captured through the use of in-depth interviews, focus groups, or application of the case method approach.

Mixed methods research is recognized as a distinct research approach where both qualitative and quantitative processes and procedures are combined to examine the topic under inquiry.[3] A fundamental assumption is that combining and integrating these two methodological approaches offers an opportunity to elucidate more fully a complex topic. Mixed methods designs vary (e.g. convergent parallel, explanatory sequential, exploratory sequential) and are chosen based on what approach will be most effective in answering the research question.[3] Mixed methods studies are rapidly becoming a standard approach in primary care and health services research as this process aligns well with the complex and multifaceted problems challenging

DOI: 10.1201/9781003394679-19

researchers today. Indeed, mixed methods approaches are well suited to provide evidence elucidating the patient-centered clinical method.

Two mixed methods studies provide research evidence that supports the universality of the patient-centered clinical method. There have been questions as to whether there is a universal desire by patients for patient-centered care or whether this varies by person and/or region. A mixed methods study by Turner and Archer[4] employed questionnaires and subsequent semistructured qualitative interviews to explore whether communication skills that they characterized as "mostly based on Western (European and American) models of empathy"[4] were culturally appropriate in the complex context of South Africa. Of the 14 items that covered technical and interpersonal aspects of the patient–clinician interaction, over 70% of respondents identified 10 of the items as important; the importance of these items was also supported by the findings from the study's qualitative interviews. Items valued by patients that are consistent with the patient-centered clinical method included "The doctor listens to what I say without interrupting" (Component 1: Exploring Health, Disease, and the Illness Experience); "The doctor is interested in my feelings and worries" (Component 2: Understanding the Whole Person); "The doctor includes me in decision-making" (Component 3: Finding Common Ground); and "The doctor tries to make me feel comfortable" (Component 4: Enhancing the Patient–Clinician Relationship).[4] These findings echo those of Little et al. in 2001 that found the vast majority of survey respondents in the United Kingdom wanted their general practitioner to provide patient-centered care that included items such as "Be friendly and approachable"; "Listen to everything I have to say about my problem"; and "Discuss and agree with me on treatment".[5]

Mixed methods research by Zulman et al. has been used to elaborate practices that promote physician presence, described by the authors as a state of awareness, focus, and attention with the intent of understanding patients.[6] This study derived preliminary practices from a systematic review, followed by qualitative interviews with physicians, patients, and non-medical professionals whose occupations involved intense interpersonal interactions such as firefighters, chaplains, and social workers.[6] They next conducted a Delphi process by a panel of researchers, clinicians, patients, caregivers, and health system leaders. The result of this research was five practice recommendations: 1) prepare with intention; 2) listen intently and completely; 3) agree on what matters most; 4) connect with the patient's story; and 5) explore emotional cues. Recommendation 2 is part of the overall patient-centered clinical method while recommendations 3, 4, and 5 map respectively to Component 3: Finding Common Ground; Component 2: Understanding the Whole Person; and to exploring patients' feelings as part of Component 1: Exploring Health, Disease, and the Illness Experience. This mixed methods research supports the universality of the importance of patient-centered care to both patients and clinicians.

EXPLORING THE PATIENT'S HEALTH, DISEASE, AND ILLNESS EXPERIENCE

Qualitative methodologies and mixed methods approaches are helpful in gaining a greater understanding of the needs and expectations of patients. The combination of qualitative and quantitative inquiry is useful for making sense of patients' illness experiences, as it gives primacy to patients' voices, to listening for meaning as well as facts, and to providing illumination of patients' stories.

The importance of focusing on patients' voices is illustrated well in a descriptive qualitative study exploring patients' emotions regarding the risk of hypoglycemia in managing their diabetes.[7] A thematic analysis of the 16 interviews revealed that patients' emotions included fear, anxiety, and frustration but also confidence and hope. With time and experience, patients could find confidence to manage their diabetes and mitigate hypoglycemia risk. The role of hope was seen as a way of tempering feelings of fear and anxiety. This research encourages clinicians to explore the complexity of patients' emotions as a first step in helping them manage their illnesses.

Qualitative and mixed methods approaches also can illuminate the concerns and experiences of both patients and clinicians and the situations in which they find it difficult to discuss the illness experience. Nowhere is this more important than when patients are reluctant to raise sensitive topics with their clinicians. A descriptive qualitative study exploring patients' perspectives on the role of primary care in obesity management found patients had clear expectations that their primary healthcare clinicians initiate discussion about weight concerns.[8] Some patients reported being at ease discussing weight and indicated that their family physician had responded to their needs and concerns. However, other patients indicated their family physicians never raised weight with them. Patients attributed this to a lack of time or their family physician ignoring the issue or not taking it seriously.

In a mixed methods needs assessment study by Filipetto et al. exploring patient perspectives on overactive bladder, participants indicated in qualitative interviews that they would prefer their provider initiate discussion about urinary symptoms because the patients found it embarrassing to raise the subject themselves.[9] This was congruent with the quantitative findings where only 42% of patients raised the issue of urinary or bladder symptoms themselves. Despite the preference by patients that providers take the lead in this discussion, only 14% of participants indicated that their physician asked about these symptoms. The study concluded that this reluctance by patients leads to delays in seeking care on average 3 to 5 years and results in unidentified and untreated symptoms.

Webb et al. tackled the reluctance of young people 14 to 25 years old to seek health care for mental health and lifestyle behavior issues.[10] They conducted a mixed methods implementation study with the goal of determining whether a health and lifestyle-screening app, *Check Up GP*, increased patient-centeredness and the likelihood of young peoples' disclosures of sensitive issues. The study's quantitative survey results found participants that used *Check Up GP* reported significantly greater disclosure of sensitive issues than the group that did not. The qualitative interviews elaborated that participants found *Check Up GP* created scope to address unmet health needs and increased the participants' sense of being prepared. Interventions such as *Check Up GP* can extend the ability of clinicians to explore patients' disease and illness experience by giving patients the space and time to comfortably disclose issues that are difficult for them to raise.

Findings from these three examples[8-10] underscore the significance of using patient-centered care to elicit the needs and expectations of people who struggle with sharing difficult concerns with their clinicians including patients' preferences for clinicians to raise potentially sensitive and contentious issues.[8, 9]

It is not only patients who are reluctant to raise difficult issues; clinicians too can find this challenging. A qualitative study by Siu explored the experiences of primary care doctors in Hong Kong regarding providing treatment for overactive bladder.[11] The authors noted that urinary problems can be considered embarrassing in Chinese culture for both patients and their doctors. Doctors sometimes avoided asking important questions needed to ascertain a diagnosis because of concern about offending or embarrassing a patient.

A study by Gewirtz-Meydan et al. interviewed physicians from different medical specialities about their perspectives on sexuality later in life.[12] They found that physicians tended to take a more biomedical approach to discussing sexual dysfunction in older adults, assuming sexual issues have a medical cause rather than, as with younger people, exploring the illness experience of sexual dysfunction. While there may be underlying physical issues in older adults, the study highlighted the need for physicians to explore their assumptions about sexuality in older patients.

Clinicians can be especially reluctant to raise potentially contentious issues that might harm the patient–clinician relationship. One such issue that clinicians worry will push patients away is discussing fitness to drive, as found in a multi-perspective qualitative study by Sinnott et al.[13] These conversations sometimes arose because of concerns about cognition and, in these cases, GPs talked about giving patients a "heads up" when cognitive problems first arose, signalling to their patients that, down the road, they may need to surrender their license. Alternately, when fitness to drive arose as a result of a patient's request for an urgent driving license medical report, GPs that had not had previous conversations with their patients described strong patient reactions including being very angry or unhappy. GPs discussed strategies they use to mitigate patients' displeasure including echoing patients' own assessments of their driving such as deciding to limit their driving to daytime or familiar locations. Still other GPs used standardized cognitive tests or national guidelines to remove the personal affect from their discussions in an effort to protect their relationship with their patients.

Clinicians as well as patients are affected by what society sees as stigmatized or contentious issues. Both can make assumptions about the other's comfort to discuss these issues. Having the courage to raise these issues with patients and asking patients about their interest in discussing these issues normalizes the topic for patients. Eliciting patient's health, disease, and illness experiences – especially concerning difficult topics – does not need to happen during one visit but can be addressed over a series of visits within a positive longitudinal patient–clinician relationship. The issue of spirituality is another area that clinicians and patients may be reluctant to discuss; more on this topic occurs in the next section of this chapter, on the component of understanding the whole person.

The research reviewed in this section demonstrates that using qualitative and mixed methods approaches yields rich understanding of the complex relationships between patients and clinicians that can affect the ability to elicit the health, disease, and illness experience.

BOX 14.1: Patients' Voices – Quotes from Select Papers

COMPONENT 1: EXPLORING HEALTH, DISEASE, AND THE ILLNESS EXPERIENCE

"I think a concerned family physician should always talk to you about your weight management, but not denigrate or harass you about it. Because you've achieved this for some reason . . . You won't change it by medicine, you'll change it by attitude and lifestyle".[8] (p. 4)

COMPONENT 2: UNDERSTANDING THE WHOLE PERSON

"I have a good relationship with my doctor because he's Samoan. He understands me and I understand him when we use Samoan language".[17] (p. 38)

COMPONENT 3: FINDING COMMON GROUND

"I simply don't have the knowledge. I just have to assume – and want to assume – that they have my best interests at heart".[25] (p. 6)

COMPONENT 3: FINDING COMMON GROUND

"If you leave the doctor's office and you feel like he wasn't paying attention, you're going to be wary to come back".[23 (p. 4)]

COMPONENT 4: ENHANCING THE PATIENT–CLINICIAN RELATIONSHIP

"They just seem to listen . . . you can go in and open up to them . . . I can just come in here and cry, and the doctor listens, and you can let it all out".[32 (p. 1060)]

TEAMS – PATIENT

"The nurse got together a dietitian, my family doctor, a social worker, a psychiatrist, a pharmacist – a whole bunch of people together . . . We had a video here [at my home], a conversation and just so everybody was on the same page with what I was doing. It was really good".[38 (p. E324)]

UNDERSTANDING THE PATIENT AS A WHOLE PERSON

Understanding the patient as a whole person invites the application of qualitative research methodologies to elicit a more in-depth picture of the larger life context. Insights acquired through qualitative and mixed methods investigations not only add to the practitioner's understanding of the specific individuals who have participated in the study, but also have the potential to be applicable in achieving a richer and deeper understanding of other patients who may share similar life contexts.

In Chapter 4, we gave consideration to the role of spirituality on patients' experiences of illness and suffering from both the patients' and clinicians' perspectives. The usefulness of qualitative findings in understanding aspects of the whole person such as spirituality is demonstrated in a qualitative literature review by Appleby, Wilson and Swinton.[14] The authors identified four categories of response by family physicians to discussing their patients' spirituality: 1) embracing – physicians who endorse the important role they play in exploring patients' spirituality in relation to their overall health; 2) pragmatic – physicians who support examining spirituality with patients who express this desire; 3) guarded – physicians who are reluctant to delve into patients' spirituality and would only do so in specific circumstances; and 4) rejecting – physicians who do not view exploration of patients' spirituality as their responsibility under any circumstance. They suggest that the extent of clinicians adopting a patient-centered approach may influence their inclination to explore patients' spirituality in relation to their illness experience. This study provides important evidence on the spiritual aspect of understanding the whole person.

Pivotal to understanding the whole person is an awareness and understanding of patients' contexts, as described in Chapter 5. The following four studies examined challenges in the delivery of patient-centered care posed by the social determinants of health (SDoH), which have long been recognized as influencing patient health. A descriptive qualitative study by Brown et al. explored the perceptions and experiences of 20 primary healthcare practitioners (family physicians, endocrinologists, nurses, dieticians, and pharmacists) regarding the impact of the SDoH on their patients with type 1 and type 2 diabetes mellitus.[15] The participants articulated two major challenges in managing their patients' hypoglycemia: socioeconomic issues (occupation type and poverty) and psychosocial issues (stage in the life cycle such as being elderly, social isolation, and mental health). This study emphasizes the need to understand the whole person in the management of a serious condition.

Another study, by Braillard et al., using a grounded theory approach revealed how the 20 family physician participants frequently felt powerlessness and frustrated in caring for patients with multimorbidity.[16] This was often due to not only the time required in managing patients' complex chronic conditions but due to being overwhelmed by the multitude of socioeconomic factors impacting the context of their patients such as financial security, cultural factors, and literacy.

Similarly, patients can experience a profound sense of powerlessness and frustration as illuminated in the Sheridan et al. qualitative descriptive study.[17] The 42 participants were older adults with multimorbidity whose residence was in the lowest socioeconomic quintile in their urban community. Most were from minority ethnic groups. While they strived to engage meaningfully with their primary care clinicians, they often felt invisible and "not heard or disregarded".[17] This lack of attention to who they were as a person and to their life context eroded their trust and hopes of "being truly understood".[17] Findings from these two studies elucidate how both patients and clinicians suffer unnecessarily when there is a failure in understanding the whole person.

In a descriptive qualitative study, Brown et al. interviewed 48 participants including physicians (e.g. psychiatry, internal medicine, family medicine), allied healthcare professionals (e.g. social work, nursing, pharmacy), and decision makers.[18] The objective of the study was to explore their experiences of caring for vulnerable patients with multimorbidity through a patient-centered interprofessional team approach. The findings revealed how social determinants of health such as homelessness and poverty often exacerbated the patients' mental and physical health requiring the team to embrace whole person care that was individualized to the unique needs of each patient. In addition, participants highlighted the importance of cultural sensitivity in addressing the multiple challenges facing these vulnerable patients with multimorbidity.

Homelessness is a global crisis that continues to increase. In a mixed methods study using an explanatory sequential design conducted in France by Jego et al., the objective was to better understand how general practitioners (GP) could provide care to homeless people.[19] Phase 1 was qualitative and explored the difficulties participants encountered in caring for homeless people. From the 19 GP interviews, three main areas were identified: (1) personal obstacles ranging from administrative issues (e.g. time, money) to the emotional toll of caring for this population; (2) care management, which was viewed as complex and particularly difficult with regard to follow up; and (3) overcoming the stigma associated with being homeless. These findings were used to create a survey, which was administered to a random sample of 150 GPs in phase 2 of the study. The questionnaire explored basic demographics and their exposure to homeless people as well as their knowledge and types of challenges in caring for this population. The response rate was 73%. The results showed that the majority of respondents had rarely seen a homeless person in their office and, of those who did, most of the patients were experiencing "moderate homelessness" defined as insecure or inadequate housing. Only 6.1% had received any training on assessing a person's "precariousness" and even fewer (1.2%) were knowledgeable about measures to screen for precariousness or access to community services for homeless people. The key difficulties identified by the survey respondents in caring for homeless people were social management, retrieving medical information, patient compliance, loneliness in practice, and the time required to care for this population. In phase 3 of the study, 14 GPs from the survey sample were recruited to participate in an open-ended interview. Their exposure and care of homeless people ranged from never to an active engagement with this population. The analysis revealed the core condition required for GPs to care effectively for homeless people was stable follow up achieved through the establishment of trusting patient–doctor relationships in which life context and patient priorities were met with non-judgmental acceptance.

Understanding the whole person is multifaceted and complex. These studies represent just a few aspects of the person (e.g. spirituality) and their context such as socioeconomic factors (e.g. financial insecurity) and social determinants of health (e.g. poverty and homelessness), which are more fully elaborated in Chapters 4 and 5.

FINDING COMMON GROUND

Finding common ground with patients presents many challenges and opportunities. Patients' perspectives on participation in all components of the healthcare process vary greatly in both the extent to which they wish to participate and how they wish to participate.[20] Qualitative research, combined with mixed methods approaches, can elicit insights into factors that achieve or impede finding common ground. The seven studies reviewed in this section illustrate that eliciting patients' values and preferences explicitly, understanding patients' individual and broader societal contexts, and incorporating patient-centered communication principles into patient–clinician interactions are essential components to finding common ground with patients around the management of their health.

A mixed methods study by Cohen-Stavi et al. employed focus groups and concept mapping with 11 nurses who provided care for 204 patients at primary clinics to identify reasons why nurses' care deviated from clinical practice guidelines for patients with multimorbidity.[21] Three broad categories of reasons (as a percentage of all reasons) were biomedical (35.3%), patient preferences and characteristics (30.4%), system context (18.3%), and unknown (16.4%). The most frequent *patient preferences and characteristics* reason was that the patient was not interested; other reasons included finding the guideline a burden, having no time, and lacking support. With patient factors being almost as common as biomedical factors, this study concludes that, for patients with multimorbidity, "patient-centered aspects are as much a part of care decisions as biomedical aspects".[21]

Consistent with the Cohen-Stavi et al. study,[21] research by Mangin et al. with patients and families concerning how their preferences are considered in medication-related discussions found that participants experienced a shared decision-making (SDM) approach when clinicians recognized the expertise of the patients and families.[22] Sixteen participants from three focus groups described expertise in two ways: as having lived experiences with chronic conditions and medications and as having sought out information on their own regarding medication management. Participants acknowledged that system issues including time limitations, coordination and communication across clinicians, and the culture of the healthcare system impact SDM. This study highlights that in order to find common ground it is necessary to understand the whole person as both an individual with lived experience and expertise, as well as an individual that manages their health within the broader context of the healthcare system.

A mixed methods study that examined SDM from the perspective of Black American patients with type 2 diabetes provides further evidence of the need to understand patients' perspectives and context as part of finding common ground concerning management.[23] Analysis of data from 32 qualitative patient interviews resulted in four main themes. First, patients wanted humanistic communication that showed empathy and built rapport. Participants indicated that using ice-breaking gestures, such as shaking hands and humor, humanized interactions. The second theme was clinicians' understanding that often patients wanted family members involved in making decisions. Third, participants felt that they did not always receive the information they needed to make care decisions. Fourth, participants commonly reported mistrust of clinicians, especially when participants reported clinicians using "autopilot communication".[23] Participants also completed the 9-item Shared Decision Making Questionnaire (SDM-Q-9). While SDM-Q-9 scores demonstrated high levels of SDM, a deeper look found lower mean scores for three questions that concerned being told about different treatment options, being asked about treatment preferences, and having their doctor weigh the treatment options with them. While discussing treatment options and preferences is essential in every patient–clinician relationship, it can be particularly important for patients from racial and ethnic minorities, and for those who have had reason to mistrust the healthcare system where the patient–clinician power imbalance can be especially problematic.

The importance of eliciting and understanding patients' values and preferences was further explored in a qualitative study of clinicians' practices and perceived barriers concerning SDM for lung cancer screening.[24] This study consisted of interviews with 24 clinicians from different healthcare specialties concerning the importance of patient values in screening decisions. All clinicians agreed the goal of SDM was to ensure that screening was congruent with patients' values; however, none indicated they asked about patients' values explicitly.[24] Rather, they depended on their past experiences with patients to guide their communication; many suggested they could usually predict how patients would respond to being offered screening. While clinicians indicated they made it clear in conversations with patients that the decision was the patient's to make, clinicians found that some patients "don't want a choice", and many are looking for a recommendation from their clinician.[24] While providing information and respecting patient choice are important components of finding common ground, it is equally important to explore what patients value and what they need from their clinicians to arrive at a decision. Sometimes, as clinicians noted, this requires providing recommendations to patients and understanding the limits of patients' tolerance for receiving and interpreting complex medical information.

An intervention study by Savelberg et al. aimed to understand the gap between the intention of clinicians to engage in SDM and the clinicians' actual use of SDM.[25] An SDM intervention for clinicians caring for patients with early-stage breast cancer was provided to breast cancer care team members. Within this study, 20 qualitative interviews determined the degree to which patients found their clinicians followed SDM protocols. Patients indicated that they received a lot of information about treatment choices; most viewed this positively, but the volume of information overwhelmed some. Patients believed for the most part that they were made aware of the two treatment options appropriate for their diagnosis and that they were provided with the pros and cons of each. In most cases what patients found lacking was being asked about their own preferences and their own values regarding treatment, with a few patients expressing fear that they lacked the knowledge to make this important decision. Regardless of their preferences not being sought, patients felt that, in the end, they made their own decision about treatment. Consistent with Melzer et al.,[24] this study illustrates that finding common ground requires patients' preferences and values be elicited and heard and that patients do not always feel equipped to share fully in decision-making about treatments.

Finding common ground on treatment can be especially difficult when the treatment is viewed differently by clinicians and their patients. An example is the arena of pain medication prescribing where patients are concerned about pain relief; whereas, clinicians are balancing weaning the medication versus dependence on opioids.[26] In a mixed methods study by Esquibel and Borkan, the authors found that in treating chronic non-cancer pain the ability to find common ground was related to the existence of a collaborative or conflictual patient–doctor relationship.[26] In the former, an effort was made to transition from focusing on pain relief to understanding the patients' perspectives and goals. This included understanding the patient as a person and the contextual issues that exacerbate or ameliorate their pain. By engaging in this dialogue within the safety of a trusting and respectful patient–doctor relationship, an adversarial stance can be avoided.

It can be seen from each study reviewed in this section that it is essential to bring together all components of the patient-centered clinical method, demonstrating the interconnectedness and dynamic interaction amongst the four components in order to find common ground.

BOX 14.2: Providers' Voices – Quotes from Selected Papers

COMPONENT 1: EXPLORING HEALTH, DISEASE, AND THE ILLNESS EXPERIENCE

"With younger adults, I expect to see sexual dysfunctions that are more psychological, whereas with older adults I assume the sexual dysfunctions are more of a mechanical dysfunction, and not performance anxiety or other psychological disturbances".[12 (p. 5)]

COMPONENT 2: UNDERSTANDING THE WHOLE PERSON

"With chronic patients, you need to see further than guidelines, see patient's resources, understand his story, see how he lives with his illness. . . . There are many facets you can't set aside".[16 (p. 5)]

COMPONENT 4: ENHANCING THE PATIENT–CLINICIAN RELATIONSHIP

"That meaningful relationship is a protective factor against burnout. You get a sense of satisfaction in what you do. You're helping someone, but also helping yourself in some way because joy is contagious. . . . That's the reason we do this. Because we want to care for people".[30 (p. 720)]

TEAMS – PROVIDER

"In cooperation with the district nursing service, we get a much better understanding of what the most profound problems are for a patient in a home situation. Sometimes this is not necessarily pain or shortness of breath, but for example, no good contact with the children anymore or loneliness or no daytime activities at all, or that the house is neglected. And that way you can take a much broader look at what that patient needs".[36 (p. 9)]

ENHANCING THE PATIENT–CLINICIAN RELATIONSHIP

As described in Chapter 7, the patient–clinician relationship constitutes the bedrock on which all care transpires. For this reason, research that uncovers the essence of the complex interactions that occur between patients and clinicians is foundational to building the theory and practice of patient-centered care. Greater in-depth understanding of the attributes of therapeutic relationships, how power is expressed in patient–clinician relationships, how caring and healing transpire, and ways of being in relationships with patients may do much to enhance the self-awareness and practice expertise of clinicians, thereby enhancing patient-centered care.

Polypharmacy in community-dwelling older patients is ubiquitous and a constant concern for primary care clinicians. Reeve, Low and Hilmer in their qualitative study conducted four focus groups with 14 older adults and 14 carers to explore their perspectives on the deprescribing of medications.[27] The participants' inclination to engage in the deprescribing process was influenced by their own personal views and beliefs about medication taking and the outcomes of withdrawal. Of equal importance was the relationship with their family physicians who they relied on for expert guidance in the prescribing and deprescribing process. The patient–clinician relationship was characterized by mutual respect and trust in the ability of doctors to take their patients' needs and preferences into consideration. In addition, finding common ground in the decisions to deprescribe was influenced by the clinicians providing information to the patients that was understandable and informed their decision-making. This study lends further evidence to the connectedness of the components of finding common ground and enhancing the patient–clinician relationship.

Using a phenomenological approach Hamilton et al., explored the lived experiences of 19 adults with chronic non-cancer pain who had been on long-term opioid therapy and specifically their perspectives on the opioid deprescribing process.[28] While they faced many barriers in deprescribing, many of which were physical, a major support articulated by the participants was a trusting relationship with their family doctors. They described how their doctors were both caring and compassionate – never abandoning them to struggle alone with their physical or emotional pain. Conversely, some participants felt judged by their family doctors while in the deprescribing process and felt desperate for education and support. This study highlights the critical role of patient–doctor relationship as we continue to battle the opioid crisis.

The phenomenological study by Woolhouse et al. explicates the sometimes-overwhelming emotional challenges faced by clinicians in their attempt to care for severely disadvantaged populations, which, in this research, were homeless women using illicit drugs, often supported by sex trade work.[29] Their findings reveal both the joys and the sorrows experienced by the physician participants in the care of this marginalized population. In order to sustain their efforts and commitment to these women, participants describe how they alter their expectations of care and engagement with this specific population and rely heavily on the support of team members. The emotional energy expended in the care of vulnerable populations is important to consider when emotional fatigue can severely affect clinicians and ultimately the patient-clinician relationship.

At a time when primary care is under siege and the burnout rate of primary care clinicians is at an all-time high, illuminating strategies to mitigate this crisis is paramount. A qualitative study using a phenomenological approach provides some answers. Hiefner et al. interviewed 20 family physicians to understand their experience of meaningful relationships with their patients and in turn what elements of these relationships offered "protection" from burnout.[30] The analysis identified a trusting patient–doctor relationship as the central element, which was enhanced by elements of providing patient-centered care leading to effective care and building continuity. Together these four elements of meaningful relationships supported the participants in forming connections with their patients and making a difference in their lives – a central reason for becoming a physician. All the participants endorsed how meaningful relationships provided protection against burnout. However, some noted how this deep caring for their patients could come at a cost as they battled major faults in the healthcare system that often intensified their patients' suffering.

In another phenomenological study by Uygur, Brown and Herbert, in-depth interviews were conducted with 22 family physicians exploring their experiences and capacity for compassion.[31] Study findings identified three interrelated concepts which were titled the Compassion

Trichotomy: motivation for compassion, capacity for compassion, and the patient–doctor relationship offering a connection point for compassion. While the authors did not focus specifically on the relationship between compassion and burnout, they did describe a "virtuous cycle".[31]

The desire to connect with their doctors within the context of a caring relationship is also expressed by patients and is supported by the following four qualitative studies. In their phenomenological study, Gillespie et al. interviewed 10 patients to explore their experience of caring. Key to "genuine caring" was the doctor's ability to listen carefully and provide the opportunity for patients to express safely their emotions.[32] Patients experienced this as respecting their individuality and being fully engaged in a therapeutic patient–doctor relationship. Similarly, the 25 patients interviewed in Murphy's and Salisbury's descriptive qualitative study emphasized the importance of feeling listened to by their doctors as well as receiving trust and respect.[33] This study was conducted through the lens of relational continuity and how clinicians' attributes, as noted earlier, can promote or breach relational continuity.

In a mixed methods convergent study, using a vignette-based survey approach and in-depth interviews, patients articulated the importance of a trusting patient–doctor relationship in the de-implementation of low value care (LVC) such as LVC-antibiotics, LVC-EKG, or a screening test for vitamin D deficiency.[34] Participants also emphasized the longitudinality of the patient–doctor relationship characterized by a physician who attentively listened, took time with the patient, and provided clear and understandable information. A valuable finding of this study was how reducing LVC could empower patients to assume increased responsibility for their own health.

In another mixed methods study using a convergent approach, patients described the qualities or actions expressed by their family physician that promoted trust in the patient–doctor relationship – expressions of empathy, clarity of information, and careful attention to the patients' problem.[35] Again, the latter two attributes demonstrate the interconnectedness of the patient–doctor relationship and finding common ground.

TEAM-CENTERED CARE IN PROVIDING PATIENT-CENTERED CARE

The final three studies described in this chapter are relevant to Chapter 8 on team-centered care, as they reveal the benefits of interdisciplinary teamwork in the provision of patient-centered care.

In a mixed methods study, Kuiper, Nieboer and Cramm examined how a patient-centered care (PCC) improvement program can enhance the delivery of primary care for patients with multimorbidity.[36] The qualitative arm of the study consisted of interviews with nine healthcare professionals (four general practitioners and five nurse practitioners) from seven practice sites affiliated with the PCC improvement program. In the interviews, participants were asked about each of the eight dimensions of patient-centered care included in the PCC improvement program. For the quantitative portion, a questionnaire was completed at baseline and at one year later by patients who had participated in the PCC improvement program in order to assess whether there was an association between patients' positive experiences and the program. In the qualitative findings, two themes spoke of the value of the team in patient-centered care. The first theme concerned *coordination of care within the GP practice*. Participants noted the need to move from working alone to a model of teamwork and acknowledged that they did not always know what their colleagues were doing for patients. Participants spoke about the importance of transfer of information with the team in order to best support patients. They also highlighted the need for team meetings in order to coordinate patient care. The second theme concerned *continuity and transition among healthcare disciplines.* In this theme, participants acknowledged the importance of multidisciplinary teamwork in strengthening continuity owing to the different aspects of care each discipline can address. Participants also indicated the importance of the transfer of information across healthcare settings, not just within the GP practice. The importance of physical proximity was raised as a facilitator of efficient patient-centered care. In the patient survey results, of the two teamwork aspects of patient-centered care, there was a statistically significant improvement from baseline to one-year post-intervention for continuity and transitions but not for coordination of care.

A qualitative grounded theory study by Brown et al. that interviewed 110 participants from 20 family health teams examined four processes of team functioning: providing patient-centered care; working to provide timely access to care; providing continuity of care within the family health team; and coordinating care (for example, for patients discharged from hospital).[37] The findings from this study illuminated how a shared goal of patient-centered care brought together the other three processes within the team. These three processes in return improved the patient-centered care that the team provided. The interaction of these components is described by the authors, "For some participants, patient-centred care was more instrumental and included improved access and maintenance of continuity within the team setting. In addition, coordination and facilitation of transitions of care were not boilerplate but geared to patients' specific needs and preferences, which are hallmarks of patient-centered care. Other participants highlighted the patient-provider relationship, articulating a commitment to caring for the whole person not just the disease, which is a basic tenet of patient-centred care".[37]

In a mixed methods study, Stewart et al. used a pragmatic randomized trial and qualitative interviews to examine the effectiveness of a patient-centered intervention for patients with multimorbidity offered through an interdisciplinary team case conference.[38] There were 86 patients in the intervention group and 77 in the control group. There were no differences in outcomes between the two groups, with the exception that the case conference improved mental health status in a subgroup of patients with annual income of less than $50,000 (Canadian) and that more follow-up hours with participants after the case conference and more providers participating in the case conference were each associated with poorer outcomes. Five themes were identified in the qualitative data analysis of the interviews conducted with 14 intervention patients: 1) valuing the interdisciplinary nature of the teams in addressing their issues; 2) feeling supported by the team in meeting their goals; 3) appreciating the advice and follow up; 4) receiving new and helpful additions to their treatment regimen, e.g. physiotherapy; and 5) attributing improvements in their health to participating in the intervention, which included an improvement in their functional ability and feeling more positive and hopeful.

These three studies[36-38] describing how teams strive to provide patient-centered care serve as a bookend to the research presented at the beginning of this chapter on patients' universal desire for patient-centered care. Collectively, these studies support a shared goal by both patients and clinicians for patient-centered care.

CONCLUSION

Much progress has been made through the use of qualitative research and mixed methods approaches to investigate patient-centered care. However, many opportunities to further advance the theory and practice of patient-centered care exist. Some of the studies were conceived to address directly patient-centered practice while others lent support to the importance of the four patient-centered components.

To date, research primarily has explored either the clinicians' or the patients' perspectives, rather than the perspective of both partners in giving or receiving patient-centered care. More direct observation and more interpretive analysis of the two-way dyadic communication that transpires to create patient-centered care will be important in the future.

REFERENCES

1. Crabtree BF, Miller W: *Doing Qualitative Research*, 3rd edition. Thousand Oaks, CA: Sage Publications, 2023.
2. Liamputtong P: *Qualitative Research Methods*, 4th edition. Melbourne, Australia: Oxford University Press, 2013.
3. Creswell JW: *Research Design: Qualitative, Quantitative and Mixed Methods Approaches*, 4th edition. Thousand Oaks, CA: Sage Publications, 2014.
4. Turner RE, Archer E: Patient-centered care: the patients' perspective – a mixed-methods pilot study. *African Journal of Primary Health Care & Family Medicine*. 9 October 2020;12(1):e1–e8, 2, 4. https://doi.org/10.4102/phcfm.v12i1.2390.
5. Little P, Everitt H, Williamson I, et al.: Preferences of patients for patient-centered approach to consultations in primary care: an observational study. *BMJ*. 2001;322(7284):468–472, 3.
6. Zulman DM, Haverfield MC, Shaw JG, Brown-Johnson CG, Schwartz R, Tierney AA, Zionts DL, Safaeinili N, Fischer M, Thadaney Israni S, Asch SM, Verghese A: Practices to foster physician presence and connection with patients in the clinical encounter. *JAMA*. 7 January 2020;323(1):70–81. https://doi.org/10.1001/jama.2019.19003. Erratum in: *JAMA*. 17 March 2020;323(11):1098, 70.
7. Brown JB, Reichert SM, Valliere Y, Webster-Bogaert S, Ratzki-Leewing A, Ryan BL, Harris SB: Living with hypoglycemia: an exploration of patients' emotions: qualitative findings from the InHypo-DM study, Canada. *Diabetes Spectrum*. August 2019;32(3):270–276. https://doi.org/10.2337/ds18-0074.
8. Torti J, Luig T, Borowitz M, Johnson JA, Sharma AM, Campbell-Scherer DL: The 5As team patient study: patient perspectives on the role of primary care in obesity management. *BMC Family Practice*. 8 February 2017;18(1):19. https://doi.org/10.1186/s12875-017-0596-2. Erratum in: *BMC Family Practice*. 4 May 2017;18(1):58.
9. Filipetto FA, Fulda KG, Holthusen AE, McKeithen TM, McFadden P: The patient perspective on overactive bladder: a mixed-methods needs assessment. *BMC Family Practice*. 14 May 2014;15:96. https://doi.org/10.1186/1471-2296-15-96.
10. Webb MJ, Wadley G, Sanci LA: Improving patient-centered care for young people in general practice with a codesigned screening app: mixed methods study. *JMIR Mhealth and Uhealth*. 11 August 2017;5(8):e118. https://doi.org/10.2196/mhealth.7816.
11. Siu JY: Communicating with mismatch and tension: treatment provision experiences of primary care doctors treating patients with overactive bladder in Hong Kong. *BMC Family Practice*. 30 October 2015;16:160. https://doi.org/10.1186/s12875-015-0380-0.
12. Gewirtz-Meydan A, Levkovich I, Mock M, Gur U, Karkabi K, Ayalon L: Sex for seniors: how physicians discuss older adult's sexuality. *Israel Journal of Health Policy Research*. 21 February 2020;9(1):8. https://doi.org/10.1186/s13584-020-00366-5.
13. Sinnott C, Foley T, Horgan L, McLoughlin K, Sheehan C, Bradley C: Shifting gears versus sudden stops: qualitative study of consultations about driving in patients with cognitive impairment. *BMJ Open*. 21 August 2019;9(8):e024452. https://doi.org/10.1136/bmjopen-2018-024452.

14. Appleby A, Wilson P, Swinton J: Spiritual care in general practice: rushing in or fearing to tread? An integrative review of qualitative literature. *Journal of Religion and Health.* 2018;57:1108–1124.

15. Brown JB, Reichert SM, Valliere Y, Webster-Bogaert S, Ratzki-Leewing A, Harris SB: A qualitative enquiry of hypoglycemia and the social determinants of health: the InHypo-DM study, Canada. *Families, Systems, & Health.* December 2018;36(4):471–481. https://doi.org/10.1037/fsh0000355.

16. Braillard O, Slama-Chaudhry A, Joly C, Perone N, Beran D: The impact of chronic disease management on primary care doctors in Switzerland: a qualitative study. *BMC Family Practice.* 11 September 2018;19(1):159. https://doi.org/10.1186/s12875-018-0833-3.

17. Sheridan NF, Kenealy TW, Kidd JD, Schmidt-Busby JI, Hand JE, Raphael DL, McKillop AM, Rea HH: Patients' engagement in primary care: powerlessness and compounding jeopardy: a qualitative study. *Health Expectations.* February 2015;18(1):32–43, 38. https://doi.org/10.1111/hex.12006.

18. Brown JB, Reichert SM, Boeckxstaens P, Stewart M, Fortin M: Responding to vulnerable patients with multimorbidity: an interprofessional team approach. *BMC Primary Care.* 30 March 2022;23(1):62. https://doi.org/10.1186/s12875-022-01670-6.

19. Jego M, Grassineau D, Balique H, Loundou A, Sambuc R, Daguzan A, Gentile G, Gentile S: Improving access and continuity of care for homeless people: how could general practitioners effectively contribute? Results from a mixed study. *BMJ Open.* 30 November 2016;6(11):e013610. https://doi.org/10.1136/bmjopen-2016-013610.

20. Haidet P, Kroll TL, Sharf BF: The complexity of patient participation: lessons learned from patients' illness narratives. *Patient Education and Counseling.* 2006;62(3):323–329.

21. Cohen-Stavi CJ, Key C, Molcho T, Yacobi M, Balicer RD, Shadmi E: Mixed methods evaluation of reasons why care deviates from clinical guidelines among patients with multimorbidity. *Medical Care Research and Review.* February 2022;79(1):102–113, 102. https://doi.org/10.1177/1077558720975543.

22. Mangin D, Risdon C, Lamarche L, Langevin J, Ali A, Parascandalo J, Stephen G, Trimble J: "I think this medicine actually killed my wife": patient and family perspectives on shared decision-making to optimize medications and safety. *Therapeutic Advances in Drug Safety.* 5 April 2019;10:2042098619838796. https://doi.org/10.1177/2042098619838796.

23. Zisman-Ilani Y, Khaikin S, Savoy ML, Paranjape A, Rubin DJ, Jacob R, Wieringa TH, Suarez J, Liu J, Gardiner H, Bass SB, Montori VM, Siminoff LA: Disparities in shared decision-making research and practice: the case for black American patients. *Annals of Family Medicine.* 7 February 2023:2943, 3. https://doi.org/10.1370/afm.2943.

24. Melzer AC, Golden SE, Ono SS, Datta S, Crothers K, Slatore CG: What exactly is shared decision-making? A qualitative study of shared decision-making in lung cancer screening. *Journal of General Internal Medicine.* February 2020;35(2):546–553, 546. https://doi.org/10.1007/s11606-019-05516-3.

25. Savelberg W, Smidt M, Boersma LJ, van der Weijden T: Elicitation of preferences in the second half of the shared decision making process needs attention; a qualitative study. *BMC Health Services Research.* 9 July 2020;20(1):635. https://doi.org/10.1186/s12913-020-05476-z.

26. Esquibel AY, Borkan J: Doctors and patients in pain: conflict and collaboration in opioid prescription in primary care. *PAIN.* December 2014;155(12):2575–2582. https://doi.org/10.1016/j.pain.2014.09.018.

27. Reeve E, Low LF, Hilmer SN: Beliefs and attitudes of older adults and carers about deprescribing of medications: a qualitative focus group study. *British Journal of General Practice.* August 2016;66(649):e552–e560. https://doi.org/10.3399/bjgp16X685669.

28. Hamilton M, Gnjidic D, Christine Lin CW, Jansen J, Weir KR, Shaheed CA, Blyth F, Mathieson S: Opioid deprescribing: qualitative perspectives from those with chronic non-cancer pain. *Research in Social and Administrative Pharmacy.* December 2022;18(12):4083–4091. https://doi.org/10.1016/j.sapharm.2022.07.043.

29. Woolhouse S, Brown JB, Thind A: Building through grief: vicarious trauma in a group of inner-city family physicians. *Journal of the American Board of Family Medicine.* 2012;25(6):840–846.

30. Hiefner AR, Constable P, Ross K, Sepdham D, Ventimiglia JB: Protecting family physicians from burnout: meaningful patient-physician relationships are "more than just medicine". *Journal of the American Board of Family Medicine.* July–August 2022;35(4):716–723. https://doi.org/10.3122/jabfm.2022.04.210441.

31. Uygur JM, Brown JB, Herbert C: Understanding compassion in family medicine: a qualitative study. *British Journal of General Practice.* March 2019;69(680):e208–e216, e681. https://doi.org/10.3399/bjgp19X701285.

32. Gillespie H, Kelly M, Gormley G, King N, Gilliland D, Dornan T: How can tomorrow's doctors be more caring? A phenomenological investigation. *Medical Education.* October 2018;52(10):1052–1063. https://doi.org/10.1111/medu.13684.

33. Murphy M, Salisbury C: Relational continuity and patients' perception of GP trust and respect: a qualitative study. *British Journal of General Practice.* 27 August 2020;70(698):e676–e683. https://doi.org/10.3399/bjgp20X712349.

34. Rockwell MS, Michaels KC, Epling JW: Does de-implementation of low-value care impact the patient-clinician relationship? A mixed methods study. *BMC Health Services Research.* 6 January 2022;22(1):37. https://doi.org/10.1186/s12913-021-07345-9.

35. Riva S, Monti M, Iannello P, Pravettoni G, Schulz PJ, Antonietti A: A preliminary mixed-method investigation of trust and hidden signals in medical consultations. *PLoS One.* 11 March 2014;9(3):e90941. https://doi.org/10.1371/journal.pone.0090941.

36. Kuipers SJ, Nieboer AP, Cramm JM: Making care more patient centered; experiences of healthcare professionals and patients with multimorbidity in the primary care setting. *BMC Family Practice.* 9 April 2021;22(1):70. https://doi.org/10.1186/s12875-021-01420-0.

37. Brown JB, Ryan BL, Thorpe C: Processes of patient-centered care in family health teams: a qualitative study. *CMAJ Open.* 1 June 2016;4(2):E271–E276, E275. https://doi.org/10.9778/cmajo.20150128.

38. Stewart M, Fortin M, Brown JB, Ryan BL, Pariser P, Charles J, Pham TN, Boeckxstaens P, Reichert SM, Zou GY, Bhattacharya O, Katz A, Piccinini-Vallis H, Sampalli T, Wong ST, Zwarenstein M: Patient-centered innovation for multimorbidity care: a mixed-methods, randomised trial and qualitative study of the patients' experience. *British Journal of General Practice.* 26 March 2021;71(705):e320–e330. https://doi.org/10.3399/bjgp21X714293.

15

Evidence of the Impact of Patient-Centered Care on Clinician Well-Being and Patient Outcomes

MOIRA STEWART AND BRIDGET L RYAN

INTRODUCTION

Research on patient-centered care and patient-centered communication has matured markedly in the past 30 years. Early research indicated some positive effects but mostly mixed effects of patient-centered care on important patient outcomes.[1-5] Research to 2014 (the publication date of our third edition) illustrated numerous well-executed systematic reviews and meta-analyses, which, on the whole, indicated that patient-centered care had a positive influence on patient outcomes such as patient adherence,[6,7] patient self-reported health and physiologic health outcomes,[8,9] and mental health outcomes.[10] Furthermore, they concluded that interventions to improve patient-centered communication were effective in changing practitioner behavior.[11,12] Finally, studies showed that patient-centered care led to lower costs of care.[13,14] All in all, this was a good news story, providing evidence that teaching and practicing patient-centered care is worthwhile. It also brought together evidence-based medicine and patient-centered medicine, in that it confirmed that patient-centered care had an evidence base.

In this chapter, we aim to update the literature, focusing on patient-centered interventions targeted at effecting change in two broad outcomes. First, we tackle the role of patient-centered care on physician wellness. Clinician stress and burnout have become alarmingly frequent, made worse by the COVID-19 pandemic.[15,16] Evidence dating back to 1995 suggests that clinicians can suffer from compassion fatigue, which may adversely affect their well-being.[17] Therefore, we want to answer the question: Do patient-centered interventions show promise for improving clinician wellness?

Second, we present a section on recent interventions aimed at improving patient-centered care with the goal of improving patient outcomes. What are their successes and limitations?

EFFECTS ON CLINICIAN WELL-BEING

Recent research suggests that what was previously labelled compassion fatigue might be stress that is not necessarily associated with compassion,[18] or empathy fatigue or empathy

DOI: 10.1201/9781003394679-20

distress.[19, 20] Some authors suggest that providing compassionate care may in fact be one means of supporting clinician well-being.[19, 20] Authors increasingly distinguish between empathy, which can be understood as the emotional resonance and the cognitive understanding of another's emotions,[21] and compassion, which attends to emotions but is active, involving finding ways to alleviate suffering.[22, 23] Compassion is an integral feature of Component 4 of the patient-centered clinical method.

There has been observational research to suggest a protective effect for clinicians when they provide compassionate and patient-centered care.[20, 24] Unlike the research on the role of patient-centeredness in patient outcomes, there have been few interventions that included clinician wellness outcomes. This current review of the literature from 2010 to 2023, including a 2020 systematic review by Haverfield,[25] identified three interventions that addressed the question: what clinician wellness outcomes have been used in trials of patient-centered interventions, and what wellness outcomes were positively affected by such interventions?

The three intervention studies were conducted in the United States, and all interventions were directed at the clinician and/or clinician learners. One study[26] focused on attending to the patient's experience, understanding the patient in their context, and attending to the relationship with the patient. The other two studies[27, 28] focused on more general professional growth regarding the patient–clinician relationship outside specific patient interactions and discussed outcomes of mindfulness, compassion, and empathy. Table 15.1 reports the types of outcome measures included in the three studies, the number of different measures used, and how many showed statistically significantly better outcomes in the intervention group compared to the control group. Given the diversity of outcomes used, comparisons are not made across the studies, but each is described separately in the following paragraphs.

One aspect of clinical care that can contribute to burnout is working with patients that clinicians believe are "difficult", with one study reporting 12 times the likelihood of burnout in physicians who held this belief compared to those that did not.[29] Edgoose et al.[26] developed an intervention to assist clinicians in handling interactions with patients that they found difficult; BREATHE OUT targets aspects of clinician self-reflection and patient-centeredness. The outcome in Edgoose's randomized prospective controlled trial was scores on the Physician Satisfaction Scale following a visit with patients that clinicians labelled as difficult. Clinicians in the intervention group were more satisfied with the encounters than were physicians in the control group.

Table 15.1 Outcome Measures for Provider Outcomes: Type, Number of Measures, and Percent of Measures Significant [n=3]

Type of Outcome Measure	Studies Using This Type of Outcome		Number of Measurements		
			# used	# and % significant	
	#	% of 3	#	#	%
Burnout	1[27]	33%	3	2	67%
Compassion	1*[28]	N/A*	Q*	N/A*	N/A*
Empathy	1[27]	33%	4	0	0%
Mindfulness	1[28]	33%	4	2	50%
Reduced stress	1*[28]	N/A*	Q*	N/A*	N/A*
Satisfaction	1[26]	33%	1	1	100%

* Findings were from the qualitative component of a mixed methods evaluation of intervention.

A small pilot study (n=28) by Quinn et al.[27] examined the impact of a 9-session 6-month curriculum for interns on the outcomes of burnout and empathy using a before and after design. The intervention was multi-pronged including didactic learning about empathy and compassion, art and improvisation training, and mindfulness and meditation training. The researchers used three measures of burnout with two being statistically significant and examined four measures of empathy with none being statistically significant.

A mixed methods study by Weingartner et al.[28] compared medical students' mindfulness score before and after an elective course based on an 8-week Compassion Cultivation Training (CCT) program,[30] which aimed to strengthen compassion, kindness, and well-being. Training included pedagogical instruction, mindfulness and meditation training and daily practice, and compassion-themed exercises. Two out of four mindfulness outcome measures were statistically significant but only in the cohort that received the full-length elective. Students reported in qualitative findings that they used CCT skills in all aspects of their lives, that it helped address stress, and that it strengthened their interpersonal interactions including with patients.

These three studies[26-28] suggest that providing direct training on being patient-centered, as well as providing training on self-awareness and mindfulness with the goal of more indirectly impacting patient-centeredness, may be effective.

The Edgoose randomized controlled trial found encouraging results suggesting that training clinicians to change their approach to patients they labelled as difficult could improve interactions with those patients. The hypothesis is that improving these particularly difficult interactions will contribute to the clinician's overall wellness.

The Quinn et al. and Weingartner et al. studies focus solely on learners, and the Edgoose et al. study included learners. It is important to provide training early in clinical learners' education so that they enter practice prepared with strategies that protect their own well-being, as well as their patients' well-being. It is important also to have an evidence base that supports clinicians already in practice to maintain their well-being.

While there is increased interest in the potential relationship between providing patient-centered care and clinician well-being, there is much left to be done to identify potential interventions and to test those using rigorous designs and sufficient sample sizes.

IMPACT ON PATIENT OUTCOMES*

A review of 16 papers was conducted to answer the question: what successes and limitations exist for interventions aimed at improving patient-centered care? What patient outcomes have been used in trials of patient-centered interventions, and what outcomes were positively affected by such interventions?

All papers chosen reported pragmatic randomized controlled trials since 2010 sourced from two systematic reviews[31, 32] and two recent papers that reviewed trials.[33, 34] We included only trials for which a main component of the intervention was directed at the patient–clinician clinical encounter. There may have also been components addressing the coordination of the healthcare system.

---

* This section is reproduced with permission from:

Stewart M: Evidence on patient-centeredness, patient-centered systems, and implementation and scaling of whole person health. In: Krist AH, South-Paul J, Meisnere M (Editors): *Commissioned Paper for the National Academies of Sciences, Engineering and Medicine, Health and Medicine Division, Consensus Study Report – Achieving Whole Health – A New Approach for Veterans and the Nation*, 2023. https://doi.org/10.17226/26854. Reproduced with permission from the National Academy of Sciences, Courtesy of the National Academies Press, Washington, DC.

Table 15.2 Description of Intervention Studies (Country, Intervention Type)

Country	#	%		
United States	4	25.0%		
United Kingdom	3	19.0%		
Netherlands	3	19.0%		
Ireland	2	12.5%		
Canada	2	12.5%		
Other	2	12.5%		
TOTAL	16	100.5%		
Intervention Type			**TOTAL #**	**% of 16**
Patient Level			16	100%
		#		
Patient Experience		*2		
Person in Context		0		
Discussing Goals		15		
Relationship		1		
Organizational Level			7	44%
Training			**7	44%

* Both of these studies also included Discussing Goals in the intervention.

** Not necessarily the same studies as in the Organization Level.

Table 15.2 shows that one-quarter (4 of 16) of the trials were conducted in the United States.[35-38] Three were from the United Kingdom,[39-41] and three from the Netherlands.[42-44] Two trials were conducted in Ireland[45, 46] and two in Canada.[34, 47] The remaining two were from elsewhere.[48, 49] As required by the inclusion criteria, all 16 of the interventions were directed at the patient level (the patient–clinician encounter), but seven of the 16 contained elements addressing the organizational level (coordination of care), and seven of the 16 included a training component for the clinicians. The vast majority (15 of 16) of trials aimed the intervention at improving the patient's and clinician's discussion of goals, preferences, and shared decisions; two of these 15 also had elements of improving the care of the patients' experience (thoughts and feelings). One trial addressed improving the relationship between patient and clinician (empathy, emotion, and sharing power). Given that almost all trials' interventions addressed discussion of goals, i.e. there was so little variation in the types of interventions, no comparisons could be made. Comparisons of the trials whose interventions included patient level only, patient level and organizational level, and those with training components, showed no discernable differences on outcomes.

Table 15.3 shows the types of outcome measures included in the trials as well as the number of different measures used and how many showed statistically significantly better outcomes in the intervention group compared to the control group. Four clinical status outcome measures were used in two of the 16 studies. Of these four measures only one (percent reduction in HbA1c) was significant, i.e. 25% (1 of 4).

Patient reported outcome measures (PROMs), such as activities of daily living and quality of life, were more frequently measured than were the clinical measures. Fourteen of the 16 trials used 49 PROM measurements of which 21 (43%) were significant.

Patient reported experience measures (PREMs), such as ratings of continuity and coordination of care and patient perception of patient-centeredness, were somewhat frequently reported. Five of the 16 trials measured 13 PREMs of which 10 (77%) were significant.

Table 15.3 Outcome Measures: Type, Number of Measures, and Percent of Measures Significant

Type of Outcome Measure	Studies Using This Type of Outcome		Number of Measurements		
			# used	# and % significant	
	#	% of 16		#	%
Clinical Status Measures	2	0.13%	4	1	25%
Patient Reported Outcome Measures PROMs	14	87.5%	49	21	43%
Patient Reported Experience Measures PREMs	5	31.3%	13	10	77%

One sees that the majority of trials say that patients are reporting better care; a substantial minority of trials report that patients' self-reported health is better; and only one-quarter reported improvements in clinical status measures. This suggests a mechanism of how outcomes are affected by patient-centered interventions, i.e. patients must notice that care is better (more patient-centered), then some patients may feel better as a result, and for some (but fewer) patients, feelings are translated into physiologic improvements.

The most striking point from Table 15.3 is the paucity of clinical measures of patient outcomes. Patient reported outcomes were vastly preferred by the researchers who study patient-centered interventions. This preference for patient reported outcomes aligns philosophically with a commitment to testing patient-centered innovations. In addition, the importance of patient reported outcomes is supported by a robust literature that directly connects one key patient reported outcome, self-rated health, with mortality.[50] Patient reported health outcomes are not to be dismissed as soft and unworthy. On the contrary, they represent the winning combination of both the preferred principle, given their fit with a patient-centered orientation, and the consequential construct, in that the measures show significant impact on mortality.

The review of 16 studies revealed three other themes: barriers to implementation, equity issues, and the value of qualitative findings.

Barriers to Implementation of Patient-Centered Interventions

Implementation failures have occurred because of inadequate time for training the team[47, 51] and the stressful context of practice.[41, 52] Some crucial components of their interventions were not actually implemented by some participating practices. The degree to which the intervention was created by the clinicians (and valued by the clinicians) may affect implementation.[34] Mercer et al.,[40] in particular, co-created the intervention with clinicians, and its intent was to strengthen the very aspects of practice highly valued by the clinicians; i.e. more time with the patient and continuity of care. It is worth noting that Mercer et al.'s study found strong associations with positive outcomes. It seems that an intervention may not be fully implemented unless, first, it is congruent with clinicians' values and, second, the context is helpful.

Equity Issues

Patient-centered care has been found to be a force for equity,[10] in that the care was effective across all levels of deprivation, supporting its unifying potential. However, this can only be the case if specific, mutually agreed-upon treatments are cost neutral to the patient, as was found by Stewart et al.[34]

Value of Qualitative Findings

The implementation and equity issues were not revealed by the trials themselves but by qualitative studies aligned/embedded in the trials. Three are noteworthy. Salisbury et al.'s trial[41] showed non-significant impact of the patient-centered intervention on all PROMs; but their qualitative study uncovered specific implementation failures, including participating clinicians dropping major components because of lack of staff support and pressures in the healthcare system.[52] Fortin et al.'s trial[47] showed implementation and training issues in their qualitative study.[51] Stewart et al.'s trial[34] showed effectiveness of the patient-centered intervention only for patients with an income of >$50K CAD per year; their qualitative study revealed that crucial aspects of the intervention actually accrued out-of-pocket expenses for patients and therefore were not accessible universally. These nuances regarding implementation barriers and equity in patient-centered care were only evident from robust qualitative studies accompanying the trials.

CONCLUSION

The three studies on clinician wellness suggest that providing direct training on being patient-centered, as well as training on self-awareness and mindfulness, may be effective. This area of research deserves much more attention.

The 16 studies on patient reported outcomes suggest that interventions to improve patient-centered practice, typically focusing on Component 3, were effective regarding patients' experience of care and less effective regarding patient reported outcomes and clinical status.

Barriers to research on the impact of improving patient-centeredness included confusion of terms pertaining to clinician wellness and compassion fatigue and implementation failure of some practice-based interventions.

A key aid to the research was the use of qualitative elements to help understand the nature of the impact (in clinician wellness studies) and to unpack reasons for implementation failure (in patient outcome studies).

REFERENCES

1. Stewart M, Brown JB, Donner A, et al.: The impact of patient-centered care on patient outcome. *Journal of Family Practice.* 2000;49(9):796–804.
2. Stewart M, Brown JB, Hammerton J, et al.: Improving communication between doctors and breast cancer patients. *Annals of Family Medicine.* 2007;5(5):387–94.
3. Lewin SA, Skea ZC, Entwistle V, et al.: Interventions for providers to promote a patient-centered approach in clinical consultations. *Cochrane Database of Systematic Reviews.* 2001;4:CD003267.
4. Elwyn G, Edwards A, Mowle S, et al.: Measuring the involvement of patients in shared decision-making: a systematic review of instruments. *Patient Education and Counseling.* 2001;43(1):5–22.

5. Mead N, Bower P: Patient-centeredness: a conceptual framework and review of the empirical literature. *Social Science & Medicine.* 2000;51:1087–1110.

6. Stevenson FA, Cox K, Britten N, et al.: A systematic review of the research on communication between patients and health care professionals about medicines: the consequences for concordance. *Health Expectations.* 2004;7(3):235–245.

7. Zolnierek KB, Dimatteo MR: Physician communication and patient adherence to treatment: a meta-analysis. *Medical Care.* 2009;47(8):826–834.

8. Griffin SJ, Kinmonth AL, Veltman MWM, et al.: Effect on health-related outcomes of interventions to alter the interaction between patients and practitioners: a systematic review of trials. *Annals of Family Medicine.* 2004;2(6):595–608.

9. Roter DL, Hall JA: Physician gender and patient-centered communication: a critical review of empirical research. *Annual Review of Public Health.* 2004;25:497–519.

10. Jani B, Bikker AP, Higgins M, et al.: Patient centredness and the outcome of primary care consultations with patients with depression in areas of high and low socioeconomic deprivation. *British Journal of General Practice.* 2012;62(601):e576–e581.

11. Rao JK, Anderson LA, Inui TS, et al.: Communication interventions make a difference in conversations between physicians and patients: a systematic review of the evidence. *Medical Care.* 2007;45(4):340–349.

12. Dwamena F, Holmes-Rovner M, Gaulden CM, et al.: Interventions for providers to promote a patient-centered approach in clinical consultations (review). *Cochrane Database System Review.* 2012;12(12):CD003267.

13. Stewart M, Ryan BL, Bodea C: Is patient-centered care associated with lower diagnostic costs? *Healthcare Policy.* 2011;6(4):27–31.

14. Epstein RM, Franks P, Shields CG, et al.: Patient-centered communication and diagnostic testing. *Annals of Family Medicine.* 2005;3(5):415–421.

15. Canadian Medical Association: *Commentary: Health Care Workers' Burnout: An Issue That Can No Longer Be Ignored,* 25 March 2022. Retrieved 11 February 2023. www.cma.ca/news/commentary-health-care-workers-burnout-issue-can-no-longer-be-ignored.

16. Kane L: Deaths by 1000 cuts: Medscape national physician burnout & suicide report 2021. *Medscape,* 22 January 2021. Retrieved 11 February 2023. www.medscape.com/slideshow/2021-lifestyle-burnout-6013456?src=soc_fb_210126_mscpedt_news_mdscp_cuts2021&faf=1#1.

17. Fernando III AT, Consedine NS: Beyond compassion fatigue: the transactional model of physician compassion. *Journal of Pain and Symptom Management.* August 2014;48(2):289–298. https://doi.org/10.1016/j.jpainsymman.2013.09.014. Epub 10 January 2014.

18. Sinclair S, Beamer K, Hack TF, McClement S, Raffin Bouchal S, Chochinov HM, Hagen NA: Sympathy, empathy, and compassion: a grounded theory study of palliative care patients' understandings, experiences, and preferences. *Palliative Medicine.* May 2017;31(5):437–447. https://doi.org/10.1177/0269216316663499.

19. Hofmeyer A, Kennedy K, Taylor R: Contesting the term "compassion fatigue": integrating findings from social neuroscience and self-care research. *Collegian.* 2020;27(2):232–237. https://doi.org/10.1016/j.colegn.2019.07.001.

20. Peck JA, Porter TH: Pandemics and the impact on physician mental health: a systematic review. *Medical Care Research and Review.* December 2022;79(6):772–788. https://doi.org/10.1177/10775587221091772.

21. Uygur JM, Smith SM: Compassion in family practice: do we need to go there? *Journal of Family Practice.* February 2017;34(1):1–3. https://doi.org/10.1093/fampra/cmw148.

22. Uygur JM: *Understanding Compassion in Family Medicine: A Qualitative Study* [Master's thesis]. London, Ontario, Canada: University of Western Ontario, 2012. Retrieved 11 February 2023. https://ir.lib.uwo.ca/etd/450/.

23. Phillips WR, Uygur JM, Egnew TR: A comprehensive clinical model of suffering. *Journal of the American Board of Family Medicine*. March–April 2023;36(2):344–355.

24. Hiefner AR, Constable P, Ross K, Sepdham D, Ventimiglia JB: Protecting family physicians from burnout: meaningful patient-physician relationships are "more than just medicine". *Journal of the American Board of Family Medicine*. July–August 2022;35(4):716–723. https://doi.org/10.3122/jabfm.2022.04.210441.

25. Haverfield MC, Tierney A, Schwartz R, Bass MB, Brown-Johnson C, Zionts DL, Safaeinili N, Fischer M, Shaw JG, Thadaney S, Piccininni G: Can patient–provider interpersonal interventions achieve the quadruple aim of healthcare? A systematic review. *Journal of General Internal Medicine*. July 2020;35:2107–2117.

26. Edgoose JY, Regner CJ, Zakletskaia LI: Breathe Out: a randomized controlled trial of a structured intervention to improve clinician satisfaction with "difficult" visits. *Journal of the American Board of Family Medicine*. January–February 2015;28(1):13–20. https://doi.org/10.3122/jabfm.2015.01.130323.

27. Quinn AE, Trachtenberg AJ, McBrien KA, et al.: Impact of payment model on the behaviour of specialist physicians: a systematic review. *Health Policy*. 2020;124(4): 345–358. https://doi.org/10.1016/j.healthpol.2020.02.007.

28. Weingartner LA, Sawning S, Shaw MA, Klein JB: Compassion cultivation training promotes medical student wellness and enhanced clinical care. *BMC Medical Education*. 10 May 2019;19(1):139. https://doi.org/10.1186/s12909-019-1546-6.

29. An PG, Rabatin JS, Manwell LB, Linzer M, Brown RL, Schwartz MD, MEMO Investigators: Burden of difficult encounters in primary care: data from the minimizing error, maximizing outcomes study. *Archives of Internal Medicine*. 23 February 2009;169(4):410–414. https://doi.org/10.1001/archinternmed.2008.549.

30. The Center for Compassion and Altruism Research and Education (CCARE): *About Compassion Cultivation Training (CCT)*. Retrieved 11 February 2023. http://ccare.stanford.edu/education/about-compassion-cultivation-training-cct/.

31. Smith SM, Wallace E, O'Dowd T, Fortin M: Interventions for improving outcomes in patients with multimorbidity in primary care and community settings. *Cochrane Database of Systematic Reviews*. 15 January 2021;1(1):CD006560. https://doi.org/10.1002/14651858.CD006560.pub4.

32. McMillan SS, Kendall E, Sav A, King MA, Whitty JA, Kelly F, Wheeler AJ: Patient-centered approaches to health care: a systematic review of randomized controlled trials. *Medical Care Research and Review*. December 2013;70(6):567–596. https://doi.org/10.1177/1077558713496318. PMID: 23894060.

33. Fortin M, Stewart M, Almirall J, Beaupré P: Challenges in multimorbidity research: lessons learned from the most recent randomized controlled trials in primary care. *Frontiers in Medicine (Lausanne)*. 24 February 2022;9:815783. https://doi.org/10.3389/fmed.2022.815783.

34. Stewart M, Fortin M, Brown JB, Ryan BL, Pariser P, Charles J, Pham TN, Boeckxstaens P, Reichert SM, Zou GY, Bhattacharya O, Katz A, Piccinini-Vallis H, Sampalli T, Wong ST, Zwarenstein M: Patient-centered innovation for multimorbidity care: a mixed-methods, randomised trial and qualitative study of the patients' experience. *British Journal of General Practice*. 26 March 2021;71(705):e320–e330. https://doi.org/10.3399/bjgp21X714293.

35. Boyd CM, Reider L, Frey K, Scharfstein D, Leff B, Wolff J, Groves C, Karm L, Wegener S, Marsteller J, Boult C: The effects of guided care on the perceived quality of health care for multi-morbid older persons: 18-month outcomes from a cluster-randomized controlled trial. *Journal of General Internal Medicine*. March 2010;25(3):235–242. https://doi.org/10.1007/s11606-009-1192-5.

36. Hochhalter AK, Song J, Rush J, Sklar L, Stevens A: Making the most of your healthcare intervention for older adults with multiple chronic illnesses. *Patient Education and Counseling*. November 2010;81(2):207–213. https://doi.org/10.1016/j.pec.2010.01.018.

37. Lynch EB, Liebman R, Ventrelle J, Avery EF, Richardson D: A self-management intervention for African Americans with comorbid diabetes and hypertension: a pilot randomized controlled trial. *Preventing Chronic Disease*. 29 May 2014;11:E90. https://doi.org/10.5888/pcd11.130349.

38. Wagner PJ, Dias J, Howard S, Kintziger KW, Hudson MF, Seol YH, Sodomka P: Personal health records and hypertension control: a randomized trial. *Journal of the American Medical Informatics Association*. July–August 2012;19(4):626–634. https://doi.org/10.1136/amiajnl-2011-000349.

39. Ford JA, Lenaghan E, Salter C, Turner D, Shiner A, Clark AB, Murdoch J, Green C, James S, Koopmans I, Lipp A, Moseley A, Wade T, Winterburn S, Steel N: Can goal-setting for patients with multimorbidity improve outcomes in primary care? Cluster randomised feasibility trial. *BMJ Open*. 3 June 2019;9(6):e025332. https://doi.org/10.1136/bmjopen-2018-025332.

40. Mercer SW, Fitzpatrick B, Guthrie B, Fenwick E, Grieve E, Lawson K, Boyer N, McConnachie A, Lloyd SM, O'Brien R, Watt GC, Wyke S: The CARE plus study – a whole-system intervention to improve quality of life of primary care patients with multimorbidity in areas of high socioeconomic deprivation: exploratory cluster randomised controlled trial and cost-utility analysis. *BMC Medicine*. 22 June 2016;14(1):88. https://doi.org/10.1186/s12916-016-0634-2.

41. Salisbury C, Man MS, Bower P, et al.: Management of multimorbidity using a patient-centered care model: a pragmatic cluster-randomised trial of the 3D approach. *Lancet*. 7 July 2018;392(10141):41–50. https://doi.org/10.1016/S0140-6736(18)31308-4.

42. Nijhof SL, Bleijenberg G, Uiterwaal CS, Kimpen JL, van de Putte EM: Effectiveness of internet-based cognitive behavioural treatment for adolescents with chronic fatigue syndrome (FITNET): a randomised controlled trial. *The Lancet*. 14 April 2012;379(9824):1412–1418. https://doi.org/10.1016/S0140-6736(12)60025-7.

43. Spoorenberg SLW, Wynia K, Uittenbroek RJ, Kremer HPH, Reijneveld SA: Effects of a population-based, person-centered and integrated care service on health, wellbeing and self-management of community-living older adults: a randomised controlled trial on embrace. *PLoS One*. 19 January 2018;13(1):e0190751. https://doi.org/10.1371/journal.pone.0190751.

44. Verdoorn S, Kwint H-F, Blom JW, et al.: Effects of a clinical medication review focused on personal goals, quality of life, and health problems in older persons with polypharmacy: a randomised controlled trial (DREAMeR-study). *PLoS Medicine*. 8 May 2019;16(5):e1002798. https://doi.org/10.1371/journal.pmed.1002798.

45. Garvey J, Connolly D, Boland F, Smith SM: OPTIMAL, an occupational therapy led self-management support programme for people with multimorbidity in primary care: a randomized controlled trial. *BMC Family Practice*. 12 May 2015;16:59. https://doi.org/10.1186/s12875-015-0267-0.

46. O'Toole L, Connolly D, Boland F, Smith SM: Effect of the OPTIMAL programme on self-management of multimorbidity in primary care: a randomised controlled trial. *British*

Journal of General Practice. 26 March 2021;71(705):e303–e311. https://doi.org/10.3399/bjgp20X714185.

47. Fortin M, Stewart M, Ngangue P, Almirall J, Bélanger M, Brown JB, Couture M, Gallagher F, Katz A, Loignon C, Ryan BL, Sampalli T, Wong ST, Zwarenstein M: Scaling up patient-centered interdisciplinary care for multimorbidity: a pragmatic mixed-methods randomized controlled trial. *Annals of Family Medicine.* 2021;19:126–134. https://doi.org/10.1370/afm.26508.

48. Kari H, Äijö-Jensen N, Kortejärvi H, Ronkainen J, Yliperttula M, Laaksonen R, Blom M: Effectiveness and cost-effectiveness of a people-centered care model for community-living older people versus usual care – a randomised controlled trial. *Research in Social and Administrative Pharmacy.* 2022;18(6):3004–3012. https://doi.org/10.1016/j.sapharm.2021.07.025.

49. Nygårdh A, Malm D, Wikby K, Ahlström G: Empowerment intervention in outpatient care of persons with chronic kidney disease pre-dialysis. *Nephrology Nursing Journal.* July–August 2012;39(4):285–293. Quiz 294.

50. Idler EL, Benyamini Y: Self-rated health and mortality: a review of twenty-seven community studies. *Journal of Health and Social Behavior.* March 1997;38(1):21–37.

51. Ngangue P, Brown JB, Forgues C, Ag Ahmed MA, Nguyen TN, Sasseville M, Loignon C, Gallagher F, Stewart M, Fortin M: Evaluating the implementation of interdisciplinary patient-centered care intervention for people with multimorbidity in primary care: a qualitative study. *BMJ Open.* 24 September 2021;11(9):e046914. https://doi.org/10.1136/bmjopen-2020-046914.

52. Mann C, Shaw ARG, Guthrie B, Wye L, Man MS, Chaplin K, Salisbury C: Can implementation failure or intervention failure explain the result of the 3D multimorbidity trial in general practice: mixed-methods process evaluation. *BMJ Open.* 6 November 2019;9(11):e031438. https://doi.org/10.1136/bmjopen-2019-031438.

16

Measuring Patient Perceptions of Patient-Centeredness

MOIRA STEWART, JUDITH BELLE BROWN, BRIDGET L RYAN, AND LESLIE MEREDITH

BACKGROUND

Patient reported outcome measures (PROMs) and patient reported experience measures (PREMs) are now important components of any healthcare research program. Patient satisfaction measures, which make judgements rather than represent experiences, are exempt from consideration here. In the early 2000s, a number of patient experience measures were developed and 13 were summarized by Hudon et al. showing the number of items for each of the four components of the patient-centered clinical method described in this book.[1]

A more recent review of 16 papers, presented in Chapter 15 of this book, revealed one measure included in Hudon et al.'s review[1] (The Consultation and Relational Empathy [CARE] measure[2]) and seven other measures as follows: The Patient Assessment of Care for Chronic Conditions (PACIC) with its five subscales of goal setting, coordination of care, decision support, problem-solving, and patient activation;[3] The NHS Long Term Conditions LTC6 Questionnaire;[4] The NHS GP Patient Survey;[5] The CollaboRATE Scale;[6] The Goal Attainment Scale;[7] The Consumer Assessment of Health Care Providers and Systems (CAHPS) with subscales on access, provider communication, and clerk and receptionist communication developed by the Agency for Health Research and Quality;[8] and The Individualized Care Scale (ICS).[9]

This chapter presents questionnaire measures of patients' perceptions of patient-centeredness developed by the authors of this book over the past 30 years, culminating in the current 18-item Patient Perception of Patient-Centeredness (PPPC) English and French versions. To distinguish these current PPPC questionnaires from their historical predecessors, we refer to the 18-item versions (English and French) as the Revised Patient Perception of Patient-Centeredness (PPPC-R).

DOI: 10.1201/9781003394679-21

THE MEASURE OF PATIENT PERCEPTION OF PATIENT-CENTEREDNESS

History of the Measure Development

Based on research conducted in the 1980s by Drs Carol Buck and Martin Bass,[10] 17 items were adapted and used by Henbest and Stewart (1990) and found to be valid.[11] Deleting four poor items, the 14-item version of the PPPC was created and used in two large studies.[12, 13] The working paper for the 14-item measure[14] has been widely disseminated across the world with hundreds of requests for the use of the measure. These authors have found the measure to be reliable and valid.

In the late 1990s, pressure to create a shorter version for easy use in practice for continuous quality improvement and education led to a 9-item questionnaire in two versions: one for the patient to complete and one for the clinician to complete (see pages 356 and 357 of Stewart et al., 2014).[15]

The following sections focus on the development and testing of the 18-item English and French versions of the PPPC-R.

Factor Structure and Reliability of the Revised Patient Perception of Patient-Centeredness (PPPC-R)

The development of the PPPC-R was an accompaniment to the change to a four-component patient-centered clinical method first described in the 3rd edition of this book.[15] The factor structure of the PPPC-R (English version) was assessed using a sample of 381 patients who had completed the original items from the 14-item PPPC and an additional 11 items intended to further capture all four components of the patient-centered clinical method. This modified version was administered to patients in community-based primary care practices in Ontario, Canada, as part of a larger study exploring team functioning in interdisciplinary primary care practice.[16]

Through confirmatory and then exploratory factor analysis, a conceptually sound three-factor 18-item solution with good fit was identified.[17] Through this process, seven items were deleted, five for low loadings on all factors and/or higher loadings on a factor to which they did not belong, and two because they were too highly correlated (above 0.90) with other items, suggesting redundancy. The model fit for the final exploratory factor analysis with 18 items and its three modified factors was $\chi2$ (102) = 133.307, P<0.01; CFI = 0.994; RMSEA = 0.029 (90% CI: 0.012–0.041). The three factors were: Factor 1) health care process corresponding to PCCM Components 1 and 3; Factor 2) context and relationship corresponding to PCCM Components 2 and 4; and Factor 3) roles corresponding to PCCM Component 3. The French version of the 18-item PPPC-R (translated from the English 18-item PPPC-R) was evaluated through exploratory factor analysis using a sample of 301 adult community-based primary care patients with multimorbidity in Quebec, Canada.[18] A three-factor solution was identified: Factor 1 corresponded to PCCM Components 1 and 4, Factor 2 corresponded to PCCM Component 2, and Factor 3 corresponded to PCCM Component 3.

Inter-item reliability for the 18-item PPPC (English) was good (Cronbach's alpha = 0.89, n = 340).[17] Inter-item reliability for the 18-item PPPC (French) was reported according to the three-factor structure the authors identified (Cronbach's alpha = 0.87, 0.77, .87).[18]

The PPPC-R Items and Calculating the PPPC-R Score

The 18 items comprising the PPPC-R (English version) are shown in Table 16.1 (English version) and Table 16.2 (French version). The PPPC-R represents all four interactive components of the patient-centered clinical method. The PPPC-R measure is coded so that low scores mean positive perceptions, in keeping with other patient outcomes where fewer problems or lower scores means a better outcome. Each item has four response options scored from 1 to 4. The total score is the sum of all item responses divided by 18.

Table 16.1 The Revised (18-item) Patient Perception of Patient-Centeredness (PPPC-R)

Please CIRCLE the response that best represents your opinion.

1. To what extent was your main problem(s) discussed today?	Completely	Mostly	A little	Not at all
2. How well do you think your provider understood you today?	Very well	Well	Somewhat	Not at all
3. How satisfied were you with the discussion of your problem?	Very satisfied	Satisfied	Somewhat satisfied	Not satisfied
4. To what extent did your provider explain this problem to you?	Completely	Mostly	A little	Not at all
5. To what extent did you agree with your provider's opinion about the problem?	Completely	Mostly	A little	Not at all
6. To what extent did your provider ask about your goals for treatment?	Completely	Mostly	A little	Not at all
7. To what extent did your provider explain treatment?	Very well	Well	Somewhat	Not at all
8. To what extent did your provider explore how manageable this treatment would be for you?	Completely	Mostly	A little	Not at all
9. To what extent did you and your provider discuss your respective roles?	Completely	Mostly	A little	Not at all

10. To what extent did your provider encourage you to take the role you wanted in your own care?	Completely	Mostly	A little	Not at all
11. How much would you say that this provider cares about you as a person?	Very much	A fair amount	A little	Not at all
12. To what extent does your provider know about your family life?	Completely	Mostly	A little	Not at all
13. How comfortable are you discussing personal problems related to your health with your provider?	Completely	Mostly	A little	Not at all
14. To what extent does your provider respect your beliefs, values and customs?	Completely	Mostly	A little	Not at all
15. To what extent does your provider consider your thoughts and feelings?	Completely	Mostly	A little	Not at all
16. To what extent does your provider show you compassion?	Completely	Mostly	A little	Not at all
17. To what extent does your provider really listen to you?	Completely	Mostly	A little	Not at all
18. To what extent do you trust your provider?	Completely	Mostly	A little	Not at all

Source: English version, used in Ryan et al., 2019.[17]

USE OF THE PPPC IN DIVERSE PATIENT POPULATIONS INTERNATIONALLY

Researchers from across Canada and around the world have requested permission to use the 14-item PPPC and the more recent PPPC-R. To date we have received over 100 requests from Argentina, Australia, Brazil, Canada, China, Colombia, Germany, Italy, Japan, Korea, the Netherlands, Norway, Russia, Bosnia, Spain, Switzerland, Taiwan, Türkiye, the United Arab Emirates, the United Kingdom, and the United States.

We have worked with some of these researchers to translate the PPPC into local languages and contexts, most recently working with researchers to translate the PPPC-R into Turkish[19] and Chinese.

Table 16.2 The Revised (18-item) Patient Perception of Patient-Centeredness (PPPC-R)

Veuillez ENCERCLER la réponse qui correspond le mieux à votre opinion.

1. Dans quelle mesure a-t-il été discuté de votre (vos) principal (aux) problème(s) de santé lors de cette visite?	Complètement	En bonne partie	Un peu	Pas du tout
2. À quel point pensez-vous que le professionnel de la santé vous a compris lors de cette visite?	Très bien	Bien	Quelque peu	Pas du tout
3. À quel point êtes-vous satisfait de la discussion concernant votre problème?	Très satisfait	Satisfait	Quelque peu satisfait	Insatisfait
4. Dans quelle mesure le professionnel de la santé vous a-t-il expliqué la nature de votre problème?	Complètement	En bonne partie	Un peu	Pas du tout
5. Dans quelle mesure étiez-vous d'accord avec l'opinion du professionnel de la santé concernant votre problème?	Complètement	En bonne partie	Un peu	Pas du tout
6. Dans quelle mesure le professionnel de la santé vous a-t-il questionné sur vos buts concernant le traitement?	Complètement	En bonne partie	Un peu	Pas du tout
7. Dans quelle mesure votre professionnel de la santé vous a-t-il expliqué le traitement?	Très bien	Bien	Quelque peu	Pas du tout
8. Dans quelle mesure le professionnel de la santé a-t-il exploré ce que sera la gestion (du traitement) pour vous?	Complètement	En bonne partie	Un peu	Pas du tout
9. Dans quelle mesure avez-vous discuté avec votre professionnel de la santé de vos rôles respectifs?	Complètement	En bonne partie	Un peu	Pas du tout
10. Dans quelle mesure le professionnel de la santé vous a-t-il encouragé à prendre le rôle que vous désiriez pour vos soins?	Complètement	En bonne partie	Un peu	Pas du tout

11. Dans quelle mesure diriez-vous que ce professionnel de la santé prend soin de vous en tant que personne?	Beaucoup	Assez	Un peu	Pas du tout
12. Dans quelle mesure votre professionnel de la santé connaît-il votre vie familiale?	Complètement	En bonne partie	Un peu	Pas du tout
13. Dans quelle mesure vous sentez-vous à l'aise à discuter de problèmes d'ordre personnel liés à votre santé avec votre professionnel de la santé?	Complètement	En bonne partie	Un peu	Pas du tout
14. Dans quelle mesure votre professionnel de la santé respecte-t-il vos croyances, vos valeurs et vos coutumes?	Complètement	En bonne partie	Un peu	Pas du tout
15. Dans quelle mesure votre professionnel de la santé tient-il compte de vos opinions et vos sentiments?	Complètement	En bonne partie	Un peu	Pas du tout
16. Dans quelle mesure votre professionnel de la santé vous démontre-t-il de la compassion?	Complètement	En bonne partie	Un peu	Pas du tout
17. Dans quelle mesure votre professionnel de la santé vous écoute-t-il réellement?	Complètement	En bonne partie	Un peu	Pas du tout
18. Dans quelle mesure pouvez-vous compter sur votre professionnel de la santé?	Complètement	En bonne partie	Un peu	Pas du tout

Source: French version, used in Nguyen et al., 2020.[18]

We work with researchers to verify that the translated PPPC items maintain the fidelity of the English version; however, we recognize the differences in primary care internationally and engage in conversations to adapt items as required to ensure they reflect the country's context and will be acceptable and understandable to the patient population to which the PPPC-R is being administered.

Historically, the 14-item PPPC has been used in studies with the general population[12, 16, 20] and with specialized populations such as breast cancer survivors,[13, 21, 22] the elderly,[23] and student athletes.[24] As well as having been used with real patients, the PPPC has also been used with standardized patients.[25] Researchers requesting the 18-item PPPC-R have included those studying patients in family medicine, nursing, oncology, pediatrics, and student mental health services.

CONCLUSION

This chapter shows the versatility of the patient perception measure across different countries and patient populations. The chapter has presented an overview of the English and French versions of the revised Patient Perception of Patient-Centeredness (PPPC-R), showing their items, factor structure, and reliability.

REFERENCES

1. Hudon C, Fortin M, Haggerty JL, Lambert M, Poitras M-E: Measuring patients' perceptions of patient-centered care: a systematic review of tools for family medicine. *Annals of Family Medicine.* March–April 2011;9(2):155–164.
2. Mercer SW, Maxwell M, Heaney D, Watt GC: The consultation and relational empathy (CARE) measure: development and preliminary validation and reliability of an empathy-based consultation process measure. *Journal of Family Practice.* December 2004;21(6):699–705. https://doi.org/10.1093/fampra/cmh621.
3. Glasgow RE, Wagner EH, Schaefer J, Mahoney LD, Reid RJ, Greene SM: Development and validation of the patient assessment of chronic illness care (PACIC). *Medical Care.* May 2005;43(5):436–444. https://doi.org/10.1097/01.mlr.0000160375.47920.8c.
4. NHS: *LTC6 Questionnaire,* 2016. http://personcentredcare.health.org.uk/resources/ltc6-questionnaire.
5. Ipsos MO, England NH: GP patient survey-technical annex 2014–2015 annual report. *Normal Dot.* Reviewed 2 January 2009. gp-patient.co.uk.
6. Barr PJ, Thompson R, Walsh T, Grande SW, Ozanne EM, Elwyn G: The psychometric properties of CollaboRATE: a fast and frugal patient-reported measure of the shared decision-making process. *Journal of Medical Internet Research.* 3 January 2014;16(1):e2. https://doi.org/10.2196/jmir.3085. Erratum in: *Journal of Medical Internet Research.* 2015;17(2):e32.
7. Turner-Stokes L: Goal attainment scaling (GAS) in rehabilitation: a practical guide. *Clinical Rehabilitation.* April 2009;23(4):362–370. https://doi.org/10.1177/0269215508101742. Erratum in: *Clinical Rehabilitation.* February 2010;24(2):191.
8. AHRQ: *CAHPS Clinician & Group Survey.* Rockville, MD: Agency for Healthcare Research and Quality. Content last reviewed July 2022. www.ahrq.gov/cahps/surveys-guidance/cg/index.html.
9. Suhonen R, Leino-Kilpi H, Välimäki M: Development and psychometric properties of the Individualized care scale. *Journal of Evaluation in Clinical Practice.* February 2005;11(1):7–20. https://doi.org/10.1111/j.1365-2753.2003.00481.x.
10. Bass MJ, Buck C, Turner L, et al.: The physician's actions and the outcome of illness in family practice. *Journal of Family Practice.* 1986;23(1):43–47.
11. Henbest RJ, Stewart M: Patient-centeredness in the consultation 2: does it really make a difference? *Journal of Family Practice.* 1990;7(1):28–33.
12. Stewart M, Brown JB, Donner A, et al.: The impact of patient-centered care on patient outcomes. *Journal of Family Practice.* 2000;49(9):796–804.
13. Stewart M, Brown JB, Hammerton JH, et al.: Improving communication between doctors and breast cancer patients. *Annals of Family Medicine.* 2007;5(5):387–394.

14. Stewart M, Meredith L, Ryan BL, Brown JB: *Patient Perceptions of Patient-Centeredness (PPPC)*. Working Paper Series #04–1. London, Ontario: Centre for Studies in Family Medicine, Western University, April 2004.

15. Stewart M, Brown JB, Weston W, McWhinney IR, McWillliam CL, Freeman T: *Patient-Centered Medicine: Transforming the Clinical Method*, 3rd edition. London, UK: Radcliffe Publishing Ltd, 2014.

16. Ryan BL, Brown JB, Glazier RH, Hutchison B: Examining primary healthcare performance through a triple aim lens. *Healthcare Policy*. February 2016;11(3):19–31. https://doi.org/10.12927/hcpol.2016.24521.

17. Ryan BL, Brown JB, Tremblay P, Stewart M: Measuring patients' perceptions of health care encounters: examining the factor structure of the revised patient perception of patient-centeredness (PPPC-R) questionnaire. *Journal of Patient-Centered Research and Reviews*. July 2019;6(3):192–202. https://doi.org/10.17294/2330-0698.1696.

18. Nguyen TN, Ngangue P, Ryan BL, Stewart M, Brown JB, Bouhali T, Fortin M: The revised patient perception of patient-centeredness questionnaire: exploring the factor structure in French-speaking patients with multimorbidity. *Health Expectations*. 27 April 2020;00:1–6. https://doi.org/10.1111/hex.13068.

19. Günvar T, Başak O, Limnili G, Yurdabakan I, Güldal D: Validity and reliability of patient perception of patient centeredness scale in Turkish. *Turkish Journal of Family Medicine and Primary Care*. 2022;16(2):286–293.

20. Reinders ME, Blankenstein AH, Knol DL, et al.: Validity aspects of the patient feedback questionnaire on consultation skills (PFC), a promising learning instrument in medical education. *Patient Education and Counseling*. 2009;76(2):202–206.

21. Clayton ME, Dudley WN, Musters A: Communication with breast cancer survivors. *Health Communication*. 2008;23(3):207–221.

22. Clayton ME, Dudley WN: Patient-centered communication during oncology follow-up visits for breast cancer survivors: content and temporal structure. *Oncology Nursing Forum*. 2009;36(2):E68–E79.

23. Ishikawa H, Hashimoto H, Roter DL, et al.: Patient contribution to the medical dialogue and perceived patient-centeredness: an observational study in Japanese geriatric consultations. *Journal of General Internal Medicine*. 2005;20(10):906–910.

24. Redinger AS, Winkelmann ZK, Eberman LE: Collegiate student-athletes' perceptions of patient-centered care delivered by athletic trainers. *Journal of Athletic Training*. 2021;56(5):499–507.

25. Fiscella K, Franks P, Srinivasan M, et al.: Ratings of physician communication by real and standardized patients. *Annals of Family Medicine*. 2007;5(2):151–158.

17

Measuring Patient-Centeredness

JUDITH BELLE BROWN, MOIRA STEWART, AND BRIDGET L RYAN

Concurrent with the development of the concepts of the patient-centered clinical method and subsequent educational programs was a research initiative to support the empirical basis of the method. Central to the research program was the creation of tools to measure patient-centered care. The patients' perception measures are covered in Chapter 16 of this book. In this chapter, we cover the measures based on observation of the clinical encounter. Many methods of measuring communication have been developed since 1950 when Bales[1] first introduced the Bales Interaction Analysis.[2-6]

Advances in assessing the patient–clinician interaction have led several authors to provide comparisons of various coding schemes. In a special issue of *Health Communication* in 2001, six research teams coded the same dataset using their respective measures.[7-12] Commentaries on the results highlight what certain coding schemes can and cannot measure.[13, 14] In addition, Mead and Bower[15] have assessed the reliability and validity of various observation-based measures of patient-centered behaviors including an earlier version of the Measure of Patient-Centered Communication (MPCC) described in this chapter.

Many of these measures, while effective in assessing patient–clinician interactions, are not specific to the patient-centered clinical method as we envision it. Thus, rather than import parts of measures relevant to patient-centered care, a new research measure was created and subsequently modified – the MPCC. This chapter describes this measure.

THE MEASURE OF PATIENT-CENTERED COMMUNICATION

Development

Based on the patient-centered clinical method developed in the 1980s, 1990s, and 2000s, a method of assessing and scoring patient–clinician encounters, either audio-recorded or video-recorded, was developed. The MPCC has evolved significantly since its inception in the early 1980s. The development of the MPCC is detailed shortly. The MPCC has a couple of advantages over other methods[1-6]: (a) it does not require that the recorded interview between the patient and the clinician be transcribed; and (b) it is theory based; that is, it is derived from the conceptual framework described in Chapters 1 and 3–7 of this book.

The initial version of the coding and scoring of the MPCC was published in 1986 and used in a study of family practice residents.[16] At that time the measure only captured Component 1, Exploring Both the Disease and the Illness Experience. As a result the measure

DOI: 10.1201/9781003394679-22

underwent significant expansion, including Component 2, Understanding the Whole Person, and Component 3, Finding Common Ground, and it provided more detailed process categories as well as coding and scoring instructions.[17] This 1995 version of the measure was used in subsequent studies in family practice.[18] The 2001 version arose in response to patients' expressed needs regarding communication[19] and is detailed in the MPCC working paper.[20]

The 2001 version has been used in a number of studies with family physicians, surgeons, and oncologists;[21] family physicians/general practitioners/primary care providers;[6, 22–29] rural health workers;[30] medical students;[31–33] oncologists;[34] primary care residents;[35, 36] psychiatrists;[37] and radiation therapists.[38] These studies have been conducted worldwide in Australia, Canada, Scotland, South Korea, Türkiye, Uganda, and the United States.

The current measure incorporates coding and scoring of Component 1, Exploring Both the Disease and the Illness Experience; Component 2, Understanding the Whole Person; and Component 3, Finding Common Ground. Component 4, Enhancing the Patient–Clinician Relationship, is not included. This component evolves over many visits between a clinician and patient and may not be measured in each encounter or may not be verbalized by the clinician or patient. While always an important part of the patient-centered method, this component was not measured explicitly in our previous studies.

It should be noted that the inclusion of the concept of health now incorporated into the first component of disease and illness has not yet been added to the MPCC.

Application of the Measure of Patient-Centered Communication: Who and Where

The MPCC can be used in a variety of patient–clinician settings. In previous studies, it has been successfully used during office visits when patients are presenting with acute and/or chronic illnesses, routine physical examinations or check-ups, office procedures, and follow-up visits for previous problems. It has also been used in the emergency department where real time coding was conducted. As well as being used with actual patients, the MPCC has been employed in office visits with standardized patients.

This latter application offers the advantage of standardization but presents specific challenges because coders may work with a preset template of patient statements and expected behaviors (i.e., specific feelings, ideas, effects on function, and expectations) on the part of the standardized patient. In reality, these behaviors may not be elicited by the clinician, or the encounter may proceed in a manner that does not provide the standardized patient with an opportunity to articulate programmed statements, either at all or at an appropriate time. For example, a standardized patient may be directed to provide the clinician with a statement about the effect of a sore back on their ability to work. If the clinician moves quickly to the treatment of the problem, and it is only then that the standardized patient has an opportunity to raise this issue, the coder would normally place the statement in Component 3, coding it as part of the mutual discussion surrounding the treatment. With standardized patients, coders must decide how to handle these situations, balancing the goal of consistency afforded by standardized patients with the goal of accurately capturing the interaction. In the case of the effect of the sore back on work, the coders might decide to move back to Component 1 so as to ensure that this statement was captured in a consistent way for all standardized patient visits.

Occasionally, an additional person such as another clinician will be present during an interview. If the clinician is not an integral part of the visit, this person should not be considered as part of the interview to be coded. However, if the visit does involve two clinicians, such as a medical student and a staff physician who are taking equal part in the interview, these two people, depending on the research question, may be seen as one physician, and the interview will be coded as if these two people speak as one physician.

The other situation where an additional person may be present is when another person accompanies a patient. In this case, the coder must decide with whom the interview is being conducted. If, for example, a parent accompanies their child who does not speak for themselves, then the interview will be coded between the parent and the clinician. If, however, the child is older and is an active participant in the discussion, the interview will be coded between the child and the clinician. In the case of an adult patient, the interview will usually be coded between the patient and the clinician unless the adult patient is unable to speak independently. This can happen, for example, in the case of a patient who has severe mental illness or is cognitively impaired.

Researchers from around the world have requested the working paper[20] that describes the MPCC. Since 2001, there have been over 230 requests from researchers in Australia, Austria, Belgium, Brazil, Canada, Denmark, Germany, Italy, Japan, Korea, Malawi, Mongolia, the Netherlands, New Zealand, Nigeria, Norway, Puerto Rico, Russia, Spain, Sweden, Switzerland, Taiwan, Türkiye, the United Kingdom, and the United States.

Reliability and Validity of the Measure of Patient-Centered Communication

Interrater reliability of the scoring of the initial version of the MPCC was established among three raters at r = 0.69, 0.84, and 0.80.[16] Using the 1995 version,[17] Stewart et al. established an interrater reliability of 0.83 and an intrarater reliability of 0.73.[39] Studies that used the 2001 version of the MPCC,[20] some of which modified or adapted the measure for local contexts, reported moderate to high interrater reliability.[22-26, 29, 31, 34, 36-38]

The validity of the scoring procedure of the 1995 version was established by a high correlation (0.85) with global scores of experienced communication researchers.[39]

CODING THE MEASURE OF PATIENT-CENTERED COMMUNICATION

Coding takes place while listening to a recording (either in segments or in full) of a patient's visit to the clinician. It is often necessary to listen to all or parts of the recording a second time in order to fill in gaps in coding that were not captured on the first pass.

Coders listen for statements from the patient and the clinician that are pertinent to the patient-centered clinical method and list only those pertinent statements. Not every statement the patient or clinician makes is coded. Coders must place statements under the most appropriate component. Components 1, 2, and 3 of the patient-centered clinical method are coded. See Figure 17.1 for the coding template of the MPCC.

Coding under Appropriate Headings

Once the appropriate component is identified, the coder will list the patient or clinician statement under the most appropriate heading. In Components 1 and 3, there is a choice of headings. In Component 2, there is only one heading. The headings for each of these components are described here.

COMPONENT 1. EXPLORING BOTH THE DISEASE AND THE ILLNESS EXPERIENCE**

Symptoms and/or Reason for Visit	Preliminary Exploration	Further Exploration	Validation	Cut-Off	SCORE
1 _____	Y N	Y N	Y N	Y N	_____
2 _____	Y N	Y N	Y N	Y N	_____
3 _____	Y N	Y N	Y N	Y N	_____
4 _____	Y N	Y N	Y N	Y N	_____
5 _____	Y N	Y N	Y N	Y N	_____
_____				ST***	[_____]
Prompts					_____
1 _____	Y N	Y N	Y N	Y N	_____
2 _____	Y N	Y N	Y N	Y N	_____
3 _____	Y N	Y N	Y N	Y N	_____
4 _____	Y N	Y N	Y N	Y N	_____
5 _____	Y N	Y N	Y N	Y N	_____
_____				ST***	[_____]
Feelings					_____
1 _____	Y N	Y N	Y N	Y N	_____
2 _____	Y N	Y N	Y N	Y N	_____
3 _____	Y N	Y N	Y N	Y N	_____
4 _____	Y N	Y N	Y N	Y N	_____
5 _____	Y N	Y N	Y N	Y N	_____
_____				ST***	[_____]
Ideas					_____
1 _____	Y N	Y N	Y N	Y N	_____
2 _____	Y N	Y N	Y N	Y N	_____
3 _____	Y N	Y N	Y N	Y N	_____
4 _____	Y N	Y N	Y N	Y N	_____
5 _____	Y N	Y N	Y N	Y N	_____
_____				ST***	[_____]
Effect on Function					_____
1 _____	Y N	Y N	Y N	Y N	_____
2 _____	Y N	Y N	Y N	Y N	_____
3 _____	Y N	Y N	Y N	Y N	_____
4 _____	Y N	Y N	Y N	Y N	_____
5 _____	Y N	Y N	Y N	Y N	_____
_____				ST***	[_____]
Expectations					_____
1 _____	Y N	Y N	Y N	Y N	_____
2 _____	Y N	Y N	Y N	Y N	_____
3 _____	Y N	Y N	Y N	Y N	_____
4 _____	Y N	Y N	Y N	Y N	_____
5 _____	Y N	Y N	Y N	Y N	_____
_____				ST***	[_____]
*** Sub-total **** Grand total		GT**** ____	÷ ____		= [_____]

Figure 17.1 Coding Template of the Measure of Patient-Centered Communication*

* From Stewart et al., 2000[39]

** As already noted, Component 1 has undergone a change to include health as well as disease and illness. The current measure does not yet reflect this change.

COMPONENT 2. UNDERSTANDING OF THE WHOLE PERSON

Any statements relevant to FAMILY, LIFE CYCLE, SOCIAL SUPPORT, PERSONALITY, and CONTEXT are to be listed below:

	Preliminary Exploration	Further Exploration	Validation	Cut-Off	SCORE
2 _____	Y N	Y N	Y N	Y N	_____
3 _____	Y N	Y N	Y N	Y N	_____
4 _____	Y N	Y N	Y N	Y N	_____
5 _____	Y N	Y N	Y N	Y N	_____
6 _____	Y N	Y N	Y N	Y N	_____
7 _____	Y N	Y N	Y N	Y N	_____
8 _____	Y N	Y N	Y N	Y N	_____
9 _____	Y N	Y N	Y N	Y N	_____
10 _____	Y N	Y N	Y N	Y N	_____
				ST*	_____

* Sub-total
** Grand total

GT** ____ ÷ ____   5   =

COMPONENT 3. FINDING COMMON GROUND

	Clearly Expressed	Opportunity to Ask Questions	Mutual Discussion	Clarification of Agreement	SCORE
Problem Definition					
1 _____	Y N	Y N	Y N	Y N	_____
2 _____	Y N	Y N	Y N	Y N	_____
3 _____	Y N	Y N	Y N	Y N	_____
4 _____	Y N	Y N	Y N	Y N	_____
5 _____	Y N	Y N	Y N	Y N	_____
6 _____	Y N	Y N	Y N	Y N	_____
7 _____	Y N	Y N	Y N	Y N	_____
8 _____	Y N	Y N	Y N	Y N	_____
9 _____	Y N	Y N	Y N	Y N	_____
10 _____	Y N	Y N	Y N	Y N	_____
				ST*	
Goals of Treatment/Management					
1 _____	Y N	Y N	Y N	Y N	_____
2 _____	Y N	Y N	Y N	Y N	_____
3 _____	Y N	Y N	Y N	Y N	_____
4 _____	Y N	Y N	Y N	Y N	_____
5 _____	Y N	Y N	Y N	Y N	_____
6 _____	Y N	Y N	Y N	Y N	_____
7 _____	Y N	Y N	Y N	Y N	_____
8 _____	Y N	Y N	Y N	Y N	_____
9 _____	Y N	Y N	Y N	Y N	_____
10 _____	Y N	Y N	Y N	Y N	_____
				ST*	

SCORE

Responded Appropriately to Disagreement with Flexibility and Understanding

1 _____   Y N   N/A   _____
2 _____   Y N   N/A   _____

                                                         ST*   ☐

         * Sub-total   GT** ____   ÷ ____   =   ☐
        ** Grand total

Figure 17.1 (Continued)

COMPONENT 1: EXPLORING BOTH THE DISEASE AND THE ILLNESS EXPERIENCE

Symptoms and/or Reason for Visit

Patients' symptoms are listed using the patients' words in the upper left portion of the Component 1 coding form (see Figure 17.1). Patients' symptoms are the stated conscious expression of their physical, emotional, or social problem, usually representing their reason for the visit. While a statement of symptoms normally initiates an office visit, it may occur at any stage of the interaction. For example, a patient may say at the end of the visit, "By the way, doctor, I've also got a pain in my knee."

Symptoms and/or Reason for Visit fall generally into six categories as follows:

1. The patient initiates the description. ("I've been having a lot of chest pain.")
2. The patient responds positively to a clinician's inquiry about a sign or symptom. (The clinician asks: "Have you been having any allergy problems this spring?" The patient responds, "No, they seem to be under control.")
3. The patient responds either positively or negatively to a clinician's inquiry regarding a known problem that the patient has not presented at the current visit. (The clinician asks, "So how has it been since your bowel surgery?" The patient responds, "It's been going well, actually.")
4. The patient raises a problem or treatment issue from a previous visit. ("That medication you gave me last time didn't help at all.")
5. The clinician elicits the patient's personal and/or family history or conducts a check-up as part of the visit. (The physician asks, "Any history of heart disease in your family?" Or "Do you smoke?" or "Any hospitalizations?")
6. The patient is present to have a procedure. In this case, there may be very little conversation, but it is appropriate to code the clinician's conversation with the patient both before and during the procedure. This is where the clinician would be scored on how they handle the issue of informing the patient about the procedure and the issue of patient consent. (The patient begins, "I'm here to have this mole removed." The clinician responds, "OK, now did I explain to you what is going to happen?" The patient indicates, "Yes, we discussed that last time.")

Prompts

Prompts are listed in the patient's words in the second left-hand section of the Component 1 coding form. Prompts are signals from patients that their feelings, ideas, or expectations have not yet been explored. Prompts may be verbal, behavioral, or arise from the context of the consultation. Prompts are defined as either statements that are out of context or restatements of a problem that has already been mentioned.

Feelings

Feelings are listed in the patient's words in the third left-hand section of the Component 1 coding form. Feelings reflect the emotional content of the patient's illness. They may be the predominant aspect of the illness, as in a grief reaction, or be a contributory factor, as in the anxiety of a discovery about a breast lump. They may arise directly out of the stated symptoms and/or reason for visit, prompts, ideas, effect on function, or expectations, as when a patient who has requested a check-up discloses during the course of the interview that she is anxious (feeling) about the effects of dyspareunia (symptom and/or reason for visit) on her sexual function. Words commonly used by patients to express their feelings are troublesome, concerned, preoccupied, afraid, fearful, worried, sad, depressed, and anxious.

Ideas

Ideas are listed in the patient's words in the fourth left-hand section of the Component 1 coding form. Patients form ideas about their illness in their attempts to make some meaning or sense of their experience – that is, they develop an explanatory model of their illness. Patients' health beliefs, values, and life experiences can inform this explanatory model. These ideas may be based on prior experiences or influenced by present events such as a recent death of a friend.

Effect on Function

Effects on function are listed in the patient's words in the fifth left-hand section of the Component 1 coding form. The illness may have an effect on the patient's daily function, including the patient's capacity to fulfill certain roles and responsibilities such as a worker, spouse, or parent. Questions by the clinician may include how the illness limits daily activities, how it impairs family roles, and how it requires a change in lifestyle. Specific activities relevant to the heading effect on function include physical mobility, eating, dressing, sleeping, toileting, working, socializing, and leisure activities.

Expectations

Expectations are listed in the patient's words in the last left-hand section of the Component 1 coding form. Every patient who visits a clinician has some expectations of the visit. Patients' expectations often relate to a symptom or a concern about which patients anticipate exploration or response from the clinician. The presentation of the patients' expectations may take many forms, including a question, a request for service, or a statement of the purpose of the visit. Expectations are also reasons for the visit other than symptoms (e.g., annual health visit, request for service, request for completion of a disability form, or request for a prescription refill).

COMPONENT 2: UNDERSTANDING THE WHOLE PERSON

There are five topics specific to Component 2 and patient statements relevant to these five topics are to be listed (see Figure 17.1, second section, for the Component 2 coding form). The five are family, life cycle, social support, personality, and context (e.g., employment/schooling, culture, environment, healthcare system). Often, statements relevant to one topic may also be relevant to another. However, we do not consider it important for these topics to be mutually exclusive, and, consequently, we have not separated them by subheadings. This is a difference from the coding for Component 1 with its subheadings.

COMPONENT 3: FINDING COMMON GROUND

There are two areas specific to Component 3, Finding Common Ground: problem definition and goals of treatment – which represent (a) establishing the nature of the problems and priorities and (b) the goals of the treatment (see Figure 17.1, third section, for the Component 3 coding form).

Problem Definition

Problem definition is the clinician's statement of the nature of the problem(s). This statement is listed in the top left-hand section of the Component 3 coding form. It is not necessarily a restatement of the patient's initial presentation but is the clinician's formulation after the patient's presentation has been explored. It may be that on certain occasions the clinician does not know what the problem is but may offer a number of possible definitions of the problem. In this instance, each separate hypothesis/problem definition is to be documented under problem definition.

Goals of Treatment

Goals of treatment are the present treatment plan. These are listed in the second left-hand section of the Component 3 coding form. These goals are sometimes future oriented but are reasonable and attainable. Both the clinician's stated goals for treatment and any patient expressions of goals or patient comments on the clinician goals are listed. Goals of treatment include such things as ordering a test, suggesting an examination, prescribing a medication, or suggesting a treatment. Typically, these are instrumental suggestions on the part of the clinician.

Coding of Appropriate Process Categories

After writing the statement in the appropriate place, the coder must assign process categories to each statement. These process categories describe the clinician's response or lack of response to the patient's statements. The following two sections describe (a) the process categories for Components 1 and 2 (which are identical) and (b) for Component 3, respectively.

COMPONENT 1 AND COMPONENT 2 PROCESS CATEGORIES

The process categories include preliminary exploration (yes/no), further exploration (yes/no), validation (yes/no), cut-off (yes/no), and return (R).

Preliminary Exploration

Preliminary exploration is the immediate response of the clinician to the patient's expression of symptoms and/or reason for visit, prompts, feelings, ideas, effect on function, and expectations. A code of "Yes" is any acknowledgment that the clinician heard and accepts the patient's symptoms and/or reason for visit, prompts, feelings, ideas, effect on function, and expectations. Alternatively, when the clinician cuts off the patient, the categorization would be "No" to preliminary exploration and "Yes" to cut-off. Premature reassurance by the clinician does not count as preliminary exploration.

Further Exploration

Further exploration is the second and subsequent responses of the clinician. Further exploration means that the clinician's response facilitated the patient's further expression either with verbal facilitation or by silence allowing the patient to amplify and/or redirect the conversation.

Validation

Validation is an empathetic response by the clinician to the patient's expression. A code of "Yes" means that the clinician has acknowledged the patient's expression in an empathetic way. Validation would include phrases such as, "I understand that . . . ;" "This must be a difficult time . . . ;" "These are difficult decisions to make . . . ."

Cut-Off

A cut-off is defined as the clinician blocking the patient's further expression of symptoms and/or reason for visit, prompts, feelings, ideas, effect on function, or expectations – for example, by changing the subject, excessive focus on disease, jargon, or premature reassurance.

Return

The final process category is a specific clinician behavior called a return. The return will be indicated by an R in the margin. This occurs where a clinician has cut-off a patient but subsequently in the interview returns to the patient's symptoms and/or reason for visit, Prompts, feelings, ideas, effect on function, or expectations. With a return, the clinician is considered to have initiated preliminary exploration of the patient's problem, and this nullifies the cut-off.

COMPONENT 3 PROCESS CATEGORIES

The process categories include clearly expressed (yes/no), opportunity to ask questions (yes/no), mutual discussion (yes/no), and clarification of agreement (yes/no).

Clearly Expressed

Clearly expressed requires that the clinician clearly states in language the patient can understand what they believe is the problem or what the treatment should be. Statements are not clearly expressed if (a) the statement is garbled, incomplete, contradictory, or uses excessive medical jargon, or (b) the statement is not comprehensive enough for the patient to understand the reasoning behind the statement.

Providing an Opportunity to Ask Questions

Providing an opportunity to ask questions includes the explicit request from the clinician, "Do you have any questions about this?" It can also be the patient asking a question or the patient making a comment on the problem definition or goal.

Mutual Discussion

Mutual discussion is not achieved when the clinician describes the problem definition or goal without any evidence of the patient participating in a discussion either by asking questions or stating opinions. The patient has to provide verbal content for there to be a discussion.

Clarification of Agreement

Clarification of agreement can take two forms. The first form is where the clinician explicitly asks "Do you agree with this?" and the patient responds to the question. The second form is where the clinician encourages, through silence or the implicit tone of the interaction, the patient to express agreement or disagreement.

Table 17.1 Measure of Patient-Centered Communication (MPCC) Scores for a Sample of Family Physicians (N = 39) and Patient (N = 315) Encounters*

MPCC	Mean	Standard Deviation	Actual Range
Total score	50.77	17.86	8.13–92.52
Component 1**	50.85	19.00	0.00–97.50
Component 2	39.70	42.76	0.00–100.00
Component 3	56.26	22.97	0.00–100.00

* From Stewart et al., 2000.[39]

** As already noted, Component 1 has undergone a change to include health as well as disease and illness. The current measure does not yet reflect this change.

Responded Appropriately to Disagreement with Flexibility and Understanding

The final part of scoring the interaction concerns the clinician's response to disagreement by the patient. In our experience, such disagreements rarely occur. However, although rare, we consider the clinician's response to such disagreement to be important in finding common ground.

Scoring

After the entire interview is coded, coders assign scores on the right side of the coding sheets and calculate the scores for Components 1, 2 and 3. On the last coding sheet, an overall patient-centered score is calculated. Each of the three component scores can range theoretically from 0 to 100. The total patient-centered score is an average of the three component scores, and it too can range theoretically from 0 (not at all patient-centered) to 100 (very patient-centered). A detailed description of the scoring procedure is provided in the MPCC working paper.[20]

DESCRIPTIVE RESULTS

Table 17.1 shows the means, ranges, and standard deviations of the total MPCC and the three components as found in the observational cohort study of 39 family physicians and 315 of their patients.[39] This study established the properties of the 2001 version of the MPCC.[20]

CONCLUSION

In this chapter, we have described the development, evolution, and application of the MPCC. The most recent coding and scoring of the MPCC have been outlined in some detail.

REFERENCES

1. Bales RF: *Interactive Process Analysis: A Method for the Study of Small Groups*. Boston, MA: Addison-Wesley, 1950.
2. Kaplan SH, Greenfield S, Ware JE: Impact of the doctor-patient relationship on outcomes of chronic disease. In: Stewart M, Roter D (Editors): *Communicating with Medical Patients*. Beverly Hills, CA: Sage Publications, 1989.

3. Roter DL: Patient participation in the patient-provider interaction: the effects of patient question asking on the quality of interaction, satisfaction and compliance. *Health Education Monographs*. 1977;5(4):281–315.

4. Roter DL, Cole KA, Kern DE, et al.: An evaluation of residency training in interviewing skills and the psychosocial domain of medical practice. *Journal of General Internal Medicine*. 1990;28:375–388.

5. Stewart MA: What is a successful doctor-patient interview? A study of interactions and outcomes. *Social Science and Medicine*. 1984;19:167–175.

6. Shields CG, Epstein RM, Fiscella K, et al.: Influence of accompanied encounters on patient-centeredness with older patients. *Journal of the American Board of Family Practice*. 2005;18(5):344–354.

7. McNeilis KS: Analyzing communication competence in medical consultations. *Health Communication*. 2001;13(1):5–18.

8. Meredith L, Stewart M, Brown JB: Patient-centered communication scoring method report on nine coded interviews. *Health Communication*. 2001;13(1):19–31.

9. Roter DL, Larson S: The relationship between residents' and attending physicians' communication during primary care visits: an illustrative use of the Roter interaction analysis system. *Health Communication*. 2001;13(1):33–48.

10. Shaikh A, Knobloch LM, Stiles WB: The use of a verbal response mode coding system in determining patient and physician roles in medical interviews. *Health Communication*. 2001;13(1):49–60.

11. Street Jr RL, Millay B: Analyzing patient participation in medical encounters. *Health Communication*. 2001;13(1):61–73.

12. VonFriederichs-Fitzwater MM, Gilgun J: Relational control in physician-patient encounters. *Health Communication*. 2001;13(1):75–88.

13. Rimal RN: Analyzing the physician-patient interaction: an overview of six methods and future research directions. *Health Communication*. 2001;13(1):89–99.

14. Frankel RM: Cracking the code: theory and method in clinical communication analysis. *Health Communication*. 2001;13(1):101–110.

15. Mead N, Bower P: Patient-centeredness: a conceptual framework and review of the empirical literature. *Social Science and Medicine*. 2000;51(7):1087–1110.

16. Brown JB, Stewart MA, McCracken EC, et al.: Patient-centered clinical method II. Definition and application. *Family Practice*. 1986;3(2):75–79.

17. Brown JB, Stewart MA, Tessier S: *Assessing Communication between Patient and Doctors: A Manual for Scoring Patient-Centered Communication*. CSFM Working Paper Series #95–2. London, Ontario: Centre for Studies in Family Medicine, University of Western Ontario, 1995.

18. Kinnersley P, Stott N, Peters TJ, et al.: The patient-centeredness of consultations and outcome in primary care. *British Journal of General Practice*. 1999;49:771–776.

19. McWilliam CL, Brown JB, Stewart M: Breast cancer patients' experiences of patient-doctor communication: a working relationship. *Patient Education and Counseling*. 2000;39(2–3):191–204.

20. Brown JB, Stewart M, Ryan B: *Assessing Communication between Patients and Physicians: The Measure of Patient-Centered Communication (MPCC)*. Working Paper Series #95–2 (2e). London, ON: Centre for Studies in Family Medicine, 2001.

21. Stewart M, Brown JB, Hammerton J, et al.: Improving communication between doctors and breast cancer patients. *Annals of Family Medicine*. 2007;5(5):387–394.

22. Epstein RM, Shields CG, Meldrum SC, et al.: Physicians' responses to patients' medically unexplained symptoms. *Psychosomatic Medicine*. 2006;68(2):269–276.

23. Cegala DJ, Post DM: The impact of patients' participation on physicians' patient-centered communication. *Patient Education and Counseling*. 2009;77(2):202–208.

24. Clayton MF, Latimer S, Dunn TW, Haas L: Assessing patient-centered communication in a family practice setting: how do we measure it, and whose opinion matters? *Patient Education and Counseling*. September 2011;84(3):294–302. https://doi.org/10.1016/j.pec.2011.05.027.

25. Munro ML, Martyn KK, Fava NM, Helman A: Inter-rater reliability of the measure of patient-centered communication in health promotion clinic visits with youth. *International Journal of Community Health*. 2014;3:34–42.

26. Lundy JM, Bikker A, Higgins M, Watt GC, Little P, Humphries GM, Mercer SW: General practitioners' patient-centeredness and responses to patients' emotional cues and concerns: relationships with perceived empathy in areas of high and low socioeconomic deprivation. *Journal of Compassionate Health Care*. December 2015;2:1–7.

27. Mercer SW, Higgins M, Bikker AM, Fitzpatrick B, McConnachie A, Lloyd SM, Little P, Watt GC: General practitioners' empathy and health outcomes: a prospective observational study of consultations in areas of high and low deprivation. *Annals of Family Medicine*. March 2016;14(2):117–124. https://doi.org/10.1370/afm.1910.

28. Mercer SW, Zhou Y, Humphris GM, McConnachie A, Bakhshi A, Bikker A, Higgins M, Little P, Fitzpatrick B, Watt GCM: Multimorbidity and socioeconomic deprivation in primary care consultations. *Annals of Family Medicine*. March 2018;16(2):127–131. https://doi.org/10.1370/afm.2202.

29. Günvar T, Gürel Y, Güldal D, Başak O: Inter- and intra-rater reliability of the measure of patient-centered communication. *Turkish Journal of Family Medicine and Primary Care*. 2022;16(4):744–750.

30. Nayiga S, DiLiberto D, Taaka L, Nabirye C, Haaland A, Staedke SG, Chandler CI: Strengthening patient-centered communication in rural Ugandan health centres: a theory-driven evaluation within a cluster randomized trial. *Evaluation (London)*. October 2014;20(4):471–491. https://doi.org/10.1177/1356389014551484.

31. Lee HM, Park HK, Hwang HS, Chun MY: Patient-centeredness of medical students during a real patient encounter and a standardized patient encounter on the clinical performance examination. *Korean Journal of Medical Education*. June 2013;25(2):139–147. Korean. https://doi.org/10.3946/kjme.2013.25.2.139.

32. Teng VC, Nguyen C, Hall KT, Rydel T, Sattler A, Schillinger E, Weinlander E, Lin S: Rethinking empathy decline: results from an OSCE. *Clinical Teacher*. December 2017;14(6):441–445. https://doi.org/10.1111/tct.12608.

33. Park KY, Park HK, Hwang HS, Yoo SH, Ryu JS, Kim JH: Improved detection of patient centeredness in objective structured clinical examinations through authentic scenario design. *Patient Education and Counseling*. May 2021;104(5):1094–1099. https://doi.org/10.1016/j.pec.2020.10.016.

34. Clayton MF, Dudley WN, Musters A: Communication with breast cancer survivors. *Health Communication*. 2008;23:207–221.

35. Fenton JJ, Kravitz RL, Jerant A, Paterniti DA, Bang H, Williams D, Epstein RM, Franks P: Promoting patient-centered counseling to reduce use of low-value diagnostic tests: a randomized clinical trial. *JAMA Internal Medicine*. February 2016;176(2):191–197. https://doi.org/10.1001/jamainternmed.2015.6840.

36. May L, Franks P, Jerant A, Fenton J: Watchful waiting strategy may reduce low-value diagnostic testing. *Journal of the American Board of Family Medicine.* 12 November 2016;29(6):710–717. https://doi.org/10.3122/jabfm.2016.06.160056.

37. Campbell SR, Holter MC, Manthey TJ, Rapp CA: The effect of common ground software and decision support center. *American Journal of Psychiatric Rehabilitation.* 2014;17(2):166–180. https://doi.org/10.1080/15487768.2014.916126.

38. Dong S, Butow PN, Costa DS, Dhillon HM, Shields CG: The influence of patient-centered communication during radiotherapy education sessions on post-consultation patient outcomes. *Patient Education and Counseling.* June 2014;95(3):305–312. https://doi.org/10.1016/j.pec.2014.02.008.

39. Stewart M, Brown JB, Donner A, et al.: The impact of patient-centered care on patient outcome. *Journal of Family Practice.* 2000;49(9):796–804.

18

Conclusion

MOIRA STEWART

In the context of many societal challenges, this book makes the case that the patient-centered clinical method is an essential ingredient in the renewal of health care and the health professions. It cleaves to the basic principles of compassion and equity while integrating them with biomedical tasks.

Under one cover, based on four decades of work, this book unites theory with a practical clinical method and its teaching and research. Theory, practice, teaching, and research reinforce each other. For example, we learn from practitioners that their practice of compassion helps counteract burnout, in their view; we learn from research trials that compassionate care is related to higher practitioner satisfaction; and we learn that students benefit from learning about how to be compassionate caregivers.

If there is one key word for this book, it would be synthesis. In the clinical method, we recommend the clinician seek to understand a synthesis unique to each patient of the patient's disease, health, illness, person, and context. In education, we seek an integration of humanistic values into clinical teaching. In research, we recommend the use of multiple methodologies to synthesize an understanding of how, when, and for whom patient-centered care works. We also stress the synergies between the patient-centered clinical method and other models of care such as goal-oriented care, person-centered care, narrative medicine, evidence-based medicine, and shared decision-making.

One of the abiding strengths of this book, and its previous editions, is the presentation of the patient-centered framework in concise diagrams. Clinicians tell us that these pictures guide them even in the thick of an intense patient encounter. Educators have found them to be invaluable. However, these diagrams, even though helpful, are a double-edged sword: there are limitations. We have attempted to overcome the rather linear format of previous diagrams by creating a more circular appearance. Still, none of these representations adequately depicts the complex interactive process that weaves and extends through time, always in motion. Although extremely helpful for clinical practice, for teaching, and for clarity in research, diagrams can never fully capture the mysterious reality of a relationship between a clinician and a patient.

What are the key messages of this book and its view of the future? The key message is that the concepts of the patient-centered clinical method in today's world are both timely and timeless. The concepts are rooted in the enduring humanistic qualities of compassion and equity. They are in greater need now than ever. This book, by including case examples of a wide variety of patients from Europe, Asia, South America, Africa, and North America, demonstrates

DOI: 10.1201/9781003394679-23

that patient-centered care is a worldwide phenomenon. Looking to the future, we can expect the patient-centered clinical method to evolve and adapt to different cultures and societal circumstances.

The education for patient-centered care provides key messages of hope for overcoming the challenges in training health professionals. This book provides useful reviews and guides to learning how to deal with disease, developing a professional identity, learning to heal, and a learner-centered model of teaching. Overcoming the many challenges now and in the future will rely on role models to enact these guides.

Another key message is how important and useful patient-centered care is in many contexts in current times. This book tackled two of these contexts, demonstrating strong support in the literature for teamwork that promotes patient-centered care and for tips to increase the patient-centeredness of virtual care.

Optimistic key messages from the research on patient-centered care abound. Qualitative and mixed methods studies provide rich examples of how patient-centered practice works and how patient outcomes are influenced. Quantitative trials showed some, but not all, positive results in relation to two really important outcomes. First, clinician satisfaction and burnout were positively influenced by patient-centered interventions. Second, patient experience measures are more positive after patient-centered interventions. Another key research message is that such research is increasing by leaps and bounds – the two measures presented in this book have been used by more than 200 researchers from 25 countries and translated into eight languages. Nonetheless, there is much research yet to be done, and here are some key recommendations for future research, based on the four research chapters in this book:

- Do not become confused about the definition of patient-centeredness. Chapter 1 tells us that worldwide, after multiple review papers, the definition is clear and consistent.
- Measures addressing patient perceptions and observable behaviors exist and are widely used (Chapters 16 and 17). These measures are more balanced than others in the literature (these others tend to focus mostly on finding common ground), but still almost all measures reviewed fail to address the important fourth component, enhancing the patient–clinician relationship. Therefore, it would be useful to address the measurement of Component 4.
- Mixed methods studies are essential to a deep understanding, not only of *whether* a patient-centered intervention works (or not) but *how* the intervention has worked (or not worked) to positively influence outcomes.
- More well-rounded interventions covering all four patient-centered components may be more powerful in their impact on outcomes. The vast majority reviewed in Chapter 15 focused solely on Component 3 (Finding Common Ground) which may be limiting.
- Interventions which are co-created or collaboratively implemented with clinicians are recommended because implementation failure due to lack of clinician buy-in has been shown in studies with negative findings (i.e. no effect of the intervention).
- Equity or lack of equity inherent in interventions may be the reason for a failure of impact. One example is the intervention ought not to cost the patient out-of-pocket expenses which disadvantage some patients with lower incomes.
- Patient engagement in research on patient-centered care is recommended as a basic principle.

In conclusion, with the message ringing in our ears of how dire the situation is in health care, post-pandemic and throughout the world, let us commit to being part of a solution that espouses compassion, equity, synthesis, and integration in clinical care, education, and research on the patient-centered clinical method.

Index

Note: Page numbers in *italics* indicate a figure and page numbers in **bold** indicate a table on the corresponding page.

Printed in the United States
by Baker & Taylor Publisher Services